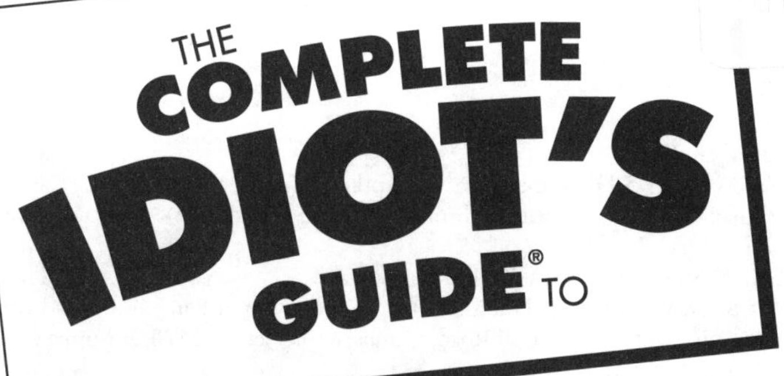

Exotic and Pole Dancing

Illustrated

by Wendy Reardon

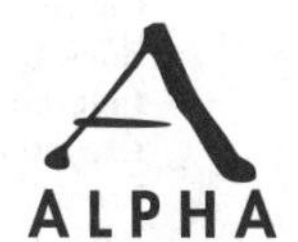

ALPHA

A member of Penguin Group (USA) Inc.

ALPHA BOOKS

Published by the Penguin Group
Penguin Group (USA) Inc., 375 Hudson Street, New York, New York 10014, U.S.A.
Penguin Group (Canada), 10 Alcorn Avenue, Toronto, Ontario, Canada M4V 3B2 (a division of Pearson Penguin Canada Inc.)
Penguin Books Ltd, 80 Strand, London WC2R 0RL, England
Penguin Ireland, 25 St Stephen's Green, Dublin 2, Ireland (a division of Penguin Books Ltd)
Penguin Group (Australia), 250 Camberwell Road, Camberwell, Victoria 3124, Australia (a division of Pearson Australia Group Pty Ltd)
Penguin Books India Pvt Ltd, 11 Community Centre, Panchsheel Park, New Delhi—10 017, India
Penguin Group (NZ), cnr Airborne and Rosedale Roads, Albany, Auckland 1310, New Zealand (a division of Pearson New Zealand Ltd)
Penguin Books (South Africa) (Pty) Ltd, 24 Sturdee Avenue, Rosebank, Johannesburg 2196, South Africa
Penguin Books Ltd, Registered Offices: 80 Strand, London WC2R 0RL, England

International Standard Book Number: 978-1-59257-560-2
Library of Congress Catalog Card Number: 2006930727

09 08 07 8 7 6 5 4 3 2

Interpretation of the printing code: The rightmost number of the first series of numbers is the year of the book's printing; the rightmost number of the second series of numbers is the number of the book's printing. For example, a printing code of 07-1 shows that the first printing occurred in 2007.

Printed in the United States of America

Publisher: *Marie Butler-Knight*
Editorial Director: *Mike Sanders*
Managing Editor: *Billy Fields*
Senior Acquisitions Editor: *Paul Dinas*
Senior Development Editor: *Christy Wagner*
Production Editor: *Megan Douglass*
Copy Editor: *Keith Cline*
Cover Designer: *Bill Thomas*
Book Designers: *Trina Wurst/Kurt Owens*
Indexer: *Angie Bess*
Layout: *Chad Dressler*
Proofreader: *Mary Hunt*

Contents at a Glance

Contents

Foreword

The Complete Idiot's Guide to Exotic and Pole Dancing Illustrated is a useful, practical guide that's bringing the sexy dance and pole moves from the exotic dance stage directly to your home. As a former exotic dancer, I spent countless hours learning how to walk in heels, how to perform pole tricks, and what to wear in my attempt to create an image of "sexy confidence," through trial and error.

Now, women just like you can learn how to move the way exotic dancers move and pole dance just as beautifully as they dance. Everything you wanted to know about being sexy, confident, beautiful, and powerful is here for you in one place.

Sexy is defined as arousing or tending to arouse sexual desire or interest. Slang. Highly appealing or interesting; attractive. It's the sultry walk, the flirtatious hair, the sensual dress. We all can learn how to be sexy.

Many women may have felt sexy and desired at a certain time in their lives, but over time, through marriage and divorce, having children and juggling multiple jobs, they have forgotten what sexy is. Others may have never known what seductive feels like and may have lived their lives believing they don't have the right to feel attractive. And there are the women who know what sexy feels like and have the gift of letting themselves feel desired on a daily basis. Let's face it—exotic dancers are sexy, and secretly you may have wondered what gives them their suggestive sex appeal.

Confident is defined as marked by assurance, as of success; marked by confidence in oneself; self-assured. Very bold; presumptuous. Having confidence in yourself is vital to having success in just about everything you do. Learning how to striptease and pole dance is no exception. From eye contact, to knowing your next move, self-assurance is very rewarding. Building on your own unique qualities, you'll learn how having confidence makes performing a striptease or pole dance less intimidating. A confident woman is a sexy woman.

Beautiful is defined as having qualities that delight the senses, especially the sense of sight. Excellent; wonderful. Every woman wants to be beautiful and be seen as a goddess. The thought of walking through a room and knowing that every person, both men and women, is noticing you is very thrilling. Now take that thought and narrow it down, by imagining being seen as stunning by your partner and feeling radiant while dancing for him. Pole dancing is a sensual art; it showcases the female form in movement on a vertical pole.

Powerful is defined as having or capable of exerting power. Effective or potent; a powerful drug. Being powerful is hot! Performing a striptease can be a very empowering experience. As the performer, you have control over your partner and their five senses, from the lighting, to the music, the scents, the textures, and the flavors they may taste. Your new sense of domination may have its beginning the first time you see yourself wearing a pair of high heels or a slinky G-string. Pole dancing is equally as powerful as you learn how to maneuver your body on the pole, entertaining others as well as yourself.

You are a real woman. Your experiences in life have brought you to this point where you have decided to pick up this book. Setting aside your profession and daily responsibilities, exotic and pole dancing are here for you to embrace. The time has come for your inner exotic dancer to be set free to move sensually to any beat and become one with the pole. You will be sexy, confident, beautiful, and powerful. Enjoy the journey.

Fawnia Mondey-Dietrich

Fawnia is the world's first known exotic dance instructor, fitness model and writer, figure competitor, and actress. Fawnia was a real-life exotic dancer who won numerous titles on the Canadian exotic dance circuit. Since 1998, her instructional DVDs and innovative use of the Internet have made her the main influence in making pole dancing a mainstream cultural phenomenon today. Visit Fawnia's exotic dance website at www.ExoticDanceSchool.com.

Introduction

You are about to rediscover your sexy side and get an amazing workout in the process.

The Complete Idiot's Guide to Exotic and Pole Dancing, Illustrated is not just a guide for women who crave a stimulating workout; it's for the soccer moms who need to feel sexy after having kids, the desperate housewives looking for fun when the pool boy isn't available, and even the retiree who refuses to let age stifle her sensual side.

The moves in this book are the very basics that I teach in my classes, and just like I tell my students, when you have a base to work from, you can add in your own personality and create your own moves and your own exotic style.

How to Use This Book

You'll find three concise parts to this book, each devoted to one of the main aspects of exotic dancing: the emotional, the physical, and the performance.

Part 1, "Boring Beige to Hot Pink: Developing Your Diva Dynamic," seeks to break down the emotional barriers most women have when it comes to appreciating their own bodies as they are, and stresses the concept of becoming someone else when you dance.

Part 2, "Let's Get Physical: The Art of Exotic Dance," teaches you the core physical exotic routine moves, including tips on floor work, chair dancing, and how to swing on the pole. This part will really get you moving!

Part 3, "It's All About You, but Include Him, Too!" shows you how to perform a seductive striptease, give your lover the most sensual lap dance he has ever experienced, and more!

Part 4, "Putting It All Together," is where you make all your hard work shine! I've suggested many different themed costumes and songs to get your creative juices flowing, so to speak. There's also a chapter with some lightly choreographed routines so you can practice with those until you feel comfortable enough doing your own dance spontaneously. But the best chapter of all is the last, where I'll show you how to put together a real performance starring you and your friends!

In the back, the appendixes give you information on where you can get the "right stuff" for your performance, as well as exotic and pole dancing lessons throughout the United States.

Follow Along Now ... What's on the DVD

Because it's sometimes easier to learn by seeing (and doing!) than just by reading, we've included a DVD with the chapters. On the DVD, you'll see me performing all the moves I've described in the chapters. You'll also watch me dance to several full songs, as well as give a man a real lap dance (which was the most fun part for me!).

Exotic Extras

Throughout this book, I've sprinkled extra bits of insight and tips. Here's what to look for:

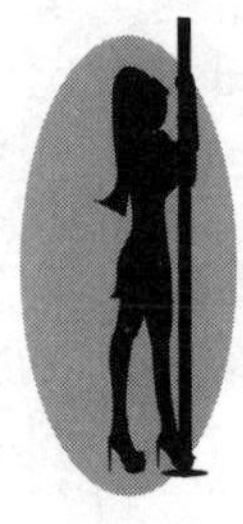

Slick Tricks

Take note of these hot tips and tricks to truly polish your performance and amaze your audience.

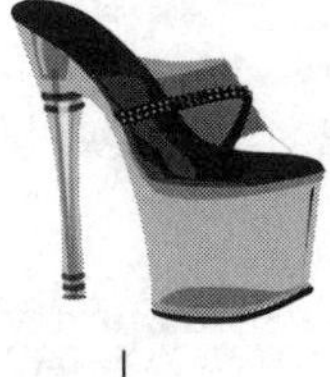

Trippin' Up

Read these notes for mistakes you don't want to make during your performance—physically or psychologically.

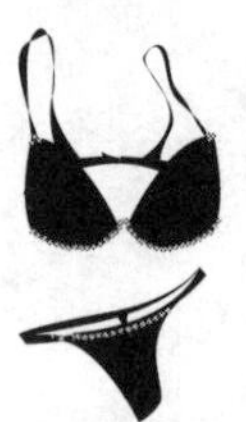

Behind the G-String

In this box, you'll find real-life anecdotes from both professional and amateur dancers.

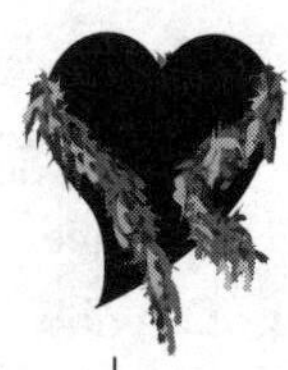

Feelin' the Love

Here you'll find insights from real students and teachers who have learned the art of exotic dancing, from how it made them feel to how their loved ones reacted to their sexy dance!

Acknowledgments

First and foremost, I want to thank my wonderful editor, Paul Dinas, for his encouragement, feedback, and belief in this project; my photographer, Eric Levin of Elevin Photography (www.elevin.net); the crew of Good Life Productions, Neil and Julia (www.Goodlifeproductions.com); Judy Roberts (www.sfbmusic.net); Josh Hoekwater at Aircraft Music Library (www.aircraftmusiclibrary.com); makeup artists extraordinaire Anna Miner and Alisa Parker (www.weddingmakeovers.com); the brilliant minds at Mijon Technologies who extracted my manuscript from my broken computer (www.mijon.com), and Mike Suss, my patient webmaster who makes my crazy changes at all hours of the night and puts up with my visiting pet rats.

Bianca laTessa deserves the utmost praise for her support and words of wisdom; my chiropractor Dr. Josh Dubin, who fixes me when I break (www.dubinchiro.com); Pia of Pia's Positive Vibrations in Hingham, where I taught my very first classes; and the Open Door in Braintree for letting me rent their yoga studio as my business grew. Thanks to Bill Taylor for believing in my vision and lending me the money to finally get a studio of my own and Tony and Larry Agnitti of Agnitti Property Management for their trust in giving me the chance to open my pole dancing studio in spite of all the suspicion a studio of my nature brings in conservative Massachusetts.

The highest of thanks and appreciation go to my faithful instructors who teach my classes and parties, without whom Gypsy Rose would be nothing today: Alena Taylor, Meredith Griffiths, Amy Beni, Amber P. Knight, Vickie Enos, Marybeth Canwell, Gabrielle Valliere, Lee Delzingo, Sheryl Sullivan, and Vanessa Carlisle.

But I wouldn't be anywhere if it weren't for those who made exotic dancing so fun for me that I became addicted: Jimmy and Big Joe at Snooky's Ventura; Duke and the late J. J. from Snooky's Simi Valley; Jim and Brad at Snooky's in Oxnard; and Jeff and JK at PJ's in Oxnard, California. Also, thanks to the late Jackquie Martine and the Rainbow Agency of London and the crew at the Satin Doll in Providence, Rhode Island.

But the best, and most important for last, this book is dedicated to my parents, Joan and John; my sister, Beth, and her husband, Neal Hughes; the best tattoo artist in all Brooklyn, my brother, John "the Dang" Reardon; Debby Pitaro; my late grandmother Marion Low; and her best friend, Marion Kenney, who, at 91 years old, still does some pretty sexy butt circles!

Trademarks

In This Part

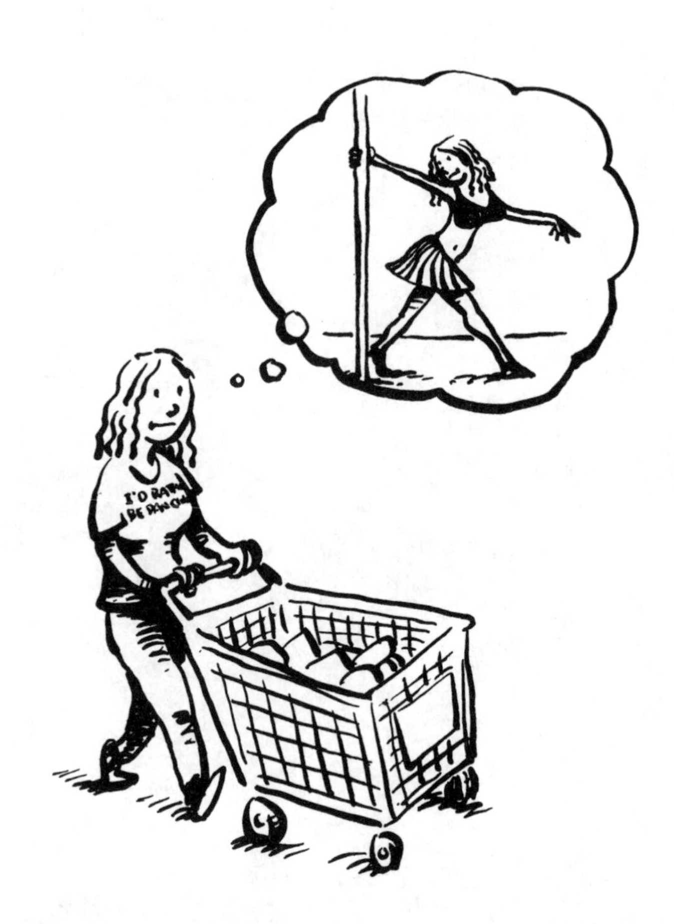

Part 1

Boring Beige to Hot Pink: Developing Your Diva Dynamic

The entire underlying concept of exotic dancing is that you become someone else; you step out of your everyday life into a fantasy world where you can look and act like you never could on a day-to-day basis. No exotic dancer wears her dancer clothing to go food shopping; in fact, we're all just regular women you'd never expect to be exotic dancers if you saw us in the supermarket or post office.

The difference between "regular women" and us is that we know how to become someone else both in our minds and our bodies, through costuming, hair, makeup, and, above all, attitude. And now you, too, can finally develop and unleash your "inner diva" and let her lead you to exciting places you never thought you'd go!

In This Chapter

- What will other people say?
- The phone-booth transformation
- You're not perfect—be proud of it!
- Men are simple
- It's all acting

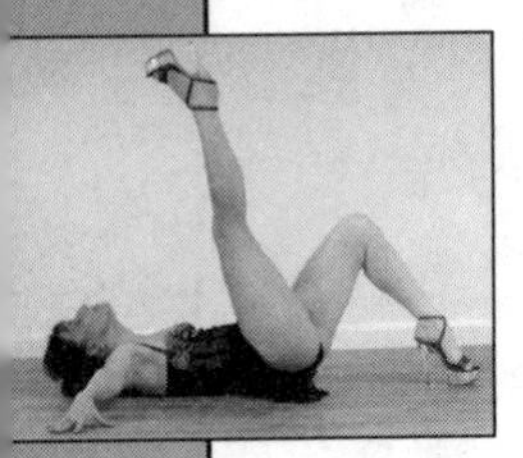
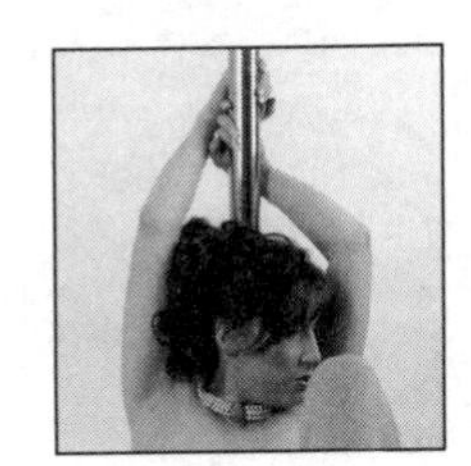
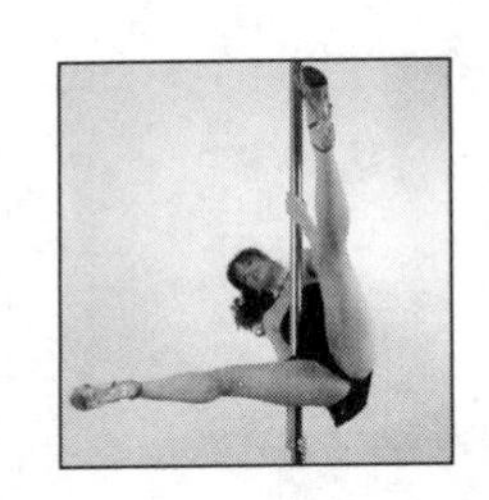
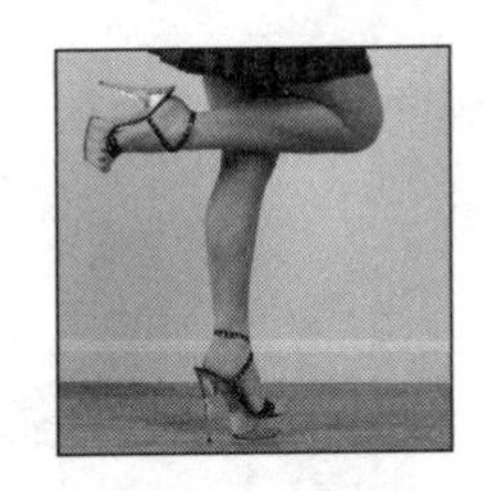
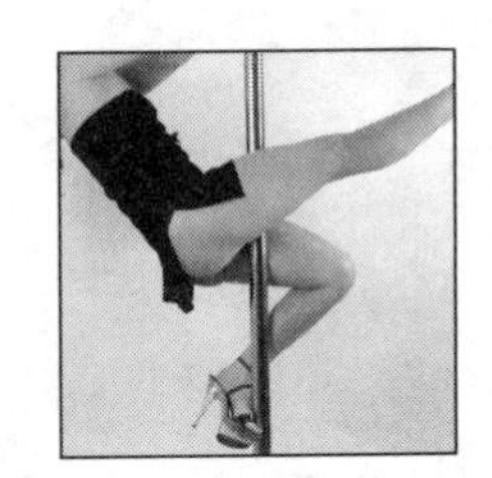
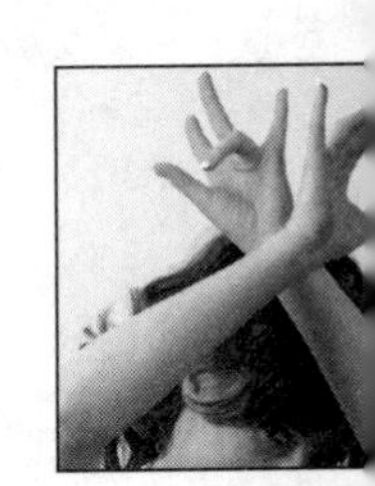

Chapter 1

Forget Your Body—It's All in Your Mind

To put on a truly amazing performance as an exotic dancer, you must start with the most important part of exotic dancing—the mind-set. When you have the correct psyche, you will look hot, even if you're wearing sweatpants! You must become someone else, and you can do several things to help you create your new, sexy, alter ego.

That's the focus of this chapter—getting your mind ready to dance. Let's go!

I've Got to Hide This Book!

You might be asking yourself, *What will people think if they knew I bought a book on exotic and pole dancing?* They'll surely think you're weird, you're some kind of perverted slut, or they'll laugh at you and tell you that you could never swing around a pole. Besides … you're not *that type*.

Most women who join my classes are housewives or women just looking to do something a little daring to throw some zing into their lives. You'd never know who's pole dancing; it could be the woman in the cubicle next to you. Believe me when I tell you I've had everyone in my classes from international bank managers to optometrists, clothing designers, high school English teachers, lawyers, doctors, retirees, swim instructors, property managers, second-grade teachers … the list goes on!

And what exactly is *that type?* Newsflash: exotic and pole dancing aren't just for "sluts" anymore! And the women who have the most issues with pole dancing are the ones who secretly wish they could do it but can't get over the immorality of the whole thing. Correct me if I'm wrong, but if a pole is horizontal, that's called gymnastics, and it's wonderful for children. If a pole is vertical, though … Heaven help us, the very moral fiber of society will collapse!

And FYI, I am a world-renowned papal scholar who wrote *The Deaths of the Popes: Comprehensive Accounts Including Funerals, Burial Places, and Epitaphs* and was quoted in the *Washington Post*, *Miami Herald*, and *The New York Times* when John Paul II died in 2004. St. Peter's did not collapse when I stepped inside in the fall of 2005 to give tours based on my book, nor was I struck by lightning. Exotic dancing put me through graduate school, and now I teach it, complete with very short skirts and platform boots.

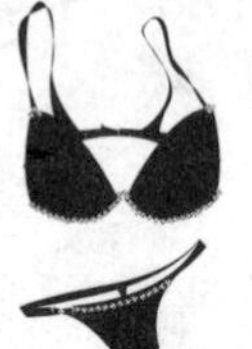

Behind the G-String

One of my clients told me she was at dinner with her 13-year-old son and husband, and as they left the restaurant, she saw an awning with a brass pole and she couldn't help herself … she swung around the pole and starting workin' it! She said people were screaming and honking their horns, but she felt really great when her son looked at her and said, "Mom, you are soooo cool!" And the best part is, she's 50 years old!

—Wendy, owner of Pole Dance Studio New York

So if an esteemed church scholar can pole dance, so can you. And forget anyone who tries to judge you for it! Besides, every few months it seems Oprah does a show on pole dancing and how empowering it is for women. So if Oprah does it … you know it's okay.

Therefore, the entire underlying theme of the book is this: *no apologies!*

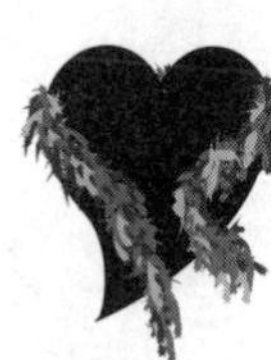

Feelin' the Love

I was so afraid to tell my mother that not only had I been taking exotic dancing lessons but was now teaching them that I lied to her for a long time about my "dance lessons." Finally, I found the courage to confess exactly what kind of dancing I was doing, and instead of being shocked and angry, she helped me design my fliers and business cards!

—Amber P. Knight, Gypsy Rose instructor

The Psychology of a Dancer

Chances are you wouldn't recognize an exotic dancer at the bank or post office or even when she's dropping her child off at school. There's a reason for this: exotic dancers are not themselves when they are onstage; they are a fantasy. They become someone else, and for most dancers, that's the only way they can get up there and do it.

Yet when I was a dancer, and even now when I perform for my students, in my mind I am not Wendy the Scholar. I am Holly, the sweet, innocent, yet incredibly confident and sexy exotic dancer. I, like all exotic dancers, have a split personality. As soon as we get into our costumes and on that stage, we become the other person.

It's just like Superman, you know—mild-mannered, nerdy, klutzy Clark Kent who steps into a phone booth only to emerge as the incredibly sexy, strong, confident Superman. It's the same concept for an exotic dancer—we enter the club as a regular gal in our sweats and T-shirts and transform into super-hot babes when we emerge from our "phone booth" (a.k.a. the dressing room). If only we dancers had x-ray vision like Superman to see how much money a customer has in his wallet!

As I state many, many times throughout this book, exotic dancing is all *acting*, and when you act, you become another person. To help yourself psychologically with this "transformation," you need a stage name to make your personality change tangible. When you have that name, you have taken the first step in becoming someone else. You have a name, and thusly another complete personality.

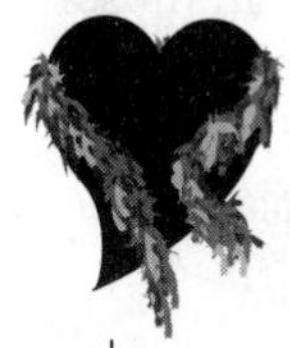

Feelin' the Love

I know how most people stereotype a girl for exotic dancing, but if they only knew the truth of it all—all us girlies have a little diva inside! We just need to let her out to play once in a while.

—"Peaches Holiday," student

You can choose an adjective that may reflect a small part of yourself, such as Spicy, Vixen, Foxy, or Cat. Standard stripper names are also always a good choice, because when you hear names like Bunny, Bambi, Candi, Coco, or Amber, you automatically think of a hot, steamy, scantily clad sexpot.

Even just a normal name you find pretty, like Brittney, Tiffany, Juliana, Veronica, or Holly can work, or you can be creative with names like Aurora, Xandra, Harley, Blaze, Saber, Gypsy, or Lace. Two names are also very sexy, such as Sexual Chocolate, Sweet Thing, etc.

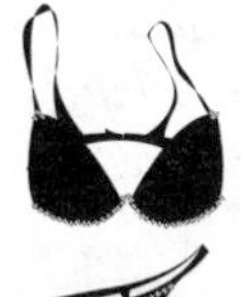

Behind the G-String

Taking a stage name is so important that in my classes, women must have one by the second class or they're automatically called Flatulence or Crusty. When my mom took my class, she called herself Miss Kitty, which was sexy in a cringing kind of way for me because she was my mother (and I had to listen to Dad's pole jokes!).

Or you could follow that old schoolyard rule of picking your stripper name using the name of your first pet with the first street you lived on. In my case, my name would have been Lolly Main. That method could backfire though if you end up with something like Ralph Butterworth!

Overall, have fun picking your stage name. Be creative. Get out your thesaurus if you need to!

The Great Wall of Diva

But how do you actually do it? How do you get out there in front of your man and dance for him without him thinking you're a stupid, silly woman trying to be sexy but failing miserably? How do you do it without cracking up laughing?

This is where I take on the role of drill sergeant (hey, now there's a sexy idea for a costume!). Imagine I am right next to you, shouting in your ear, bad breath and flying spittle to boot. There is really no other way to do this because we don't have 5 years for confidence therapy; we've got about 5 seconds! So in that case …

You put up a wall, soldier! This wall is 2 inches thick of invisible steel, and nothing, and I mean NOTHING, can get behind this wall to hurt you in any way … no strange looks, no comments, no whispers, no giggles. When you are behind this wall you are invincible, so you are GOING to stick your butt in his face, and he's going to like it whether he wants to or not. Who is he to think badly of you?

Who is a man—or woman, for that matter—to criticize you? Are they perfect? No? Then don't even THINK about letting any facial expressions or anything else from some other slob make YOU feel self-conscious. And even if someone is very handsome or prettier than you … so what? The truth is you are not perfect, and you are going to be proud of it!

Did you hear me, soldier? I said you are not perfect and you are going to be proud of it! Massage those rolls you hate! Caress those saddlebags! Look like you love them, soldier, and your audience will, too!

Okay, I'm done shouting now. I call this invincible steel shield the Great Wall of Diva. You can do anything you want behind this wall because no one or nothing can hurt you, so you let it all out; give 1,000 percent while you're dancing because that wall is there protecting you.

Even today, when beginner students watch me dance for the first time, or I've got a group of 10 to 15 giggly 20-something girls for a bachelorette party at my studio and I have to dance, up goes my steel wall. Women, as we all know, are much more critical of other women than men are, yet I, a 35-year-old woman, have to get up and do a dance down to my booty shorts and bra for a bunch of girls who have no concept of slowing metabolisms (not that I'm bitter) and who expect the large-breasted, tall, breathtaking exotic dancer stereotype. And I know they're just getting lil' ol' me.

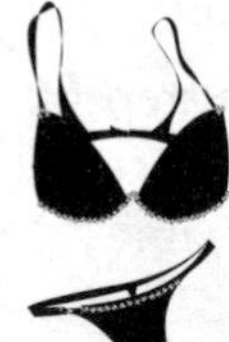

Behind the G-String

When I was a dancer at Ventura Snooky's, a very pretty girl named Misha went before me, and I thought to myself, *I can't compete with that.* But then a little voice said very clearly, *Then don't,* and since that day I have never worried or become insecure if a woman is prettier than I am. I just accept it and move on—and I've been a lot happier ever since!

Yet I do it. I do an exotic striptease for the most critical segment of the population, and I'm sure they're saying in their minds, *Her boobs aren't very big, she's not petite, she doesn't have that Las Vegas exotic dancer look,* etc. But you know what? Screw 'em! Yep, I *do* have small boobs, I'm *not* a toothpick, and I *don't* look like a Vegas stripper … what's it to ya?

And when I'm done with my dance, all those little critical girls are whooping and hollering and declaring to each other how amazing I was and that they could never dance like that! So you see, it really is all in the mind.

The man you're dancing for is on your side. He wants you to succeed and be sexy. He wants to see that you are proud of yourself! And the more you dance, the more you'll realize that confidence is sexier than any perfect body.

Men Are Easy to Please

Men think differently than women do. They are so visual, but in a simpler way. They don't pay attention to our hair or clothing or see the cellulite, saddlebags, or other imperfections we, as women, magnify to a degree that it destroys our self-esteem. We are trained to recoil in disgust and to be completely ashamed of any flaws we may have. Women are "trained" from a very young age that we should be perfect, that we should be thin or look just right or no man will want us.

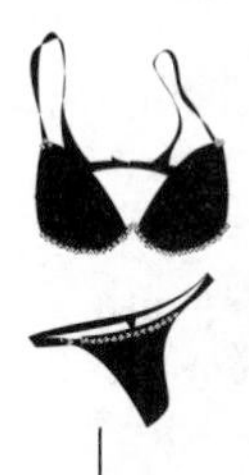

Behind the G-String

I'm a small B breast size, yet I get more compliments for having real breasts rather then oversized large fake ones. And that's not just in places like Providence, Rhode Island. That's in London and Los Angeles, too.

Well ladies, guess who created all those problems? *We did!* Women did! We are responsible for beating that idea into ourselves because then we can sell ourselves makeup and weight-loss plans and plastic surgery and everything else that's available to make us look—and feel—better. Then the women who make all the money off us are the ones who can really afford to have all that plastic surgery done, and so they continue to look great, while we, the average women, continue to beat ourselves up because we don't look like them.

Men don't think that way. Men are actually much easier to please visually than we are. In fact, they are so simple that if you tell them something is sexy they'll believe you. For example, when you're dancing, massage the part of your body you most dislike, whether it be your stomach, your thighs, or whatever. Act like that is the sexiest part of your body, like you love it, show it on your face that you are in absolute ecstasy as your caress your stretch marks. He will see this confidence, he will see that you *want* your own body, and he'll think, *Oh yeah … that's so sexy!*

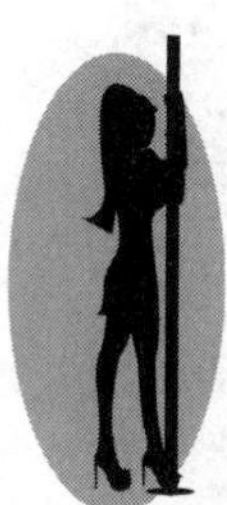

Slick Tricks

Act like you love every part of your body, especially your flaws. If you look like you think it's sexy, he will, too!

When I was a dancer in clubs, I worked with *many* different shapes, sizes, ages, and races of women, and believe me when I tell you, you don't have to be super skinny, and young with big breasts for a man to find you attractive. They don't like bone-racks; they like real women.

Don't get me wrong—guys love to look at pretty women with an hourglass figure and big breasts, but don't we like to look at muscular men with large biceps, too? Most women, however, prefer a man with some imperfections over one of those complete muscle-heads. (Okay, were I to find a muscle-head guy in my bed, I wouldn't kick him out, but work with me here …)

You Are the Queen

This is *your* show. *You* are the queen. If you just want to walk back and forth across the room for your dance you will, and he will like it, whether he wants to or not.

You put on your sexy face, your costume, and your attitude, and you take control! Suck in that attention and use it. This kind of attitude often takes years of therapy to achieve, but we don't have *years* of therapy. We have a few minutes. So in those few minutes, *you will be confident when you dance, you are the queen, you are the sexiest woman who ever walked, you are going to dance for yourself, and he is going to like it!* Learn to turn it on and off like a light switch.

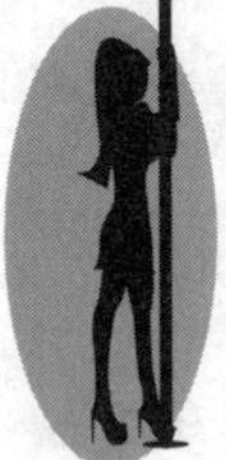

Slick Tricks

I danced with a pretty but very heavy girl named Amber at Oxnard Snooky's who made more money than most of the other dancers. Why, you ask? Because of her confident attitude.

Remember, you are dancing for *yourself,* not performing for *him.*

Period. That's it. No talk. (Wendy puts her hand up to block your protest.) Nothing more to say on the subject. Done. Closed. You are sexy, confident, and a great dancer. End of discussion. You have no choice in the matter. *You just are!*

Take Your Sweet Time

Now that you know you're dancing for yourself and that you're in control, you must not *tell* that to your audience. You must show them. And one of the most powerful tools you have to do this is timing.

Everything you do in your dance, particularly your introduction, must be done at your pace. This is your show. You'll do what you want, when you want, and *your audience will like it* because quite frankly, *they don't have a choice.*

Do important businesspeople rush out to meet you at a meeting, or do they make you wait? They make you wait. This is an excellent subliminal trick because the longer you have to wait, the more important the other person appears to be. They want you to feel "beneath" them, that they are not going to drop everything to rush right out to meet you because you're just not that important. The same principle applies here. Take your time. Let them know who's in charge, all without saying a word. Your timing will tell it all!

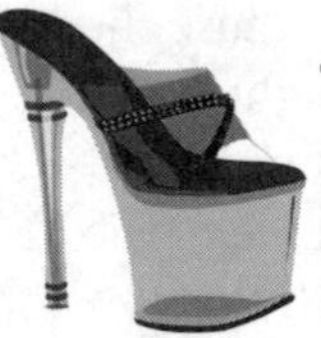

Trippin' Up

You are in control of your show, so act like it! If you rush out to start dancing or hurry through your dance, subliminally you are showing your audience that they are not in control and instead are trying to please them, which breaks down your confidence.

You need to sustain the overall mood through your performance. You are sexy and you know it, and you could care less whether your audience lives or dies, because you're enjoying yourself too much to stop for them.

So take your sweet time. When you spread your legs, keep them open for at least 3 seconds because it's the shock of the move that gets the audience. If you end in any kind of a pose, like from a shoulder roll turn or a mud flap pose, keep the pose for a few seconds. Let your audience admire you. You'll move on when you're good and ready.

No Club Dancing!

Before I turn you loose, let me leave you with this thought: *no club dancing*. Club dancing moves themselves are okay if they're slower, more sensual, and go with the undercurrent of the song. Even a faster, club-type song should be danced to via the undercurrent, never the surface beat. Your pulsating may be a little faster for a faster song, but that's okay so long as you're not club dancing!

When you club dance, your audience will lose the sense that this is all about how sexy you are, and you will end up performing for him, subliminally saying, "Look how well I can dance!" instead of, "I know I am *soooo* sexy!" You'll lose the whole focus of the dance if you fall into just flat performance club dancing.

So remember to do this for you. Yes, you can let him watch, but this is your dance. You're in control. You're the queen.

The Least You Need to Know

- Onstage, you are an entirely different person, with a personality all her own. Be able to turn your personality on and off.
- Exotic dancing is all about you, not him. Let him watch, yes, but dance for yourself.
- Exotic dancing is an act. You don't have to believe it, just act it out.
- Men are not as critical as we think they are. They're happy to watch as long as you act like you're happy to dance.

In This Chapter

- It's all about attitude
- Let your eyes and body speak for you
- Touching yourself: very sexy

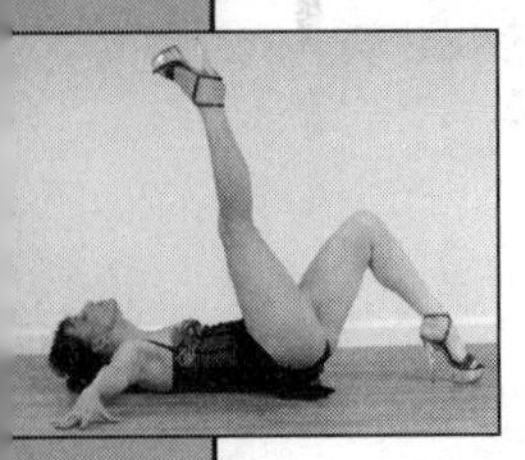
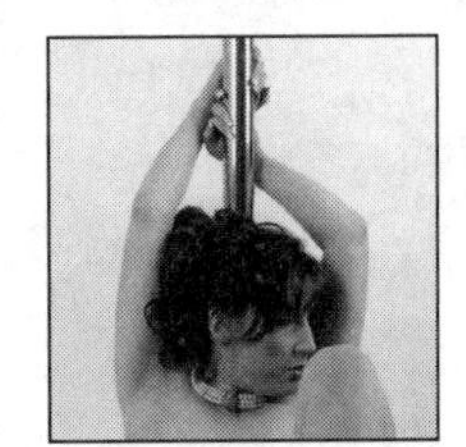
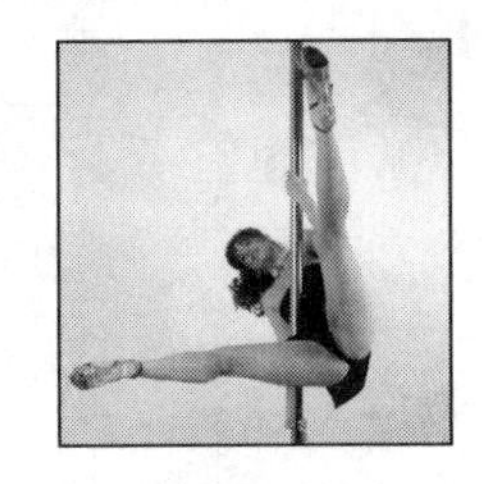
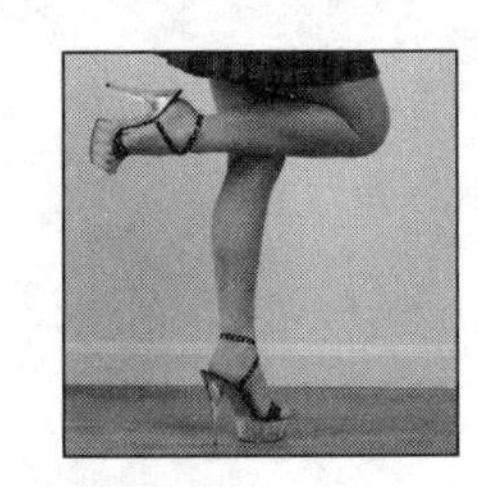
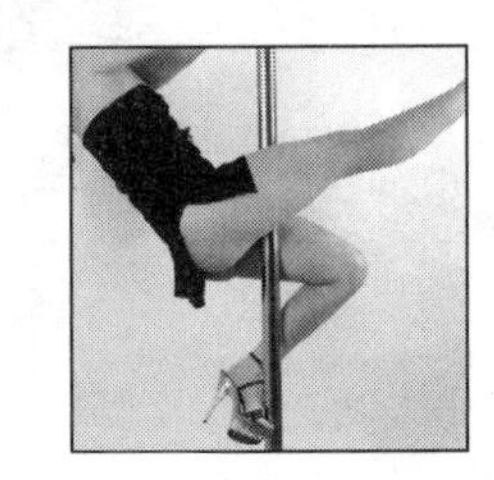
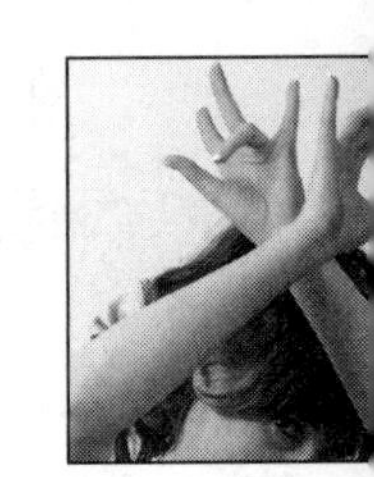

Chapter 2

Show, Don't Tell

Actions speak louder than words, and that's especially true when you're exotic dancing. You're using dance as a medium to express your sexuality to your audience—and to yourself. Exotic dancing is more than just the physical moves you make with your body, though. You also have to think about the emotion you show by your facial expressions and by how you caress yourself. (Believe it or not, there are right and wrong ways of caressing!)

This might sound like a lot to think about, but trust me: when you get the hang of it, you'll be able to dance like the pros do! Let's see how it's done.

90 Percent Attitude

I've danced with girls who are gorgeous and have perfect bodies but who don't make any money because they look bored and uninterested when they dance, like they'd rather be anywhere but performing onstage. Believe me, if you're not excited to be dancing, it shows!

Yet the girls who looked like they were having fun, made eye contact, and appeared to be truly enjoying themselves—whether they had perfect bodies or not—made the most money. Why? They got the attention and money because of their attitudes, not their physical bodies.

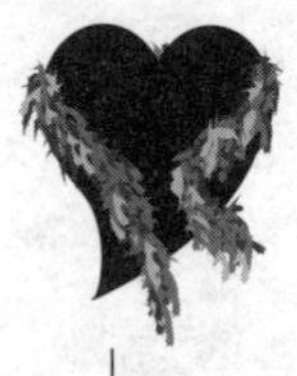

Feelin' the Love

When you're dancing, keep this math in mind:

90 percent of your dance is in your attitude and facial expression.

10 percent is your physical dance.

0 percent is your body appearance.

The Eyes Have It

When you smile, your eyes light up. When you're upset, your eyes reflect that, too. Your eyes are the most powerful and seductive tool you have, so use them! That attitude I talked about earlier? Make your eyes a billboard for what you're feeling.

Look at yourself in the mirror with a sexy look. (Don't even tell me you don't have one! Every woman does!) It's kind of a cat-who-ate-the-canary look, an I-know-something-you-don't-know expression or a you-want-me-but-you're-not-going-to-get-me attitude. Practice that look in the mirror, and keep that expression on your face while you dance.

Try it a while, and you might be surprised how a facial expression can help you believe you are truly someone else when you perform—not to mention help define you as a sexy dancer!

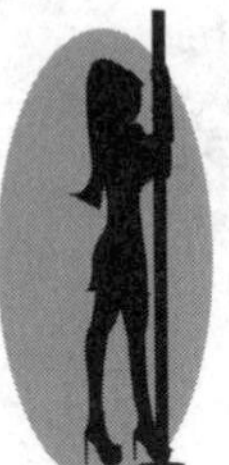

Slick Tricks

Always have a sparkle in your eye when you dance. The more you look like you're enjoying yourself, the more your audience will, too!

To add more drama to your dance, roll your neck and shoulders, close your eyes, sigh, and appear to be in your own world.

That expression is also a subliminal control thing. Your audience is going to think, *What does she know that I don't know?* or *Why is she so smug?* That will show them *you* are in control. Your confidence will show in your eyes.

Move Your Mouth

While you dance, be sure to move your mouth, too. You essentially want to look like you're so into your dance, the music has taken over, the passion is overwhelming you, and you're becoming so turned on by dancing for your man that you're in complete ecstasy! Yes, I'm being serious—you really do want to be *that* dramatic.

A good way to be sure your face doesn't go blank when you dance is to lightly lip-sync the song you're dancing to. Now, you don't have to lip-sync every word or really articulate your mouth, but do it is almost as if you are whispering the words as you dance. Even if you only know the chorus or a few key words, you can still "sing" the song to your significant other. This not only makes you feel more in to your dance, but it shows your audience that you're dancing that specific dance to that song, you're not just doing moves to music.

You can also animate your face by licking your lips, biting your lip, grinning, blowing kisses, using a prop like a lollipop, and winking.

Helping Hands

Guys think it's so wonderful when a woman touches herself, so be sure to caress yourself as you dance. When I was a club dancer, we were not allowed to touch our breasts or groin area. Instead, I used my fingers to caress around them or delicately frame them—a tease in its own right!

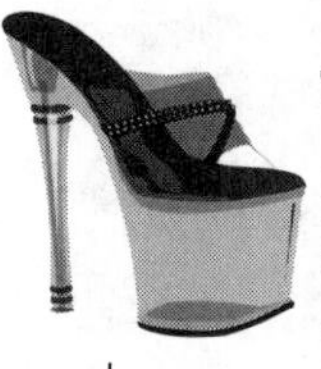

Trippin' Up

Never let your hands or arms just hang down. Always keep your hands caressing, massaging, or moving gracefully when you dance.

There is an art to caressing yourself, however. You don't want to rub your hands all over your body quickly. That's what you do when you're cold, and that's not sexy.

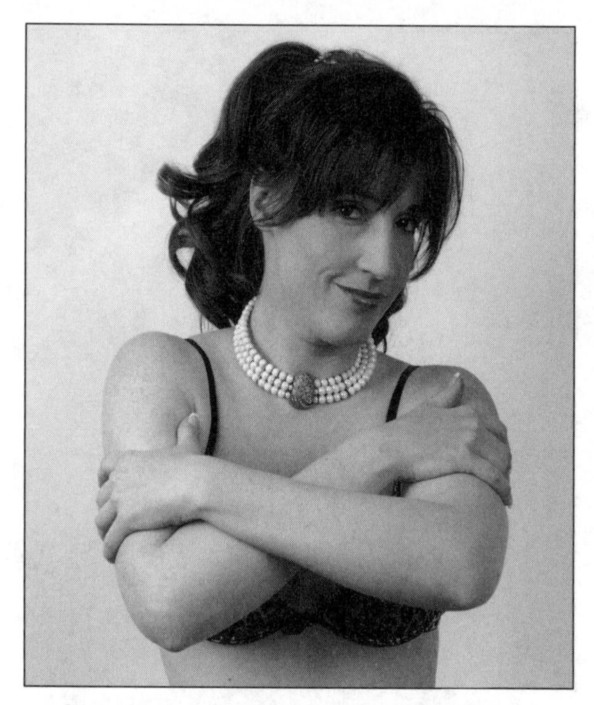

This is the incorrect way to caress yourself. I look cold, not sexy

You want to show your audience you are caressing every part of yourself because your body is beautiful and you know it! (Again, even if you don't believe it is … act like it!) Therefore, move your hands *slowly,* even if you're dancing to a fast-paced song. Move with the undercurrent of the song, not the surface beat.

To caress yourself properly, start by holding your arms out straight and then bend them at the elbows so your hands are on the opposite elbow. (Picture the *I Dream of Jeannie* pose.) Place just your middle fingers on your elbows so your other fingers aren't touching your arms at all. As your fingertips glide around your body, you may end up with more of your finger than just the tip. That's okay; your audience isn't going to say, "Hmmm, the inside of her knuckle on her right hand was touching her arm, instead of just her fingertips. I'm going withhold my tip." (If they did, you'd kick their beer over on them.) That's the kind of detail that although important, you shouldn't dwell on it.

Put pressure on your middle fingers (to keep you from going to fast—remember, you're sexy, not cold!), and slowly draw them up your arms to your shoulders, across your breastbone, around your breasts, down your side, and basically massage your torso like it's gold!

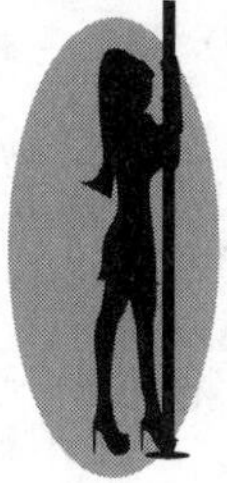

Slick Tricks

Keeping pressure on your fingers when you caress yourself is essential. The pressure forces you to move your fingers slowly—a silent way to prove to your audience that *you know you are sexy.*

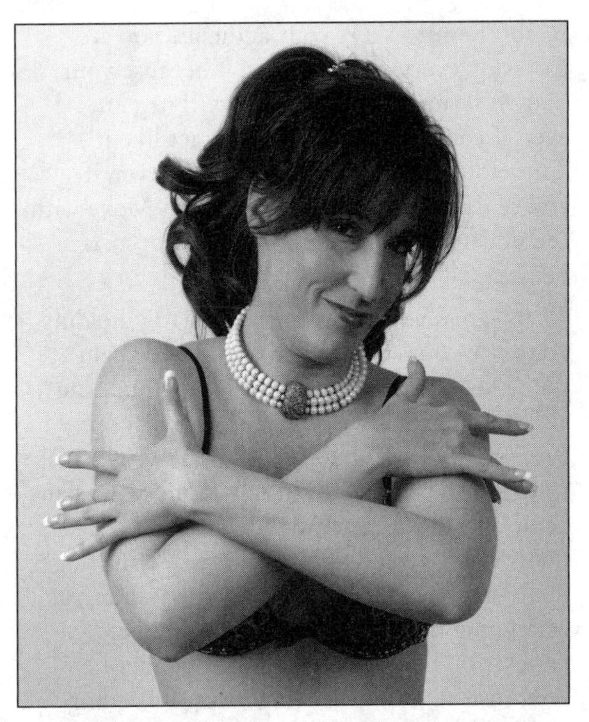

Imagine your body as that of your lover's. You know how you love to drag your hands all over him! Remember to do it like you mean it!

Okay, now I know you're laughing at this and thinking, *Oh, I can't do that! This feels silly touching myself—it's so not like me!* I don't care how silly it feels, because it looks great. And remember, *this is all acting*. The more dramatic you are, the sexier you'll look to your audience. That is, after all, what you want, right? You want to look sexy!

You can also use your hands artistically by rolling them delicately over your body.

Put your hands up in front of you, your palms facing each other. Bend in your thumbs and middle fingers so they create a *C*. Loosen your other fingers so they're not totally straight and delicately frame the *C*.

Roll your wrists, cross your hands in front of you with your elbows bent, and continue to roll your wrists until your hands move gracefully. (Fun fact: this is actually a belly-dancer hand move.)

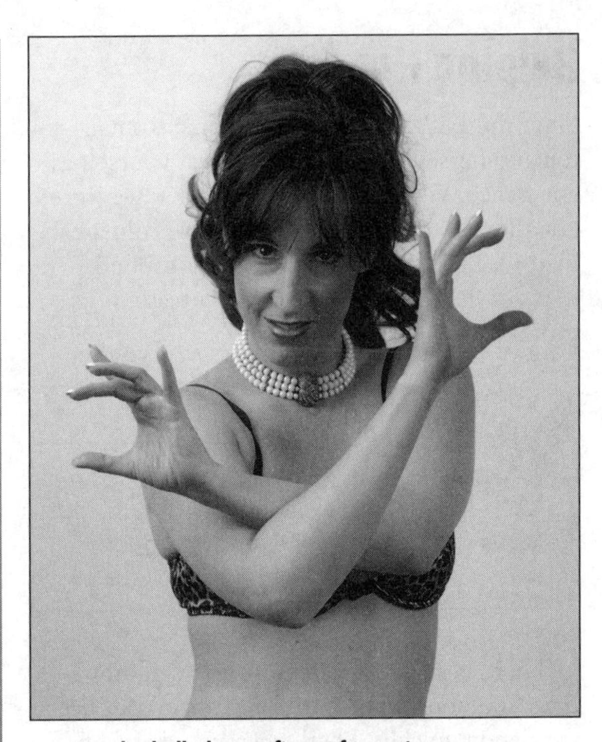

Use the bellydancer finger formation to appear delicate.

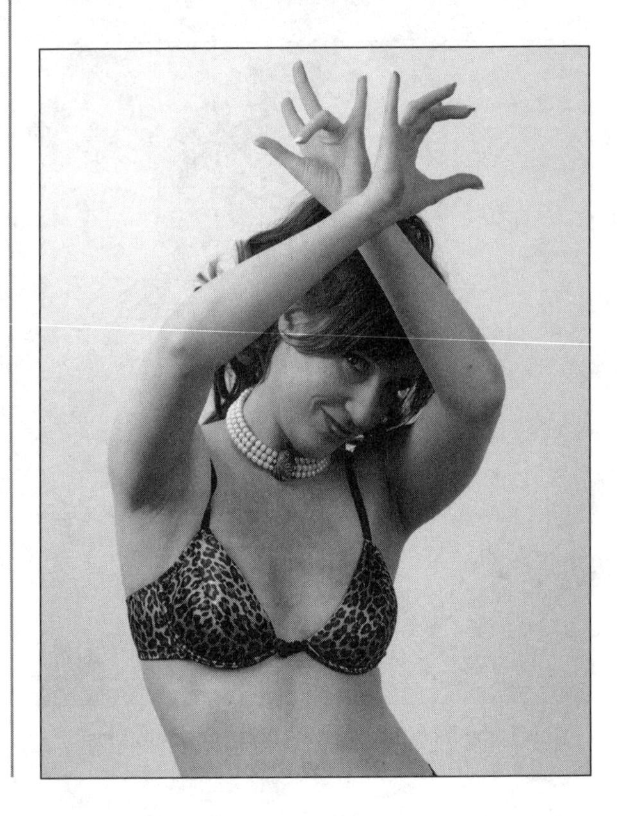

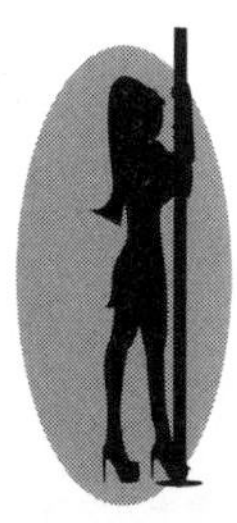

Slick Tricks

Keep your fingers in a delicate pose as you caress yourself. Hands are an important detail, essential to a strong performance.

Dance with your hands above your head, in front of your groin (so it appears as if you're touching yourself, but you're not), and even behind your back in front of your butt.

You can also "feather" your fingers as you do this, which is moving all your fingers back and forth quickly in a feathery motion.

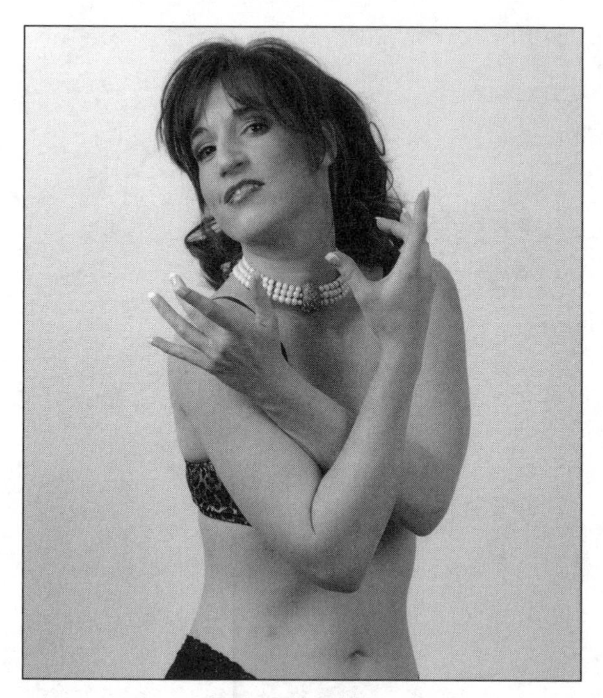

When you bring your hands over your head, be sure to bend your elbows so you don't just flap your hands like a bird.

Be sure to always keep your hands caressing, massaging, or moving gracefully, never flat. Flat isn't sexy.

You'll get the hang of this the more you practice and the more you watch yourself in the mirror.

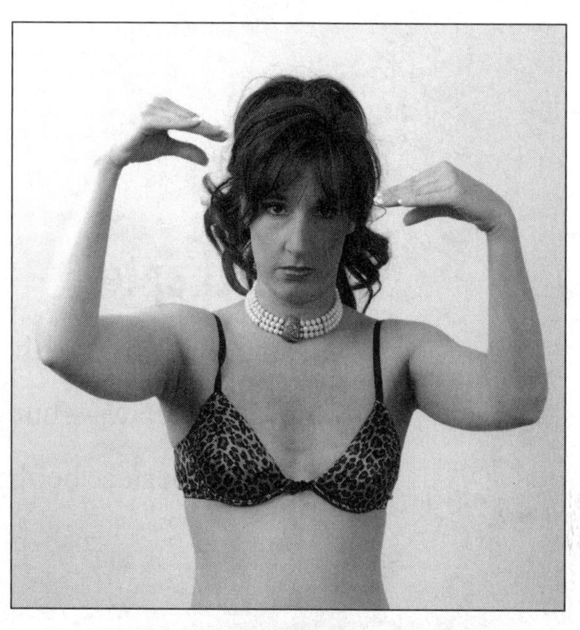

Be sure your fingers and hands aren't too stiff.

The Least You Need to Know

- Be sure to keep a sparkle in your eye while you dance.
- To keep from having an "I'm bored" stone-face expression, lightly lip-sync the music you're dancing to, blow a kiss, lick your lips, etc.
- Put pressure on your fingers when you caress. This keeps you from moving too quickly and shows your audience that you're so sexy, you can't keep your hands off yourself.
- Be dramatic when you dance and especially when you caress yourself. That's what this is all about!

In This Chapter

- Using makeup to enhance, not overwhelm
- Love your flaws—but cover them, too
- Building perfect boobs
- Hair and nail brush-ups

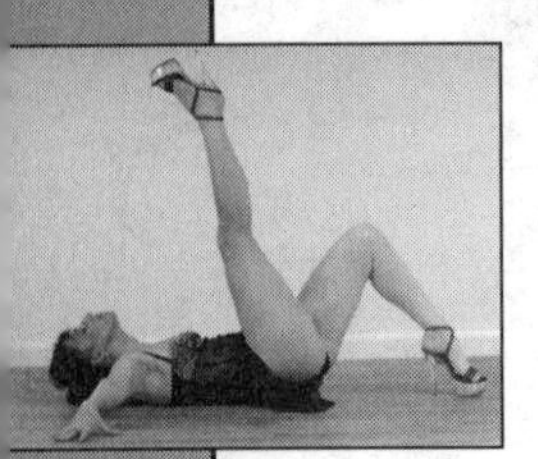
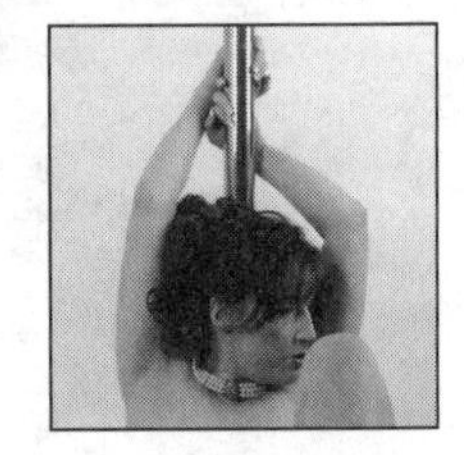
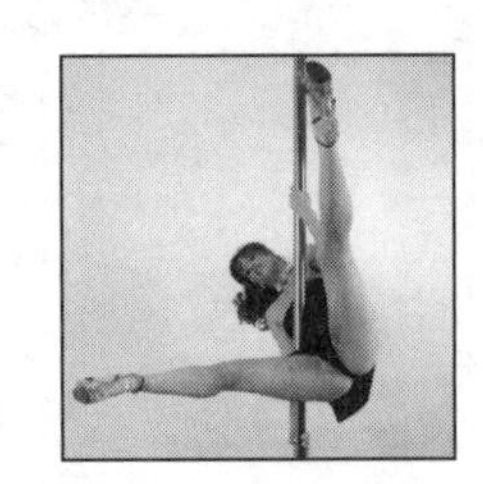
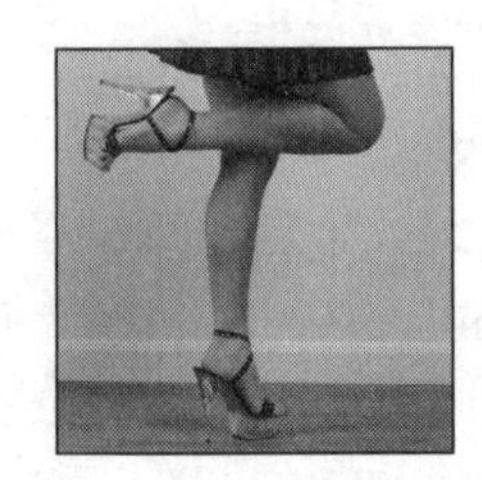
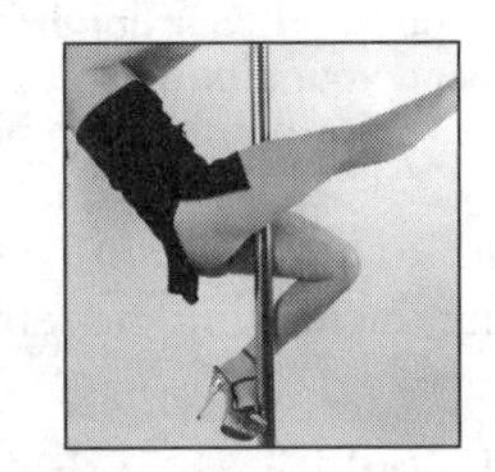
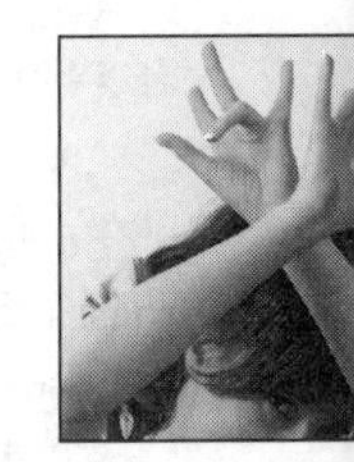

Chapter 3

The Cinderella Syndrome

To truly feel sexy, confident, and able to get the desired results from this book, it's essential that you learn to step out of your everyday life and really dress the part of an exotic dancer, not unlike our good friend Cinderella (though she didn't pole dance—that we know of!). And like Cinderella, you must have a fairy godmother and pet rats to help you dress if you are to believe the Disney version of the story. Luckily, I happen to have pet rats, so I'm all set there, but I don't have a fairy godmother (I don't even think I had a godmother, come to think of it) so that fairy godmother must be … you!

Yes, you! You must wave your magic wand and transform yourself into a glamorous, if not somewhat loose-looking princess. Your makeover is not restricted to just face makeup, though. It includes all of you, because the dance is really in the details, which includes hair and nails. You need to feel like a completely different person. You might feel overornamented at first, but when the whole new you is put together, you'll see that it's a perfect balance for the new, sexy you—and that it feels good!

Take me, for example. Normally I'm just a plain woman, but toss on a hot dress, platform heels, sexier makeup, and long hair, and—voilà—you've got Holly, Exotic Dancer. If I can make such a dramatic transformation, so can you!

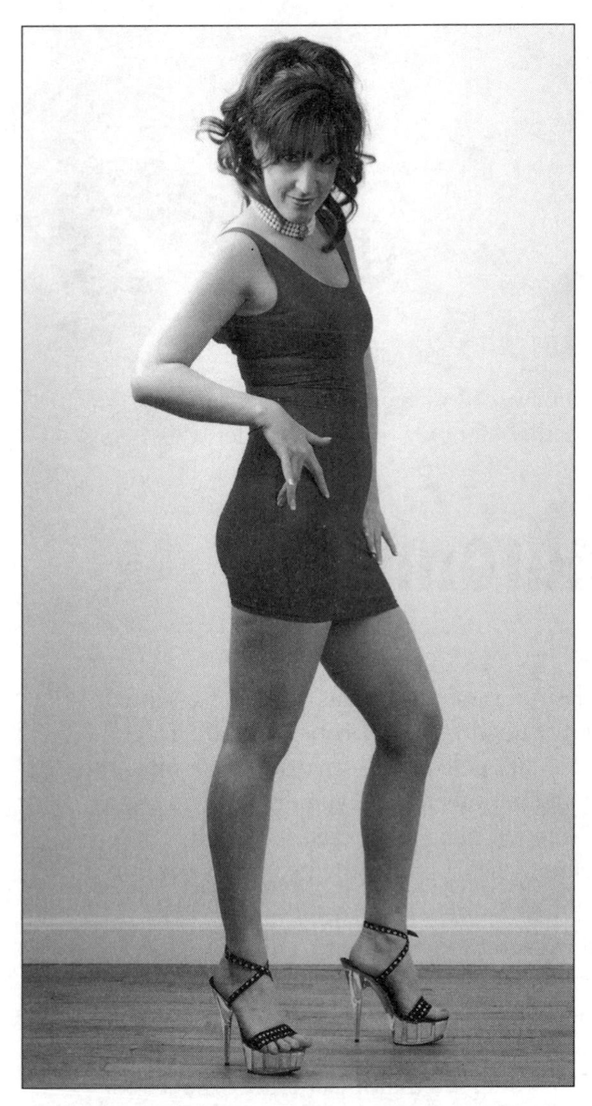

With just a little bit of effort, I can make myself look great and feel really sexy!

It's impossible to feel sexy—and, therefore, practice exotic dancing—while wearing workout clothing, no makeup, and sneakers. If you're going to do this, do it right!

Getting All Made Up

By "sexy makeup," I do not necessarily mean "heavy makeup." You want your makeup to be dramatic, not distracting! You do want to wear a little more than usual, but you don't want him to see the makeup first. Makeup is only for enhancing, not masking.

Whatever base makeup you normally wear should work, although I prefer the spray-on airbrush makeup by ERA because of its incredibly even coverage and lightweight feel. Spray it directly over your face and neck and then pat it down with a fluffy makeup pouf. While it's drying, blend in around your eyes and nose. Then use a concealer under your eyes or wherever you may need to conceal; blend that in as well.

You don't even need to powder over the spray-on, although I like to powder my nose just a bit to absorb any shine that may appear.

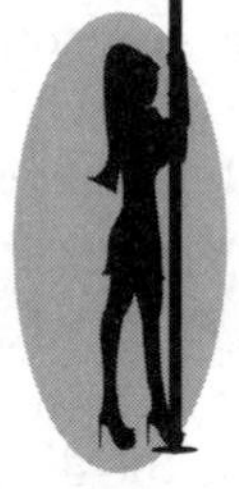

Slick Tricks

Brushing blush horizontally under your chin will make any pudge in that area less noticeable.

Bedroom Eyes

And now for your eyes. I've got dark brown eyes, so I start with a dark brown shadow in the crease of my lids. (Depending on your eye color, you can use whatever eye shadow colors you want.) Then I add cream-colored eye shadow to my lids and my brow bone. I use black liquid eyeliner in the thinnest line I can get right on the eyelash line on top of my lids. While the liner is still wet, I take a separate eye shadow applicator and smudge the liner ever so gently so it doesn't look like a hard line.

Then I take a pointed foam eye shadow applicator, dust it in the dark brown eye shadow, and apply it lightly over the black liner to soften it. I use a little bit of the black liquid eyeliner in the outside corners of my eyes and about an eighth of the way across my bottom eyelash line and then do the same thing with the smudging and brown eye shadow to soften. (Remember to always soften everything with eye shadow. You don't want any hard lines anywhere.) Then, for the rest of my under-eye area, I use just brown eye shadow as an actual liner.

Using an eyelash curler, curl your eyelashes. To make them look really long, place the curler as far back as you can so you can feel your eyelashes being pulled a bit when you apply pressure to close the curler. Hold that for 3 seconds. Then coat the top of your eyelashes with black mascara. Now apply mascara as you normally would, going from underneath your lashes out to the tips. I usually apply two coats of black mascara (but only one on the top of my lashes).

If you don't have particularly long eyelashes, try the fake ones. They'll really make a difference, and you'll be amazed at how they can really open your eyes.

Blushing Blush

Next, apply your regular blush to the apple of your cheek. Just be sure you don't end up with red streaks!

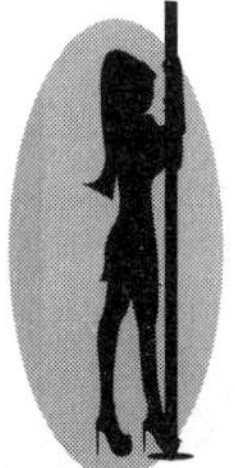

Slick Tricks

Brush some blush vertically between your breasts and extending up about 4 inches to give the illusion of shadow. This makes your breasts look bigger in the dim light!

Luscious Lips

For your lips, start by powdering them with either compact or loose powder; this helps the color stay on. Then use a darker lip liner to contour your lips, and then color them in.

Use a lipstick a shade darker than you normally do for dramatic affect and then use a very very light lipstick to highlight your bottom lip. Just run the light color over the dark one a few times until it's several shades lighter.

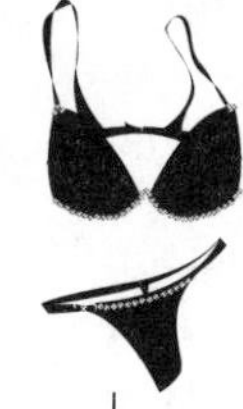

Behind the G-String

There's no need to go out and buy a $10 lip liner, because the 99¢ ones do the same thing. Besides, your audience is not going to know the difference!

Concealing Weapons

We all have flaws, and although we love them, we are going to cover them. I find that Dermablend (which you can get at department stores) is the best body makeup. It's a little pricey, but it's worth it because it lasts forever and it works.

Use just a little concealer to cover any scars, acne, varicose veins, or light stretch marks that make you uncomfortable.

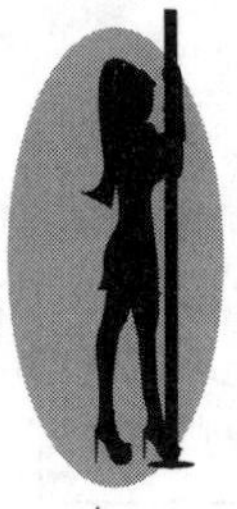

Slick Tricks

Don't go overboard with the concealer. Remember, you'll be dancing in dim light or by candlelight, which will naturally conceal these wonderful characteristics. And if you can't cover it, then be *proud* of it!

I am blessed with very very dark leg hair and extremely fair skin, and I find it very annoying when I can see the black hair below the surface of my skin. Your audience isn't going to notice this, but as a woman, I know it's there, and it bothers me.

So I apply Dermablend, particularly around the bikini area, to cover up my lovely see-through skin. I then cover it with a light coating of the sealing powder. The end result? My skin looks completely flawless!

Enhancing You

Nowadays you could create a complete person with everything fake, from boobs to eyelashes, from nails to hair. And that's the point of exotic dancing, right, to make a whole new you?

Let's look at some of your enhancement options.

Are They Real?

You don't need surgery or implants to get bigger (better?) boobs! Just head to Victoria's Secret or your favorite department store's lingerie section! You can get super-duper padded bras, blow-up bras, rubber breast thingees to put in your bra … there are all kinds of fun enhancements you can try!

And when it comes time to strip it all off, secretly slide out any enhancements you may have—or proudly face him, take out one at a time, and fling them away. Yes, you used them, and you're proud of it!

Fabulously Fake Nails

Every detail on your body counts when you are dancing, even down to your fingernails. You could get a manicure, but if you're lazy like me, you can get glue-on nails at your nearest pharmacy. I prefer Broadway Nails; they're about $6 and look extremely real. You just glue them right over your own fingernails and they last for about a week before they start to pop off.

The look you're going for dictates what style nails you want to get. For the very sensual look, I'd go for the forever classic French nails. Sparkles and nail art are lovely, but for pure, classy, timeless look, go for the basic French. If you're going for a harder or more fun dance, then by all means go for the long nails!

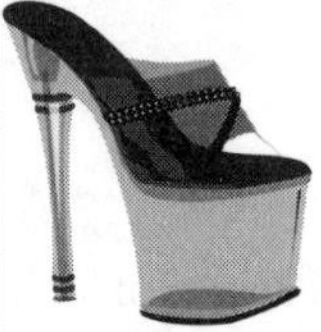

Trippin' Up

Sexy nails does not have to mean *long nails!* If they're too long, and if you're not used to long nails, they'll distract you when you're dancing and you'll be conscious of them—which will throw off your whole performance.

Be sure to paint your toenails, too. Red is a sexy color to paint your toes. Plus it's so cheerful to wake up in the morning and see bright red toes smiling back at you! Just be sure to touch them up or remove the polish when that fun red starts to chip off.

Hair Today, Gone Tomorrow

I'm one of those women whose hair simply will not grow long, and ladies, as much as I hate to admit it, men really do like long hair. But that's okay, because for your dance, you can have the long hair you've always wanted! Isn't it wonderful living in the twenty-first century!

You will be *amazed* at the difference the hairpiece can make. It will really, truly make you feel like someone else and will change your look entirely.

Plenty of online stores sell hair pieces, although I prefer to see it first so I can match the color to my own hair. Most beauty supply stores carry Revlon hair pieces in different styles and colors and are fairly inexpensive—which is good if your hair is going to be used at only certain times.

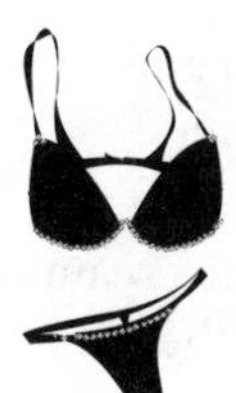

Behind the G-String

A hairpiece or wig should look natural, so if you've got dark features and you get a blond wig, it's going to look silly and be distracting to your audience.

For those of you with super short hair that can't be put into a ponytail, try a headband wig. These clever inventions make it look like your long, luxurious locks are simply pulled back into a headband. This can be kept in place with bobby pins.

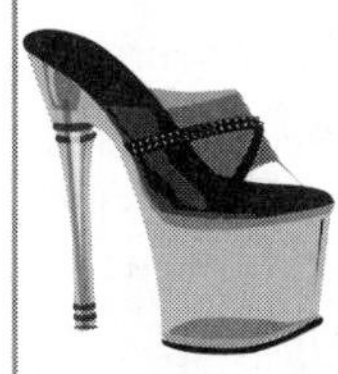

Trippin' Up

Always secure your hairpiece to your head. Don't just toss on a wig, because it will slide or fall off.

If you decide to go for a headband wig, or even another other look, be sure you have a salesperson help you. And tell that salesperson to be honest! Don't let her tell you something looks great unless it really does, just so she can make a sale. Ease her mind by telling her you will definitely be buying a hairpiece if she is honest enough to help you pick out the perfect one.

Dealing with "Female Stuff"

It's fun being a girl, getting to dress up, curl our hair, use makeup, and accessorize with jewelry and adorable shoes … but then there's the Dark Side. The Dark Side, as I'm sure you can figure out, is the annoying part of being female that we only whisper about to each other, if we can even bring the subject up at all.

Maybe you have some questions about dancing while you're on your period or just what the best method of hair removal is. Never fear. In this section, I answer FAQs about such unpleasantness.

What About "That Time"?

When I was a professional dancer, we had to dance during "that time," because it was our job and we still had to go to work. You can dance, too, if you want to. Just use a tampon, but cut the string in half and tuck it up.

Wear a black sheer or solid dress that covers your tummy if you're bloated, because remember you can still just tease or go topless. You don't have to take it all off; you show him what you want to, when you want to. He will want you more knowing he can't have you now.

Hair Removal: Waxing vs. Shaving vs. Cream

Ah, hair removal. The bane of being a female at times. You have many options when it comes to hair removal. You might want to try out a few methods and decide what you like best.

Some girls swear by a Brazilian wax, which entails going to a salon and having someone wax it all. This hurts only for a second, and they get everything. Also when you wax, the hair doesn't grow back as quickly and eventually grows back thinner.

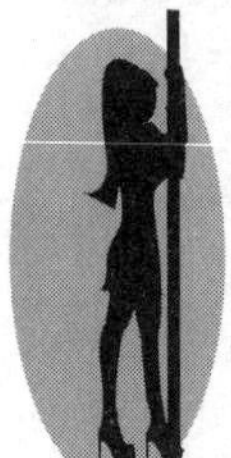

Slick Tricks

Wipe an alcohol pad over the area you're going to wax and let it dry before you apply the wax. This clears up any natural skin oil and will allow the wax to stick better and remove more hair.

I wouldn't recommend trying a Brazilian on yourself unless you know exactly what you're doing. I cannot think of anything more painful if you were to, um, miss. Also you have to wait for the hair to grow longer before it can be waxed.

Shaving can work well if you're going to dance that night. Try to use a fresh razor, but not a disposable one; they don't offer the control and protection a normal razor does. Start in the front and shave down in the direction the hair is growing. Next, shave it from the right side to the left and then from the left to the right. Finally, shave up, in the opposite direction of hair growth. Try to do the same underneath and around, although it's more difficult, so shave it as you can. And don't forget your butt, too.

Razor burn (the red bumps that appear in the bikini area after you shave) is not only annoying, but very unsightly and can be painful. Luckily though, you can prevent the burn. I find that Tend Skin works best. When you get out of the shower, apply in areas you shaved that are not used to being shaved. Or you can use hydrogen peroxide on the affected areas (it doesn't sting) and follow it with Neosporin.

I prefer to use creams as my method of fuzz-removal because it's easy and painless, albeit a bit messy and stinky. Slather the cream where you want the hair removed, and follow the directions as to how long to leave it on. (Some creams only require 4 minutes.) Just don't go more than a minute or so over the time or use it on any broken skin.

Use a washcloth to remove the cream and store the cloth in a baggie until you can do laundry because cream removers have a very powerful odor. Also be sure not to let the cream get on any fabric, because it will bleach the material. And just to be safe, follow the same razor-burn rules I gave a few paragraphs up an hour or so after you remove the cream.

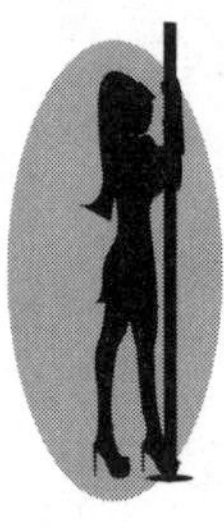

Slick Tricks

Use cream remover the night before your dance to ensure there's no trace of the bleachlike odor.

More Hair Removal: Arms, Fingers, Feet (and Mustaches)

Arms, fingers, and feet: these areas get fuzzy too, gals. Just because it's not the "focus area" as we would think, these areas, if hairy, can be a turnoff to a guy. It's almost like a guy's hairy back—that doesn't bother him in the slightest, but it makes most women cringe. These areas can be taken care of with either cold wax strips or body wax you can get at the drug store, or you can use creams or even shave. Of course, you can also go to a salon.

The female mustache, as much as we all detest them, is a real phenomenon and just one more annoying thing women have to deal with. Waxing is definitely the way to go here, because shaving makes the hair grow back thicker and hair-removal cream on your face … well, after you get your first whiff of it, I'm sure you'll agree that you don't want it directly under your nose.

Bleaching isn't a very good idea for a 'stache, because it will simply look like a fuzzy blond mustache. Just because it's not dark doesn't mean they can't see it—or feel it.

Spritz the Pits

Armpits can get pretty stinky, as we all know. Normal deodorants work well, but if you have a real problem with underarm odor, I highly recommend Certain Dri, which you can get at any drugstore. One application will actually last you about 2 days!

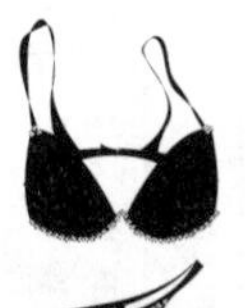

Behind the G-String

The directions on Certain Dri indicate, "Do not use immediately after shaving." I didn't think they meant me, so I used it after I shaved. Apparently, they did mean me, because within minutes, my pits turned bright red and began to burn. And it didn't go away for hours! Lesson learned: always follow manufacturer directions.

Tattoos … on You!

Temporary tattoos can be fun and a bit daring, particularly if you've got a reputation for being very … how shall I say it … "beige." You can find temporary rub-on tattoos almost anywhere, so choose one that fits your personality, the essence of your song, or better yet … the essence of the new you! Have a friend put it on to be sure it is even and centered.

A lot of men find a woman with tattoos sexy, especially if those tattoos are on the small of her back, the inside of her thigh, or just on the top of her breast so that when the tease begins, all he can see is a hint of a tattoo. Trust me ladies, the more conservative you are in your daily life, the hotter he's going to get when he sees that tattoo!

Now look at yourself … dramatically made up, imperfections covered, beautiful flowing hair, gorgeous hands with classic fingernails, a sly and sexy tattoo. The transformation is almost complete. Are you beginning to feel excited about your new alter ego? I am!

The Least You Need to Know

- Use makeup to help transform into a whole other persona. And here's a helpful hint: brush blush between your cleavage to make your boobs appear bigger!
- Practice dancing with your hairpiece and nails on to be sure they don't get in the way—and stay on!
- The more details you add to this "other you," the more exotic you'll feel!
- Try temporary tattoos for extra excitement! He'll love being surprised by the art as you expose more skin!

In This Chapter

- Dressing to complement your body
- Fun with costumes
- Fun with footwear
- Shopping!

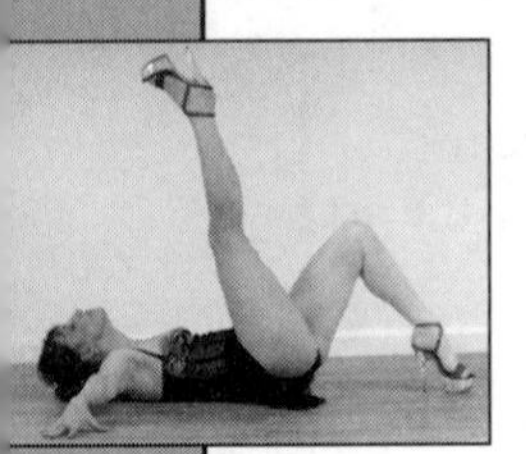
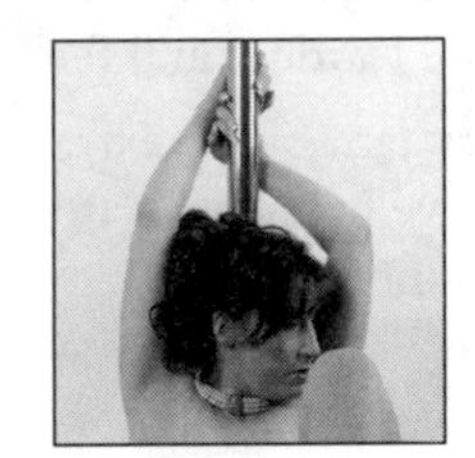
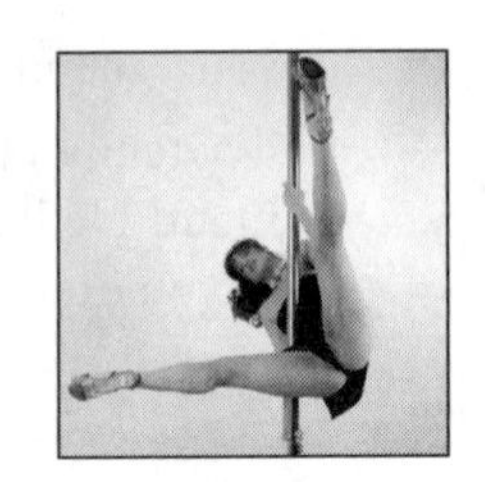
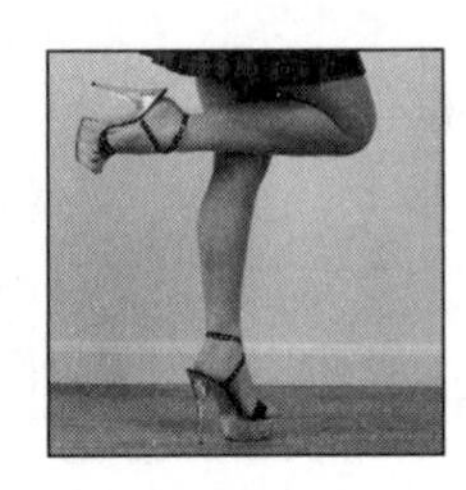
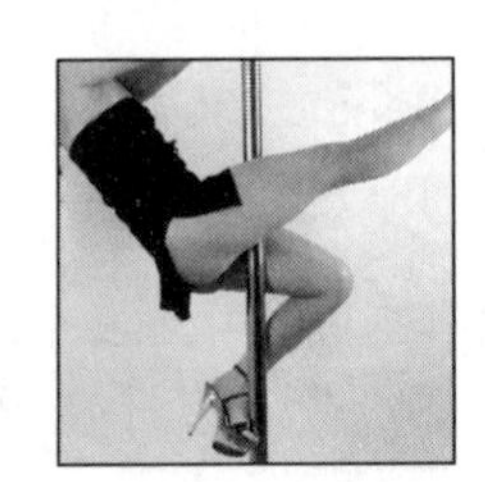
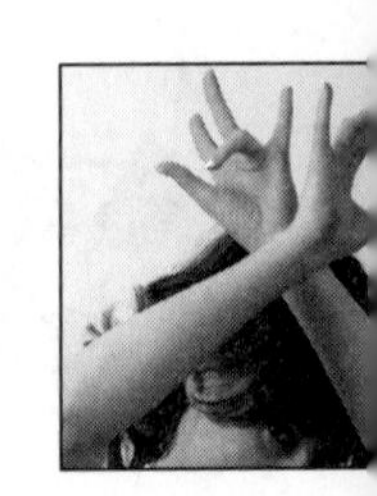

Chapter 4

See-Thru Shirts and Hot Short Skirts

It's the age-old question we face every morning: what should you wear? You want to look sexy and maybe even slutty when you dance, but not trashy. You might even want to look cute and innocent—or dark and devilish! The whole idea here is to have a little fun, to step out of your everyday life. Now's your chance to wear something crazy, to spice things up a bit!

Whatever look you're going for, you want to be sure you complement your body so that you can be comfortable—physically as well as psychologically.

Become Becoming—Dress *Your* Body Shape

Women come in all shapes and sizes, and who's to say what size is right? It's up to each woman to decide what her body should look like. She gets to decide how to dress to make her body shine! I just offer a little advice here.

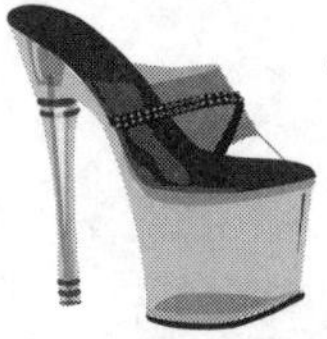

Trippin' Up

There's nothing worse than seeing a woman (or a man, as far as that goes!) in clothing so tight it shows every little bump and roll. That is *not* sexy! You want to always complement your own body shape, and "tight" may not do it. Very few women can wear something tight and look good in it—those naturally skinny women who can't seem to gain weight, or those unassuming 20-something girls who have no concept of metabolism and how when they hit 30 they're not going to be able to eat anything they want and stay skinny (not that I'm bitter …).

Dressing for Success

Some of us are top-heavy, and others aren't so much. Many women with large breasts are ashamed of them and want to hide them, but girls, please don't hide them when you're dancing! If you've got 'em, show 'em off! Be happy you have them, because not all of us do.

If you're not well endowed, you can wear a bra one cup size smaller than you normally wear to make your breasts look bigger. Be sure to keep your band size the same, though. Otherwise, it will be too tight and your skin will hang over.

And you can never have enough under wire or padding. That's why so many women love the Wonderbra! Have fun, choose sparkly bras, lacey bras, animal print, cupless …anything crazy and fun!

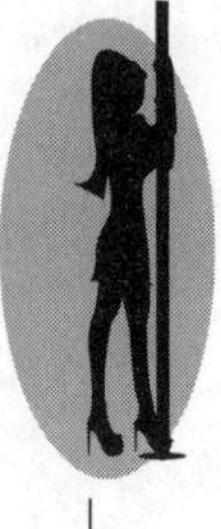

Slick Tricks

If you have any kind of wardrobe malfunction while you're dancing, act like you meant for it to happen, acknowledge it, and move on. Nothing you do in your dance is ever a mistake! Instead, consider it a preview or a quick peep show!

G-Strings and Other Underneath Things

As far as underwear goes, thongs are a no-no unless you have one of those 20-something bodies that laughs in the face of metabolism. Thongs are just not complementary to any body shape but a perfectly thin one.

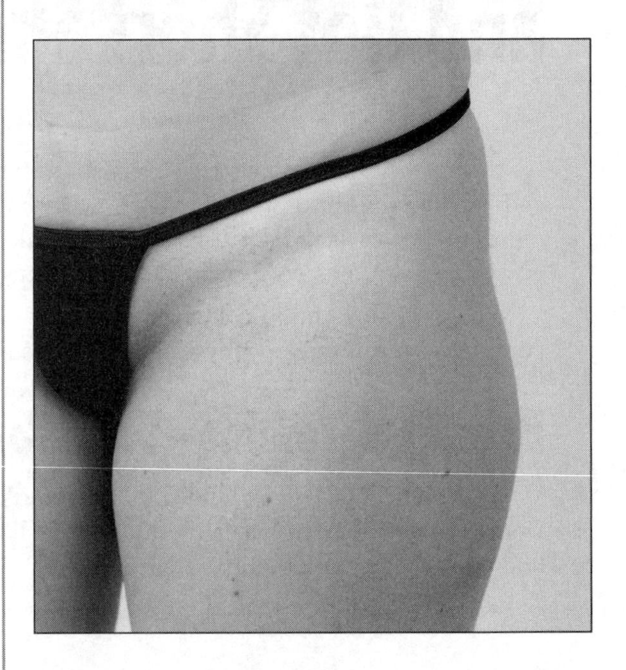

I have an hourglass/pear shape, and so V-cut boy shorts work best for me and other women with this body shape. The V cut creates the illusion that you're thinner than you are, no matter what your shape. Plus, it looks delicate and pretty!

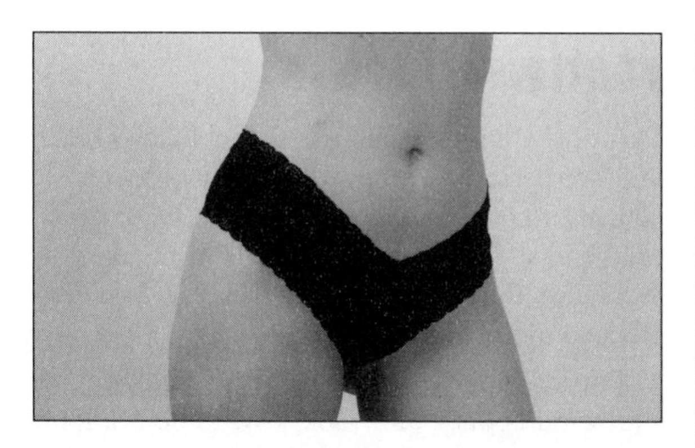

Many men love to see a garter on a woman, but if men had to try to put them on, I guarantee garters would be outlawed! They are such a pain, but they do look good and are worth the effort. Beware, though, that depending on how you move your body while you're dancing, garters will most likely pop off. I don't think any guy will mind this, though, because it actually looks sexy!

If your legs are bigger, be sure you get the correct size nylon and only pull it up far enough so that it rides smooth with your skin. Just because you have on garters or thigh-highs doesn't mean they need to be all the way up to your crotch.

Other Clothing Considerations

Now for the overthings. Whether you wear a costume or just some of your own clothes, remember to keep it sexy! Skirts are often soft, feminine, and delicate, and those that flare out when you twirl are sexy and also tons of fun! Even longer skirts/dresses are sexy. You can tease with them when you dance just as you would a shorter skirt.

Also realize that elasticized skirts can be uncomplementary, even if you don't consider yourself "fat." If you have a skirt with an elastic waistband, be sure it's a wider elastic, which is more forgiving.

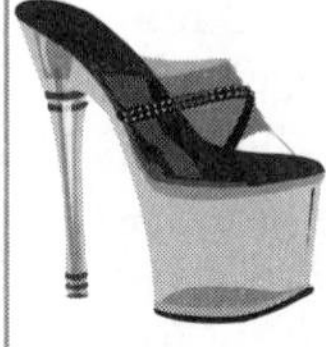

Trippin' Up

Elastic bands on any part of your costume should be flush with your skin, not "choking" it so something hangs over the edge.

Corsets are also lots of fun, although stripping out of them can be a pain because of all the clasps—unless you get some help getting out of it! For a flawless strip, get a corset made with both clasps and zippers. You can still get him to help you out of it if you want!

Who Do You Want to Be?

Now that you've got an idea of what to wear, what do we wow them with at first? What kind of mood are you in? What kind of song do you want to dance to? What message are you trying to get across?

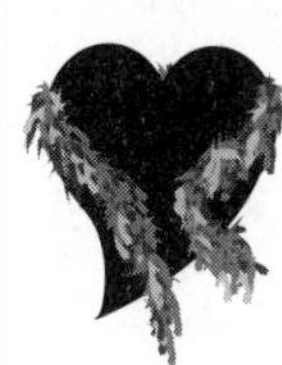

Feelin' the Love

I do dances for my boyfriend whenever I can. He loves the different costumes and the moves that play up my attributes.
—Katy, student

Costumed Capers

I always found it fun to try to match my costumes with my songs, like a cute schoolgirl outfit for Aerosmith's "Ragdoll," or a sailor outfit for "Take Me to the River." Your song doesn't necessarily have to match your outfit, and not all songs have outfits that "go" with them, so it depends on how you're feeling and what you feel sexy in (and what you can get out of gracefully!).

Pure Erotica

If you're thinking about something a little more sensual, you might not want to wear a hot pink racer outfit, but something that matches the mood. Try a lace camisole with matching lace boy shorts, lace dresses, or simple lingerie.

With erotica, you're going for soft and feminine, so choose clothing that's less tight in the butt area. It's better for the tease!

Slick Tricks

See Chapter 12 for more ideas on what to wear (and what not to wear) for your dance. I offer some fun theme ideas there, too, and some suggested music to dance to. If you're not sure what you want to do exactly, you're sure to get some creative juices flowing after reading that chapter!

Foot(wear) Fetish

Part of the fun of dancing is to feel like you're another person—a strong, confident, sexy person. Your costume and makeup help accomplish that, and shoes do, too. Platforms will make you feel taller, thinner, sexier, and truly like you've stepped out of yourself.

I'm sure you've seen some crazy high-heel shoes and boots. Some look sexy; some just look stupid. A $1\frac{1}{2}$- to 2-inch platform with a chunky heel, in either shoe or boot, is enough to be sexy—and still safe for you. Platforms over 2 inches high are not sexy; they're just too tall.

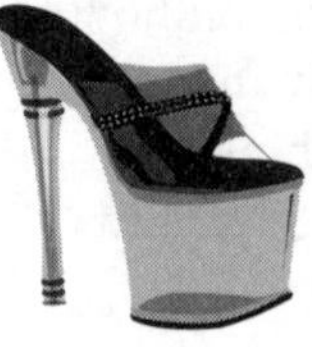

Trippin' Up

You want to impress your man with your moves and attitude, not the fact you can walk on stilts. Too-tall platforms will not only make you unsteady, they could also throw off your performance because you'll be preoccupied with not falling over. He'll notice that, not your sexy moves, and that will ruin the whole mood of your dance.

Although stilettos look very, very sexy, you can find shoes and boots with a chunkier heel. Now, I'm not talking about a 5-inch-square heel; that's not sexy. You want the heel to be sexy and not too heavy, but you want to be able to walk and dance comfortably and not break your ankle.

If you don't normally wear heels, I wouldn't go over a 3-inch heel without a platform. Anything else will really make your feet uncomfortable because they will be at such a high tilt. If you're comfortable in platforms, go for the 5-inch-tall heel because that platform adds 2 inches, making your heel angle only 3 inches.

I danced in platform shoes when I was a club dancer and didn't discover the joy of boots until I actually began teaching. Both platforms and boots have their own advantages and disadvantages.

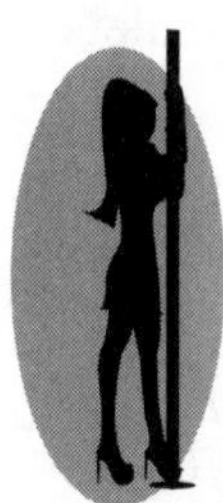

Slick Tricks

Practice walking in your shoes to break them in before you do your dance. You must be *completely* comfortable moving in your shoes to put on a star performance!

The Best of Boots:

- Boots are secure on your feet, so you don't have to worry about them flying off or crunching your toes on the floor.
- Boots help your ankle grip around the pole without pinching your skin (which you might do until you're totally comfortable with the pole).
- Boots help protect your shins from bruises.
- Thigh-high boots protect your knees when you're on a hard floor—and they look ultra sexy!
- Boots are ideal for a "hooker" dress or tough-girl look.

The Worst of Boots:

- Boots can be annoying to take off after your dance.
- The tube socks usually worn underneath make quite a fashion statement!
- Boots can make your feet stinky, so keep a hidden spray can of deodorant handy, just in case he goes near your feet.

The Joy of Shoes:

- Shoes look more delicate and feminine than boots.
- Shoes look great with any outfit.

The Despair of Shoes:

- Shoes can fly off when you're swinging around the pole. To avoid this, be sure to wear shoes that have an ankle strap.
- Open-toed shoes don't protect your toes when you do floor work, so you're conscious of your feet; that might affect your dance.
- You have to be sure your toenails are painted and your feet aren't hairy.

If you can't decide which to wear, you might be able to combine the two and get a pair of platform boots—the best of both worlds!

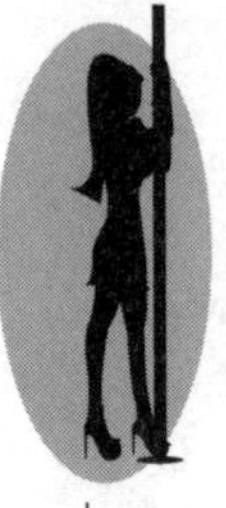

Slick Tricks

Always cut off all price tags from your clothes before you dance. (I broke my own rule here on the DVD. I forgot to cut the tag off the sweater in the lap-dance sequence. Notice how it stands out.) That includes price stickers on the bottoms of your shoes or boots, too!

Going Shopping!

Although it's become easier to find exotic dancewear and adult costumes in stores now then when I was a club dancer in the mid-1990s, the Internet still has the best selection for costumes and club wear. (Lingerie and undergarments can be bought inexpensively at local stores.)

Some dancers I worked with would spend exorbitant amounts of money at Victoria's Secret, getting bras and underwear for work. I found that a huge waste of money because we were just sliming all over the dirty floor, so I got my bras and underwear at Wal-Mart. Let me tell you, *men do not know the difference.*

Besides, your man will be admiring your whole performance and your tease, not the brand name of the bra. And the Wal-Marts of the world are now selling nice, sexy lingerie for half the price of Victoria's Secret. However, for a special occasion dance, by all means indulge yourself with a trip to Victoria's Secret!

If you can't find what you want in a brick-and-mortar store, several online stores might have what you want. Here are a few I frequent for my costumes and shoes (and none are paying for an endorsement, either):

- **www.wmsclothing.com** offers wholesale lingerie, costumes, and shoes.
- **www.catdancerz.com** has any fantasy costume you can imagine, and their prices are very reasonable.
- **www.teddyshoes.com** have the most incredible variety of shoes and boots you will ever see!

See Appendix A for more great shopping websites.

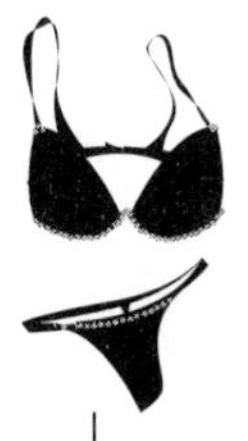

Behind the G-String

Practice all you can in your entire outfit—hair, nails, shoes, and costume—so you can eliminate any problems before your real performance.

The Least You Need to Know

- Toss the thong! V-shaped boy shorts are much more complementary.
- Avoid skin-tight clothing—unless you have a perfect body.
- When deciding on a platform heel, don't go over 2 inches tall. And use a chunky heel if you're not used to wearing heels.
- Save money when shopping. He won't know the difference between Wal-Mart and Victoria's Secret lingerie!

In This Chapter

- Creating your own home club—complete with a pole!
- Rugs, floors, or countertop—you decide
- Mood lighting to put you both in the mood
- Choosing music that moves you

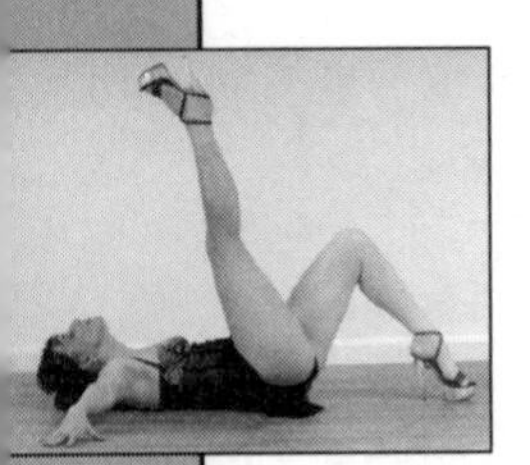
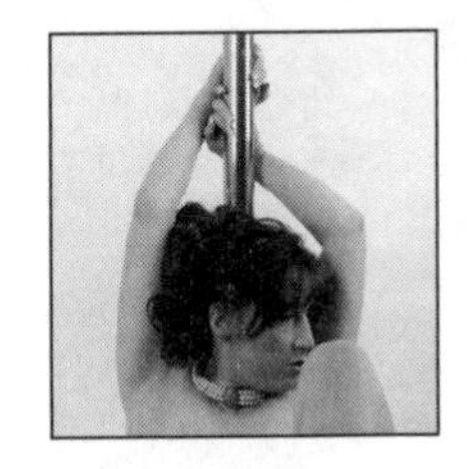
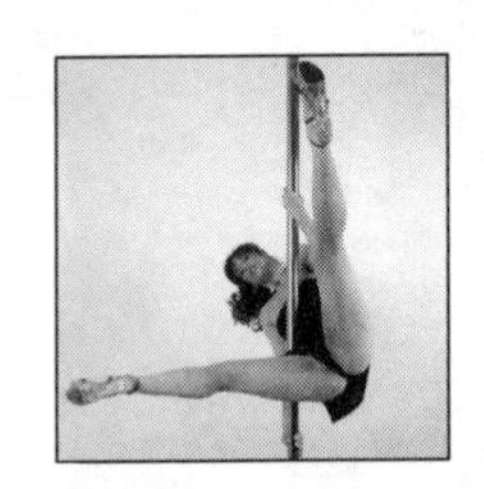
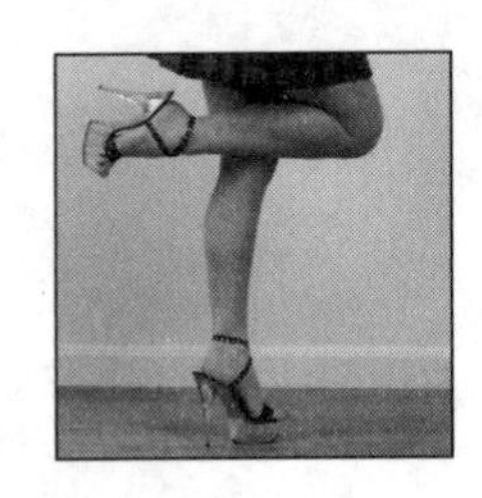
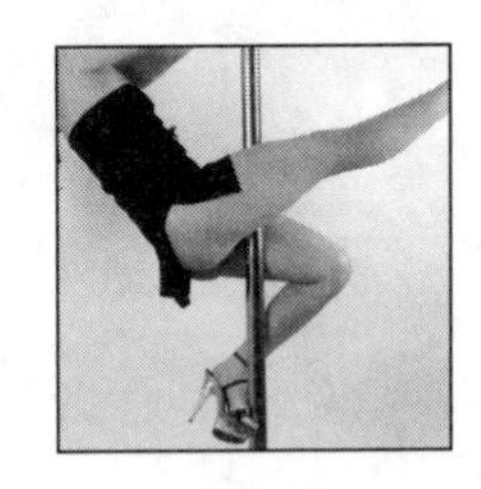
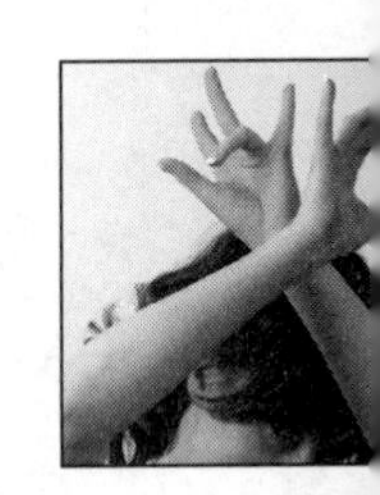

Chapter 5

Club *Moi*

Sure, shopping for your costume and shoes and thinking about the music you want to dance to are the fun parts of preparing for a dance, but you also have to think about *where* you're going to dance. In your living room? In the bedroom? Somewhere else? You need to think ahead about your dance space so that you don't have to worry about it when you're dancing.

This gives you a chance to set up your performance area ahead of time so that you can practice and become familiar with the area where you'll perform. The more you practice in this space the way it will be during your dance, the better, so by all means rearrange the furniture to where it will be when you do your dance. You don't want to perform a sexy dance move … only to bump into the coffee table, crash into the big-screen TV, or worse!

Setting the Stage

Choose an area with an empty wall or even an empty door you can slide down. You really don't need a lot of space, but be sure you've got enough room so that you don't swing your legs up and knock something off—including your man's head. An area about 6 feet by 6 feet (if you don't have a pole) in front of where he will be sitting should do it, preferably with that clear wall nearby. With a pole, you'd need about double that size.

Location, Location, Location

Where do you want to do this? What do you want the setting to be? The bedroom is always a romantic choice. If he's a car fanatic and you've got a sexy racer suit, accost him in the garage when he's working on his car. Does your living room have a nice feel to it? Even use the kitchen for true adventure or if you're going to be a Sexy Chef. (You could even do your floor work on the kitchen table if it's sturdy enough.)

Be creative when thinking about where to dance. It doesn't always have to be in the bedroom, but be sure it's a place you're comfortable, where blinds can be drawn (or not, if you're in to that sort of thing), and where you won't be tripping over children's toys (or your own).

Slick Tricks

Be sure you have a stereo with a remote handy so you can start your song from across the room if that's where your entrance will be. You don't want to have to stop, run over, and manually press play. And you want the music to be loud, but not so loud as to be distracting or wake the kids. (Otherwise, there may be some unpleasantness, most likely involving the Department of Social Services.)

Rug or No Rug?

Rugs definitely help protect your knees when you do floor work, and they're definitely warmer to dance on, but they come with some pitfalls, too. You run the risk of getting rug burn during certain moves. And shoes and boots don't slide very well on some carpet, so it's harder to turn and use any of the sliding moves.

Also if you are going to dance in a room with a wood or otherwise noncarpteted floor, put down an area rug even something as simple as a larger fluffy bathroom rug or silk sheet to lay on as you do floor work; that can look incredibly sexy.

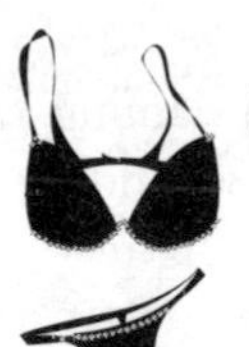

Behind the G-String

I worked with a dancer in Snooky's Simi Valley (California) who would bring a fluffy pink bath rug onstage with her and enchant the men with a long, sensual rendition of Prince's "Purple Rain." The rug added another intensely sexual dimension to her dance!

Reserved Seating

Okay, now you know where you're going to be, but where do you put him? Have him sit in the middle of a loveseat is ideal because then you've got leg room on both sides when you do a lap dance. If possible, move the loveseat away from the wall so that you have room to walk around it.

If you don't have a loveseat, any chair *without arms* will work just fine, as will the edge of the bed or even on the floor.

Sitting him on the floor has its advantages because then you're standing over him, you're in the dominant position. You're showing him that this is *your* show. Plus it's much less stress on your neck when you're crawling.

The Importance of Lighting

You don't have to be a rocket scientist to know that you wouldn't use normal white lights during your dance. White light to a dancer is like sunlight to a vampire—when faced with bright light, we recoil in pain and horror, cover our faces, and hiss until the lights go dim again.

Okay, well, maybe not. But still, white light is not the most flattering light to dance under.

Red, White, or Blue?

Candlelight is best for softer, romantic dances. Just be sure the candles aren't located anywhere (or on anything) that may get bumped, thus knocking over the candle and starting a flaming inferno. Colored red or blue lights are second best, but black light—oh, glorious black light—is a dancer's best friend!

Black lights not only hide all your flaws—bless them—but they make your white clothing, jewelry, shoes, and even your teeth glow bright white, too. Plus it makes all of us beautiful pasty white girls look incredibly tanned!

You can buy colored lights and black lights at any party or discount store.

Spot or Backlight?

Attention! *Never, ever put a spotlight on yourself!* If you do, you might as well be holding up a large sign that says "Please, look at all my wrinkles, stretch marks, scars, and ingrown hairs!" And as if I have to say it: that's not sexy!

If you backlight yourself, your audience will see just your silhouette, which could be sexy for awhile. However, with a backlight, your audience won't be able to see your face, which is an intricate part of your dance. Be sure to move so that your face can be seen during your dance.

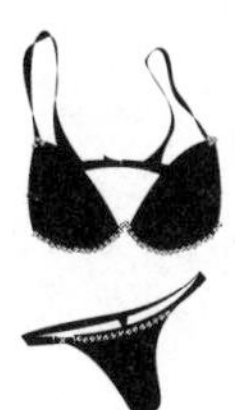

Behind the G-String

Several pubs where I danced in England put a bright white spotlight on the girls onstage. That's when your personality really has to sell you.

Getting Serious: Lighting Accessories

If you want to get fancy with your lighting, you're in the right place. You've seen disco balls and other interesting lighting in clubs, and you can have them in your own club, too.

Disco balls are great because when the spotlight shines on them, they throw great little shadows of light on the wall that add depth to the room and will truly make your room feel like a completely different place.

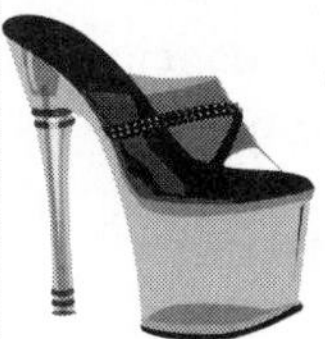

Trippin' Up

I have a disco ball in my studio, and when I first used it during class, the rotating lights made me so nauseous my Ramen noodles almost made a second appearance. Luckily I recovered so that much … unpleasantness … shall we say, was avoided and I didn't have to enforce my rule: "If you puke you clean it up, and if I puke, you clean it up, so it's a win/win situation for everyone!"

What about strobe lights? Use them if you have a real head-banging song that's not too long, but try not to use them for long stretches of time. And I would practice like crazy with the strobe because you need to know whether you can do the whole song with that flashing light and without getting a headache.

Lighting and other fun room décor is a lot less expensive than you think. www.coolstuffcheap.com has a huge selection of the most fun lighting and ambience equipment I've ever seen, with excellent prices and delivery.

A Little Night Music

What song should you dance to? For starters, one that moves you. It's got to make you feel sexy. I don't care if he wants you to dance to his favorite song—if it doesn't make you feel sexy, it will be very difficult to pull off. You'd be better off dancing to a song that really moves you because then you will become infused with the music when you dance, and it will be a stronger, sexier performance. After all, *you are dancing for yourself.* (Well, okay, you're doing a show for him, but the more you look like you're dancing for yourself and not performing for him, the more turned on he'll get.)

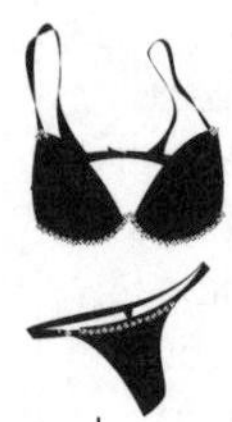

Behind the G-String

Everyone laughed when I announced I would be dancing in my recital for my students to "Safety Dance" by Men Without Hats. That song makes me feel sexy, and it was one of the strongest performances I've done!

Vixen, one of my instructors, chose to do Kenny Rogers's "The Gambler" for one of my recitals, and there was much snickering about it. Yet when she was done, everyone in that room needed a cigarette!

Be sure you get enough practice with the song. I can't stress enough how important it is that you know your song forward and backward as well as all the lyrics. The more familiar you are with the song, the more your body will switch to "autopilot" when you dance. Your brain can be doing the acting while the song tells your body what to do. If your song truly motivates you, and you really feel it deep down, it will move your very soul, and you will truly become one with the song ... one being, one entity in harmony with the cosmic universe, nay ... dare I say, you will have reached ... Nirvana.

All right, that's a bit dramatic, but it's true. You will be able to feel it if a song moves you. If it doesn't, trying to dance to it is like pulling teeth.

Paula Cole's "Feelin' Love" is 5 minutes, 30 seconds—pretty long for a song. But because that song moves me and makes me feel ultra sexy, it feels like maybe 2 minutes at best.

For more song suggestions, turn to Chapter 12.

Installing the Pole

Poles are just so much fun ... and good exercise, too! You can get removable poles that leave nothing but a hook in the ceiling or that have a fake smoke detector over the installation area. Regardless, you want about a 5- to 6-foot radius around your pole, and your pole must be secured into a beam in the ceiling. If you don't have a beam, you can do what I did in my studio: put up wood braces across the ceiling and the walls so I had a solid base for the top of the pole.

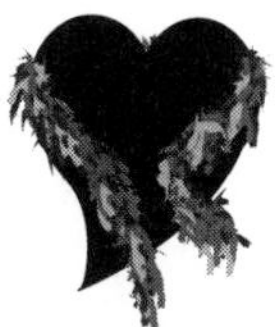

Feelin' the Love

Be careful if you try to do your pole moves on a post in your basement that holds the house up. Unless you have a huge hand, you cannot keep your hand on it and, in the middle of a launch, will end up on the floor with a severely bruised elbow, hip, and ego. Hubby still appreciates the effort, but .... It is far better to invest in a real pole ... or stick to chair routines.

—Tara Storm, student

And you don't even have to screw your pole into the floor, because removable poles come with slide-resistant pads for carpet or flooring and can hold up to 200 pounds.

I highly recommend Lil' Mynx removable stripper poles. They are very nice, their customer service is impeccable, and the poles are great quality. You can find them at www.lilmynx.com.

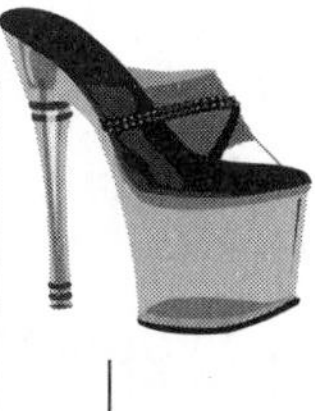

Trippin' Up

If you let your friends play on your pole, be sure you have homeowner's insurance. You wouldn't think your friends would sue, but you never know ....

The Least You Need to Know

- Be sure you have adequate space to perform your dance—without harming anything or anyone around you!
- Never put a bright white spotlight on yourself. Opt for a black light instead. These wonder lights hide all flaws.
- Choose only music that really moves you. It'll make all the difference in your dance.
- Practice as much as you can in the room before you actually do the dance. There's a reason for the saying "practice makes perfect"!
- Be sure your pole is safely installed with a clear 5- or 6-foot radius around it.

In This Part

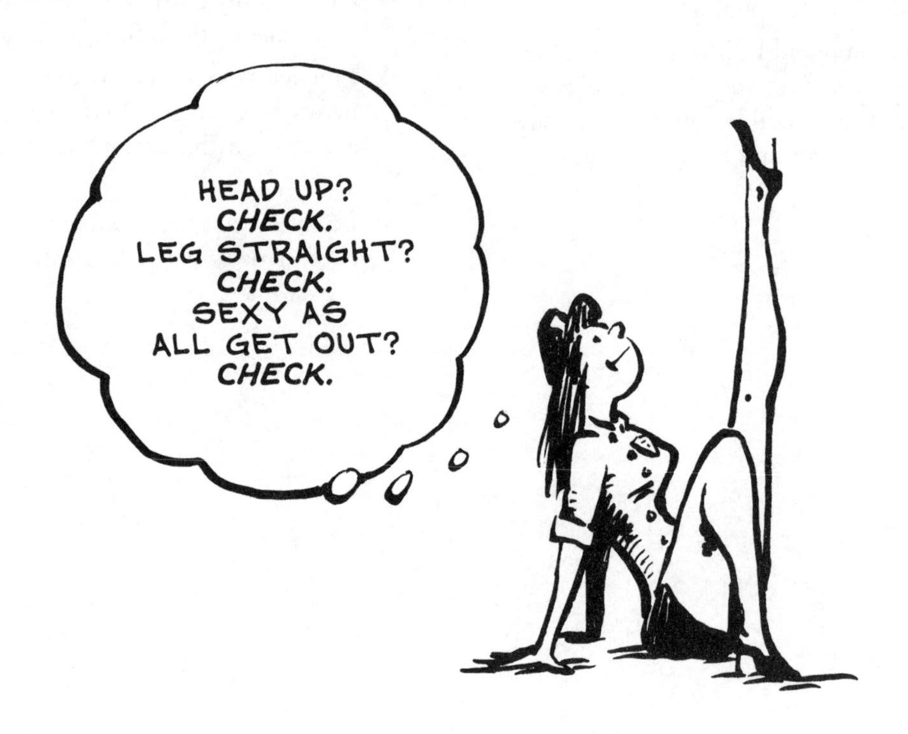

Part 2

Let's Get Physical: The Art of Exotic Dance

There is no right or wrong way to dance exotically, but a few basic moves guide the physical dance, and facial expressions help portray your inner emotions. It's almost like the physical aspect of exotic dancing is the yin and the psychological aspect is the yang. You need both to create a strong, impressive performance. Exotic dancing is just as much psychological as physical, and it won't work if you have one and not the other.

I've been told that a lot of my physical routine work includes Pilates or yoga moves, which was news to me. I just did what made me money when I was a dancer. The psychological aspect, which is all acting, just sort of happened over the years because I found that men reacted strongly (i.e., tipped more) when I looked like I was truly enjoying my dance for them.

And that is your goal—to create an empowering performance that will leave your audience needing a cigarette when you're done. After you master these physical moves, you'll feel confident enough to begin adding your own special touches. Before you know it, you'll have developed your own signature exotic dance style!

In This Chapter

- Predance stretching
- Walking, strutting, and skipping
- Transitional turning
- Wall dancing
- Transitioning to the floor

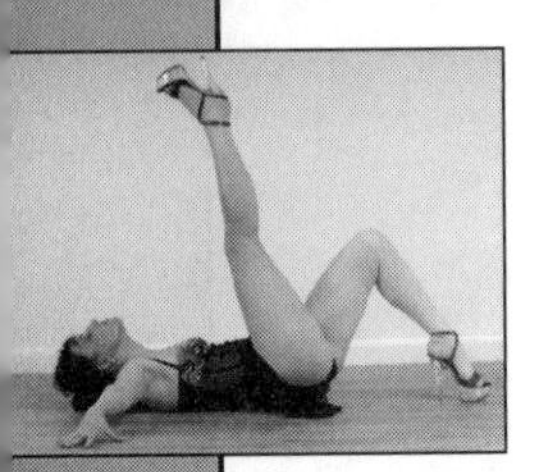
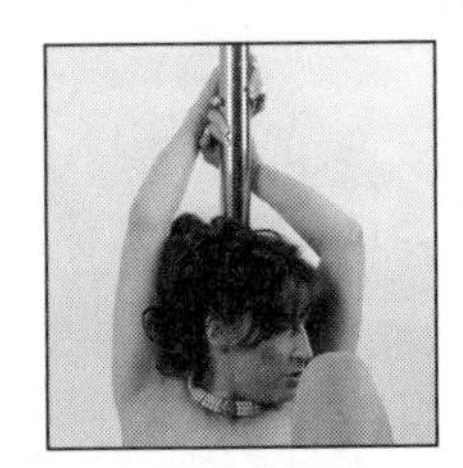
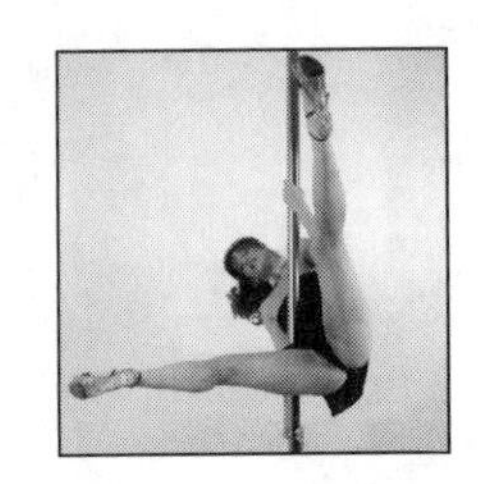
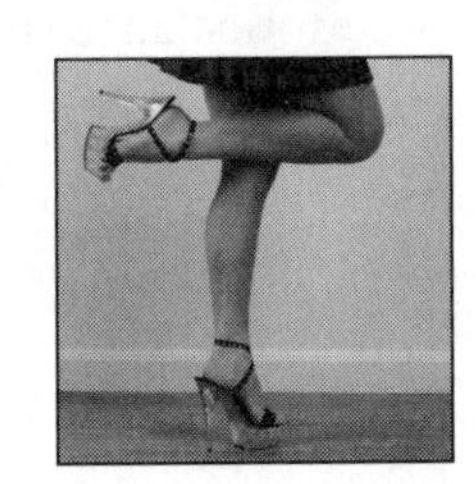
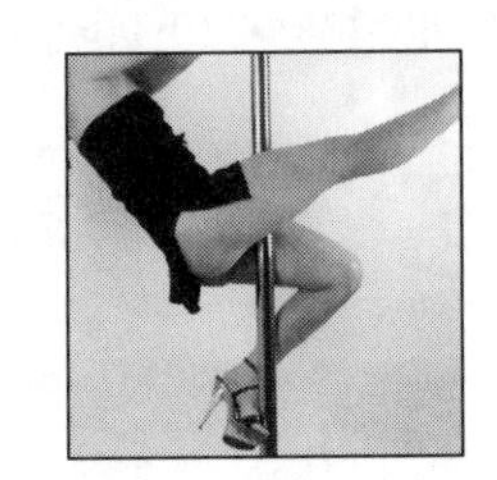
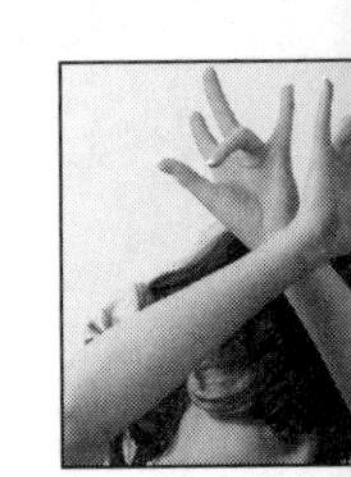

Chapter 6

On Your Feet, Woman!

I bet you can't wait to get started, and I can't either; but first, as annoying as it is, you've got to warm up. Dancing is an exercise. You wouldn't go out and run a mile without stretching first, would you? No.

Then the fun stuff! In this chapter, I show you how simple exotic dancing really is, starting with some basic "stand up" moves and transitions to get you on your way!

Before You Get Hot, You've Got to Warm Up: Stretching

The first part of your preparation is for your body's benefit. You're going to want to warm up before you actually start practicing your sexy moves so you don't pull any muscles or hurt yourself. Even if you work out regularly, you'll find yourself using muscles when you're dancing in ways you've never used them before. Let's get those muscles moving, ladies!

Upper Body

First, stand with your legs about 2 feet apart and stretch your arms as high as they can go. Now bring them out to the sides and into a wide circular motion—big, big arm circles.

Feels weird, doesn't it? Well get used to it, because when you're an exotic dancer, you use all the space around you. You don't just stay in one little area.

Lower Body

Now sit on the floor with your legs spread wide. With both hands, reach out as far as you can for your left foot and feel your back muscles stretching. Now lean for your right foot, stretching as much as you can.

Now bring your upper body between your legs as far down as it can go. Don't be upset if you can't get it too far toward the floor. At least you're warning those muscles that they're about to get called up for duty!

The Cock of the Walk

We've all seen supermodels strutting down the catwalk and everyone clapping and taking pictures of them. They feel strong, and it shows in their walk—a powerful walk, a walk that tells the world "I'm the queen, I'm the hottest thing that ever walked the face of the earth, and I know it!" That's the kind of attitude you want when you walk.

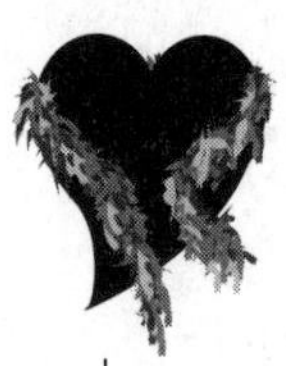

Feelin' the Love

Whenever my sisters and I are out together and Beyoncé's "Crazy in Love" comes on, we all have that knowing look in our eyes and "the Walk" soon follows!

—Maureen, student

One thing you don't want, however, is the blank expression models are trained to set on their faces. You never want to take exotic dancing too seriously. I mean, you're in your underwear or less, and there's nothing funnier than that!

When I strut, I have a sly grin on my face, like the cat who ate the canary, like I've just done something wrong and I know it but I don't care, or even an expression of "I know something you don't know …." You want the attitude of the supermodel, but not her blank expression. Show the sparkle in your eye! (I talked about your facial expression in Chapter 2, so turn back there if you need a refresher.)

This kind of attitude will show on your face, and your body will automatically move with that kind of attitude. Often you won't actually have to think about the walking.

The Supermodel Strut

Let's practice your strut. Choose a place that's fairly long if you can, and wear heels as you do this. (Sneakers or bare feet just won't work. It's virtually impossible to do this walk and really get the correct psychological feeling you must have from plain sneakers or just feet.)

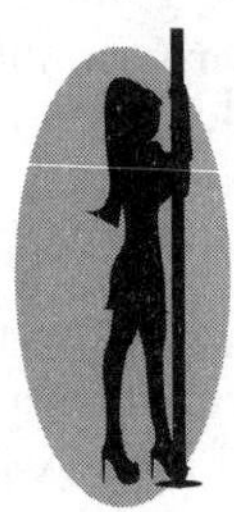

Slick Tricks

A great music choice for practicing the strut is En Vogue's "Free Your Mind." That's a very powerful song and really captures the attitude you want to have.

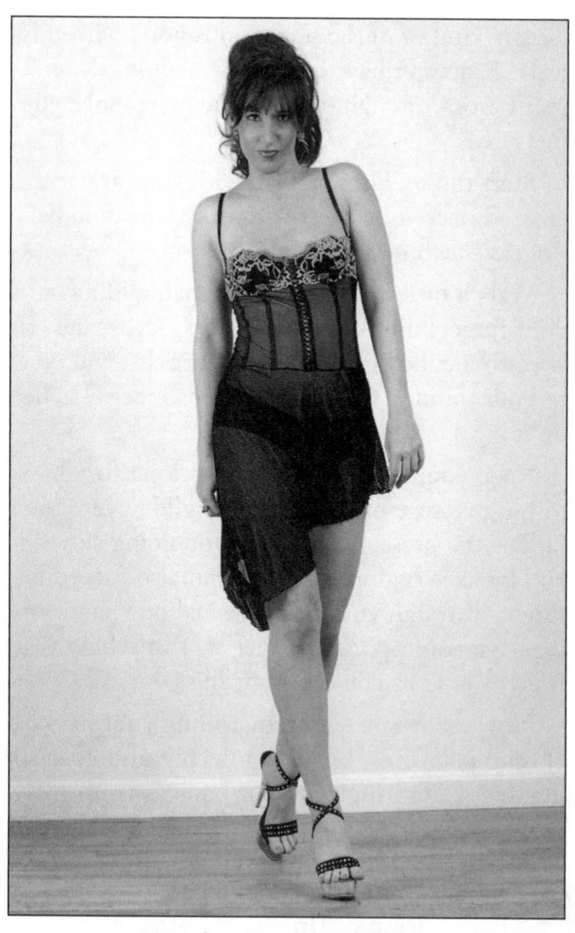

You know you're sexy ...

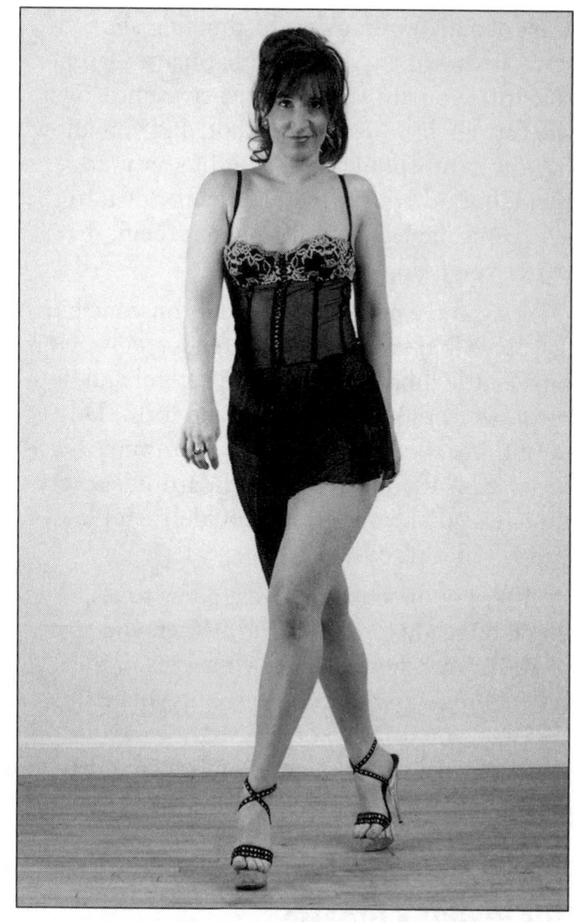

You know you're a supermodel ... Make him see it, too.

Also be sure no mirrors are nearby at this point, or cover them up for now.

Walk across the room like you would normally, and then walk back, this time adding in your I-know-something-you-don't-know grin.

Walk across the floor again, this time picturing yourself as a supermodel as you walk. No mirrors are around to show you you're not actually a supermodel, but if in your mind's eye you can see yourself strutting down a catwalk, your body will react accordingly to match what your brain is thinking. So think, *I am the hottest thing on Earth!* Now cross your legs a little more as you walk—but do not make your steps smaller.

Concentrate on your attitude as you walk, and think *only* that you are a supermodel, not about the physical walk itself. Remember "less is more," and don't try too hard.

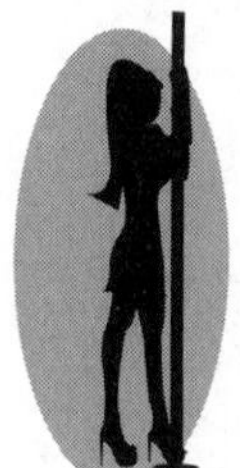

Slick Tricks

You are controlling the situation with your sly grin because it's as if you know something he doesn't know, and that, dear girl, puts him subliminally "below" you.

A lot of my students tell me they don't know what to do with their arms when they walk.

First of all, you shouldn't be thinking about your arms—or anything for that matter—other than that you are a supermodel strutting down the catwalk in Milan, you're hot, and you know it! Your arms should have a bit of a sway to them, but otherwise, they can hang down to the sides. But the less you think about them, the better you'll do.

You can try putting your hands on your hips as you walk if you want. This tends to give your hips a little more swing, but be careful and do *not* move your shoulders back and forth. Don't even think about them, in fact. Just think, *I'm a supermodel!* If you have the right attitude, everything else (like your arms, shoulders, and legs) will fall into place naturally.

After you practice this strut a few times, you'll be ready for the mirror. When you strut to the mirror, however, use your eyes in the reflection as your target. By seeing yourself this way, you can also decide what works for you and what doesn't, what is more comfortable with your arms, etc. But just keep thinking *Supermodel! Supermodel! Supermodel!*

The Walking Orgasm

Okay, you don't really have an orgasm when you do this walk, but you want to look like you are. This slower, more sensual walk focuses on body language and facial expressions, as opposed to the tough supermodel strut that's done for your audience's benefit. You need to convince your audience that you are truly in love with yourself.

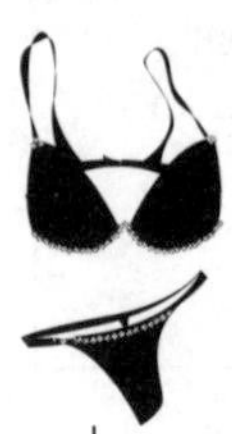

Behind the G-String

Acting is such an important aspect of this walk that I make students walk back and forth across my studio until they convince me they are in love with themselves—and I can see it in their eyes.

Any kind of music selection is good with this walk. It doesn't have to be slow necessarily. To really work, though, your music must make you feel sexy.

Start the walking orgasm with your arms crossed over your chest with only your middle fingers touching your elbows.

Walk a little slower than normal, gliding your fingers up to your shoulders, across the breastbone, down around your breasts, and on to your tummy, where your hands meet. Then do it again.

Keep your hands moving, but don't forget to put pressure on them as they glide over your body—the pressure will keep you going slow and looks very dramatic. You can also run your fingers through your hair, use just one hand to massage your opposite upper arm, anything you want as long as you are admiring yourself.

Now really spice it up by rolling your neck, closing your eyes, breathing deeply, and looking down admiringly at your body as you sexily saunter across the floor.

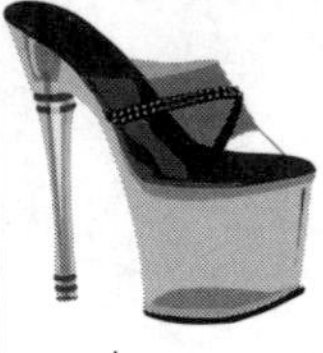

Trippin' Up

Never just rub your hands all over yourself to do something with them. Always put pressure on the fingers and caress deliberately.

It will seem silly and stupid as you do it, and you'll want to giggle because it feels strange to truly admire yourself. But I'm telling you, the more acting you put into it, the more convincing your walk will be—and the more your audience will admire you!

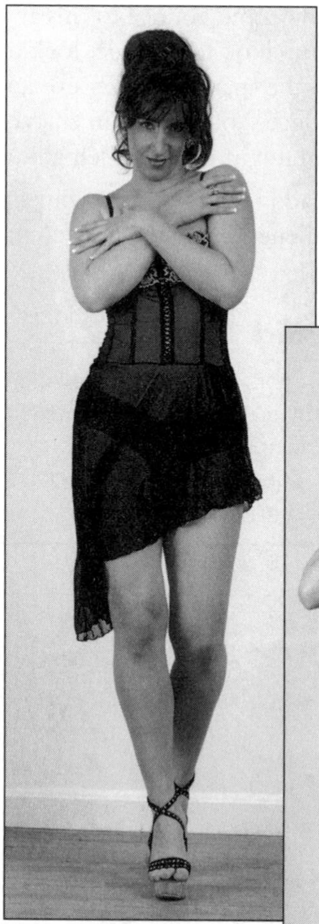

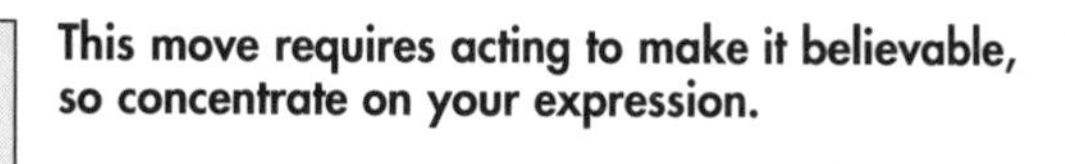

This move requires acting to make it believable, so concentrate on your expression.

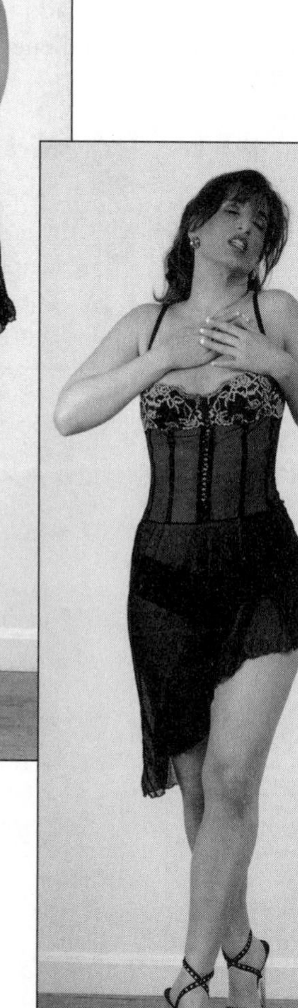

Don't worry about the walk itself. This is all about sexual drama.

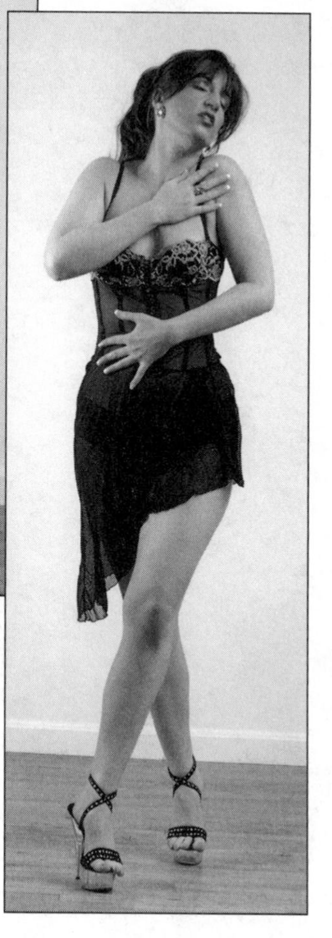

Follow your walk through until you're ready to move on.

The Cutesy Walk

Now not all of us are seriously sexy vixens; some of us are better at the irresistible girl-next-door look, which is just as sexy as the vixen look, but with a dash of devilish innocence.

The cutesy walk is a complete character walk. You have to really imagine yourself as that cutesy girl—see her in your mind's eye—and your body will conform to that character and do things you aren't even aware of to capture the girl-next-door character.

To do the cutesy walk, clasp your hands behind your back and walk forward, pivoting your toe inward as you step to about a 45-degree angle. Add some bounce to this and look around … look up, look to the side, look down coyly, but keep the sparkle in your eye and the sly grin on your face. You'll be so in character with this walk, you might find yourself almost skipping.

Now add in a wink, bite your lip, or blow your audience a kiss to really complete the act.

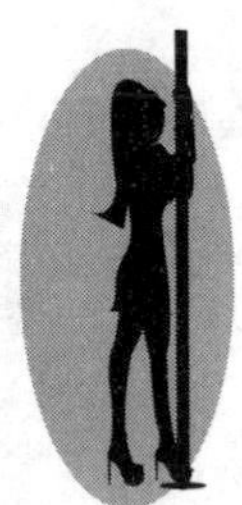

Slick Tricks

There is always something to do, something to accentuate. Something as simple as lifting your arm in the air and caressing it with your opposite hand is a move.

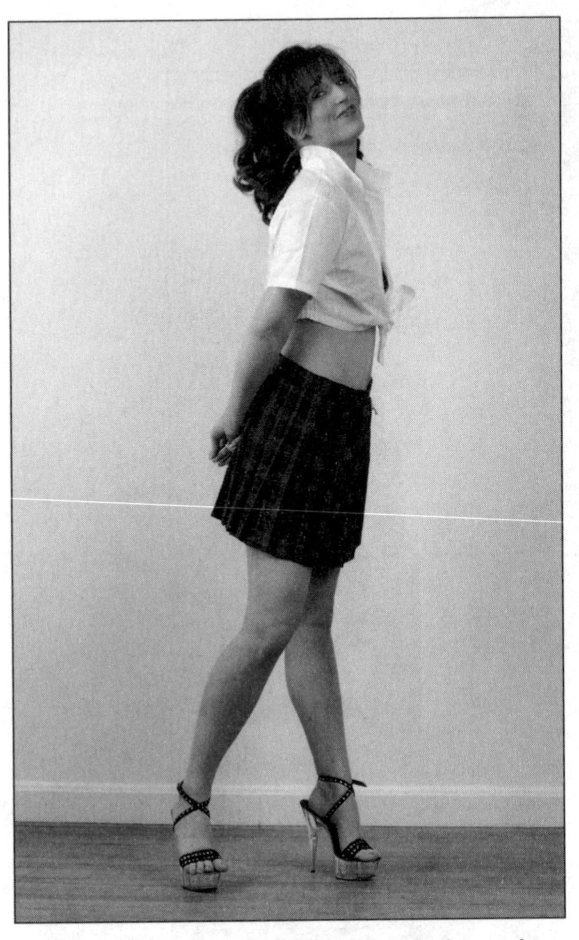

It's the look on your face that will make him melt!

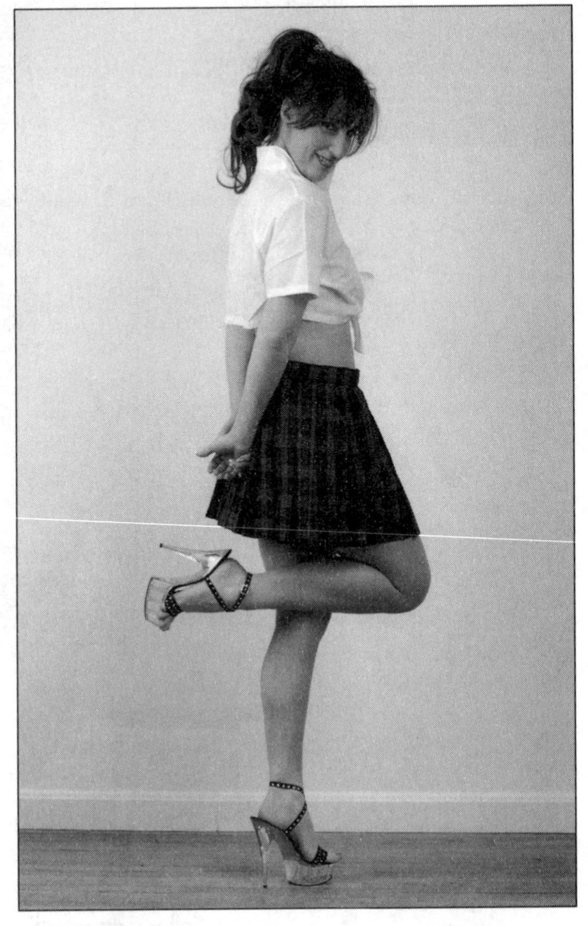

Let the character take over as you walk.

Turn It Right Round!

Every little detail in your dance counts, including turning. There's very little skill to turning, and it's very simple. When you're in your song, you won't even be thinking about turning. It will just happen. Practice these turns, but remember: you don't have to do everything exactly as I do. I want you to add your own personal style to your dance. Make it *your* dance!

Half-Turn

Start by facing the mirror with your legs about a foot apart. Put your right foot out, cross it in front of your left foot, and let your body turn around with a simple toe pivot with your left foot.

Now do it again until you get it nice and smooth, but don't look at your feet, look straight ahead. You can dress this up by using your arm as well.

As you step with your right foot, swirl your right arm up, and as your body turns, your right forearm should brush against the top of your head.

Follow this through with your right hand drawing dramatically down the right side of your face and on to your chest.

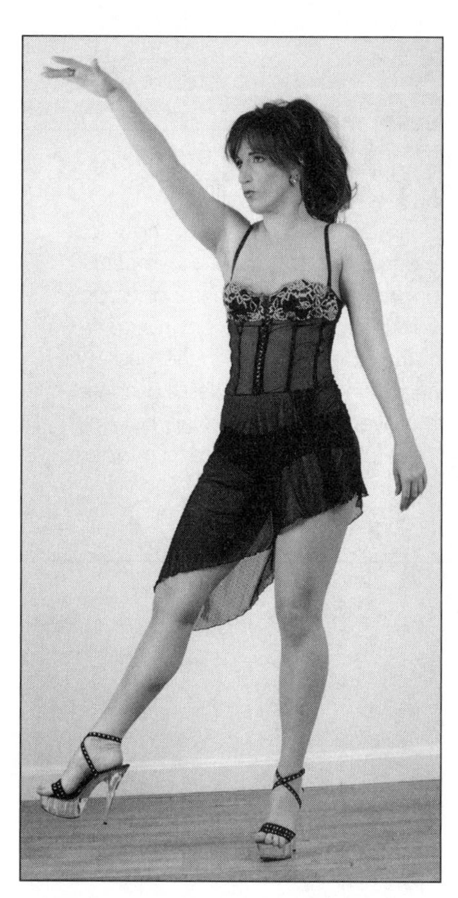

Start by sweeping your arm over your head as you step into your turn.

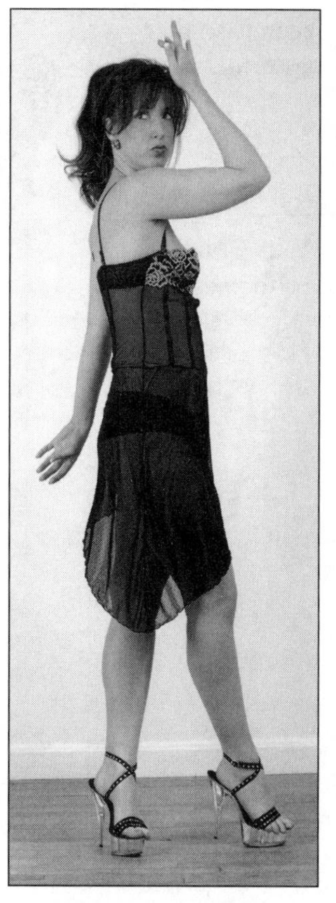

Your arm should draw down over your face and neck as you turn.

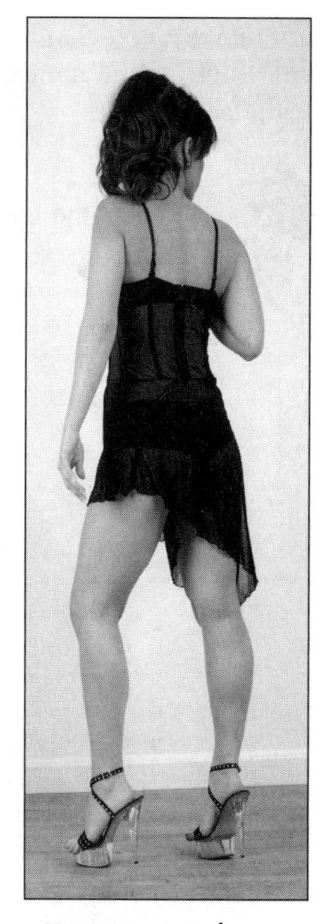

Keep your arm close to you as you end your turn. Don't let it fling out to the side.

Shoulder Roll Turn

Another easy and popular half-turn is the shoulder roll turn. Start by rolling your shoulders backward one at a time. Don't do this as an exercise; roll them because your shoulders are sexy!

Roll them deeply, almost all the way up to your ears. When your left shoulder rolls back, simply follow it around with your body so you're facing in the opposite direction. When you do this correctly, you can feel your body following your shoulder around. When you come around, let your right shoulder roll up as it naturally wants to do, but then stop it as it comes down, and you will find yourself in a sexy pose.

Hold that pose for at least 2 seconds so that your audience can admire your beautiful, strong feminine form.

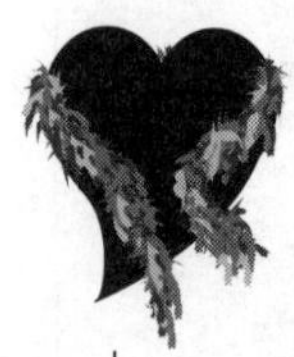

Feelin' the Love

Somehow, as girls, we are taught to be uncomfortable with our bodies. Less so now, and more so years ago. But generally, we aren't told athleticism is important, and we lose something in the process.

—Katy, student

Full Turns

I don't normally do full turns because they're too close to "regular" dancing, like you're actually *performing* for someone. (Remember, as an exotic dancer, you are performing for *yourself;* your audience is just lucky to be there!)

If you do want to do a full turn, here's one of the ways I do it: I kick my right leg out catercorner to the right and then swing it around hard to the left so that it crosses my left leg and pulls my whole body completely around.

This takes a lot of practice before you can do it without losing your balance. If you do lose your balance, follow it through as if you meant to do whatever you did and keep dancing.

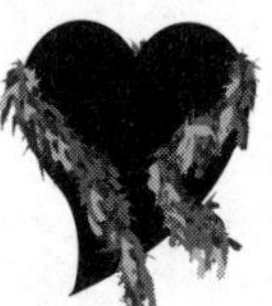

Feelin' the Love

Being slinky and seductive makes you feel sexy and confident, but it's more—we are learning how to let ourselves go, about movement, dance, and being adaptive through space and how to interact with the environment—the room, the pole, the music, the audience, etc. … and being comfortable and confident with movement and learning how our bodies move and react in a certain way is incredibly sexy!

—Tartlett, student

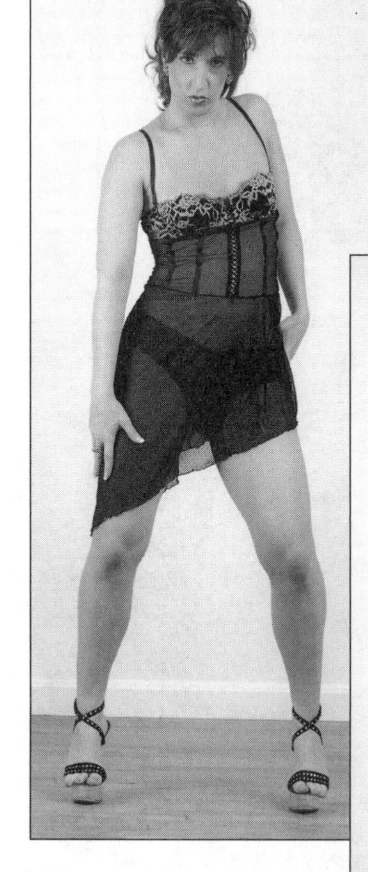

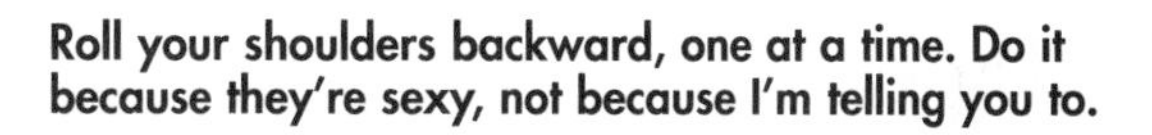

Roll your shoulders backward, one at a time. Do it because they're sexy, not because I'm telling you to.

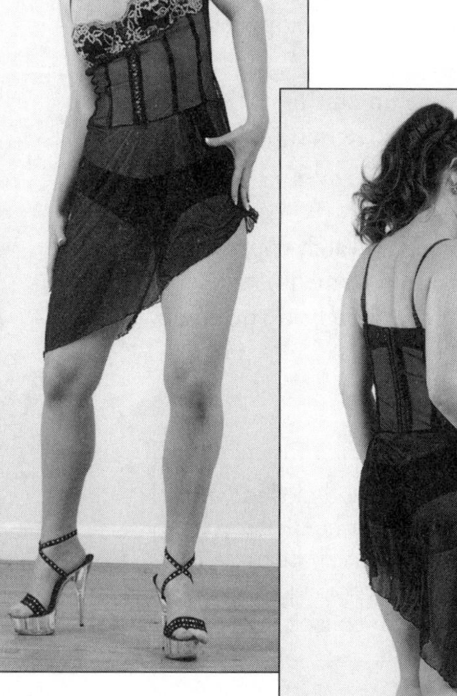

Follow your shoulder as it takes your body around.

Your body will automatically roll into a sexy pose.

Body Rolling

Rolling your body may take a little practice to get it perfect, but trust me, it's worth it!

Start by standing sideways to a full-length mirror with your right leg forward. Raise your arms so that they're above your head yet delicately bent at the elbows.

Roll your pelvis forward then back slowly, as if you are doing a butt circle (see Chapter 7), but in a forward motion as opposed to the usual side-to-side motion. Now bend down at the knees so you're in a crouching position.

Open your left leg out so your body turns to the left and then bring your right knee over so that you are now squatting in the opposite direction.

Lean forward and come up butt first (this is also an excellent way to practice butt up first; see Chapter 7) and let your arms draw up your thighs slowly.

Begin the body roll again. Watch yourself in the mirror to be sure your movement is graceful and smooth, and repeat the crouch so you come up on the other side.

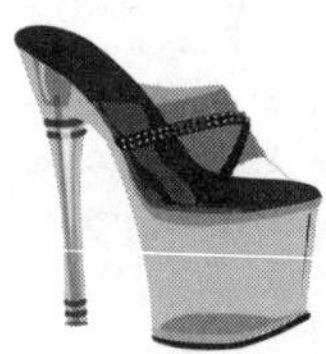

Trippin' Up

Never use the floor to balance yourself. Always put your hands on your knees to steady yourself, because when you use the floor, it looks like you aren't really in control.

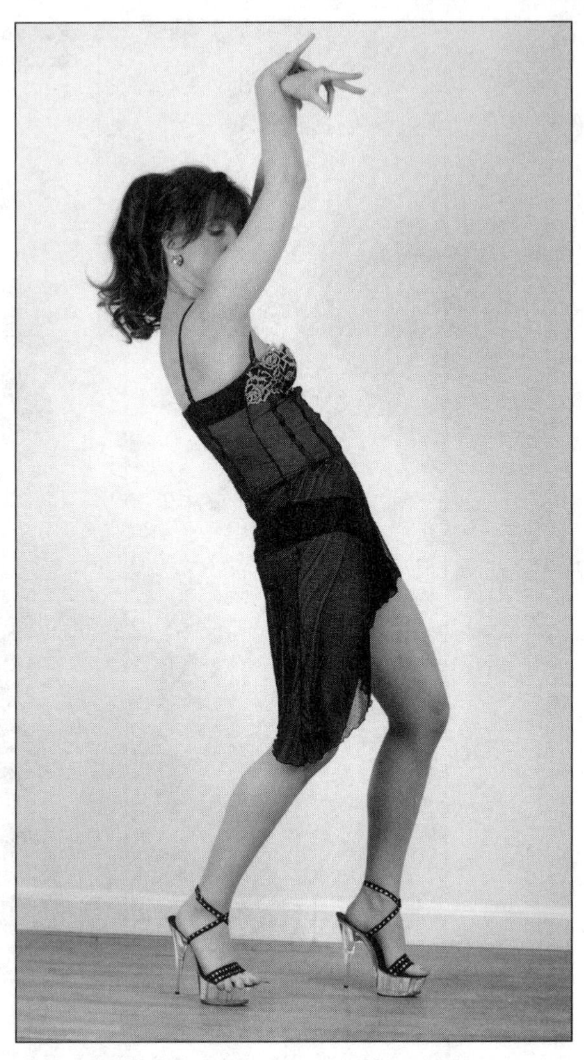

Roll your body in a wavelike motion.

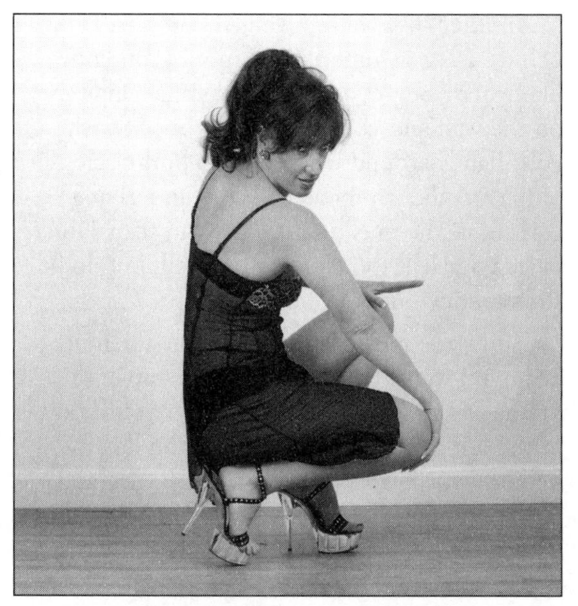

Be sure your feet are close together, and don't use the floor to balance. Keep your hands on your knees.

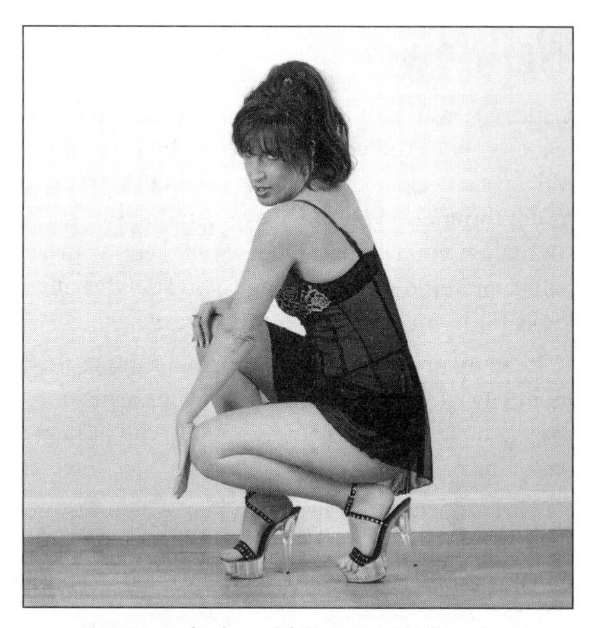

Open one thigh and follow it with the other.

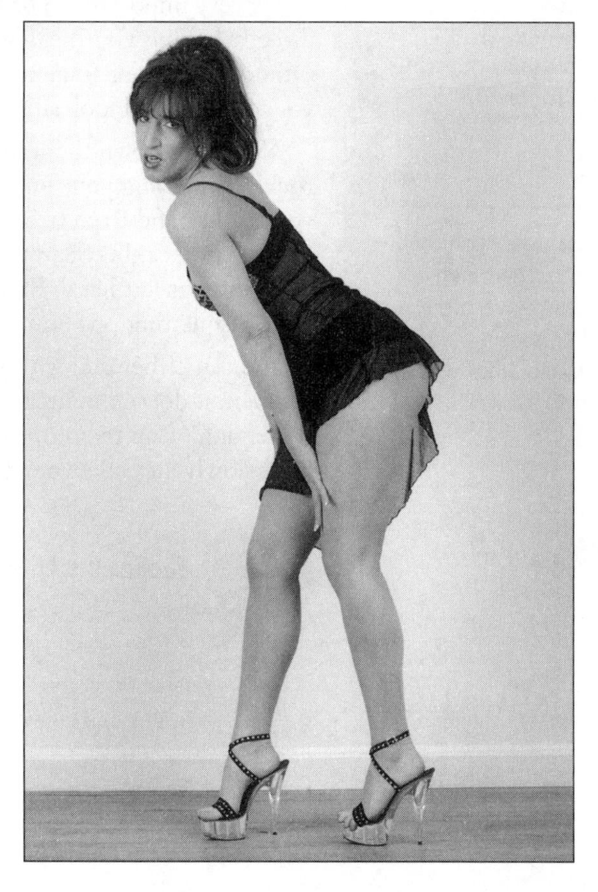

Stand up butt first—and be sure you take your time!

Wallflower

Using the wall as a prop in your dance can be just as sexy as the chair or pole, so be sure your wall space is clear of any plugs, switches, frames, or anything else you may have hanging on it. And when you slide down the wall, keep your palms and elbows in. Having them sticking out looks both uncomfortable and unsexy.

Lean against a wall with your butt about 3 inches away from the wall. Place your arms up over your head with a slight bend in the elbows and your palms out.

Turn your hands inward and cross your arms delicately over your face as you begin to slide down the wall, gently moving your butt from side to side.

Continue to slide your hands to above then around your breasts so your fingers point downward and your hands glide off over your hips.

By this time you should be in your squatting position with your back against the wall.

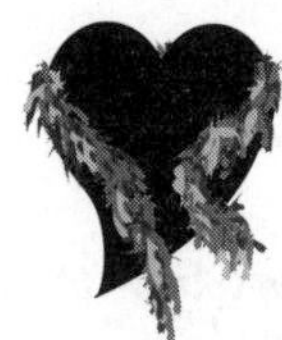

Feelin' the Love

Providing exotic dance instruction is such a crucial service to women; through this form of dance we are able to feel good when we're always barraged with information that we're not young/skinny/daring/hot enough … so thank you!

—Sasha, student

Another sexy wall move is if you start from behind … so assume the position! (You know, like when you get arrested and your hands are on the wall and your legs are spread.) Swish your hands around while you do butt circles, but remember to move with the underlying current of the music so it's soft and sexy. Don't place your feet too close to the wall, but do be sure to stick out your butt.

When the music is right, like on a definite beat, you want to turn around yet stay in the drama of the song. To do this, turn your body to the left and bring your right hand down behind your head as you do the full turn and face the opposite direction so your back is now up against the wall. Let your left hand sweep across your tummy as your face is turned completely to the left and your eyes are either shut or almost shut.

It's very important to bring your right hand directly behind your head when you turn. Otherwise, if your fingers are sticking out over your head, you'll look silly.

Now slide down the wall (don't drop like a rock!) by moving your butt side to side and slide your right hand from behind your head down over your neck, between your breasts and down to meet your left hand. By this time, you should be in a squatting position.

You can either end with your knees together or open, it doesn't matter. Just when you're there, don't clap them open and shut quickly … do it slowly and take your time.

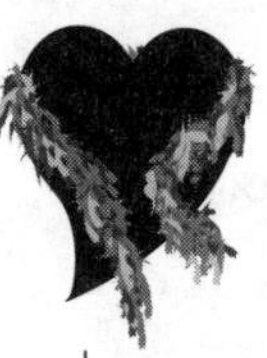

Feelin' the Love

It's all about good acting skills when you're dancing!

—Katy, student

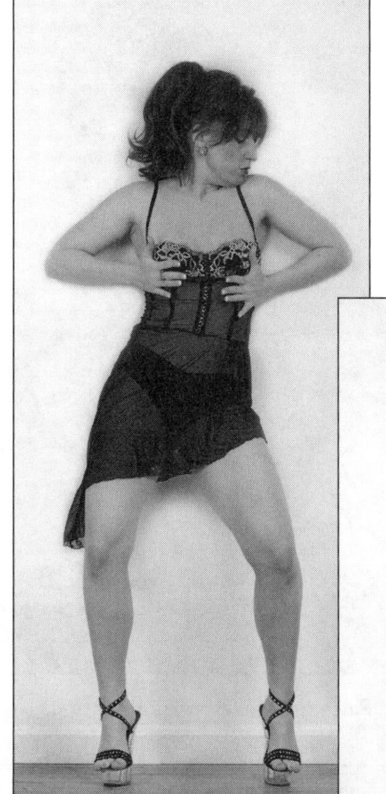

Keep your head tilted and your expression in the drama as you descend.

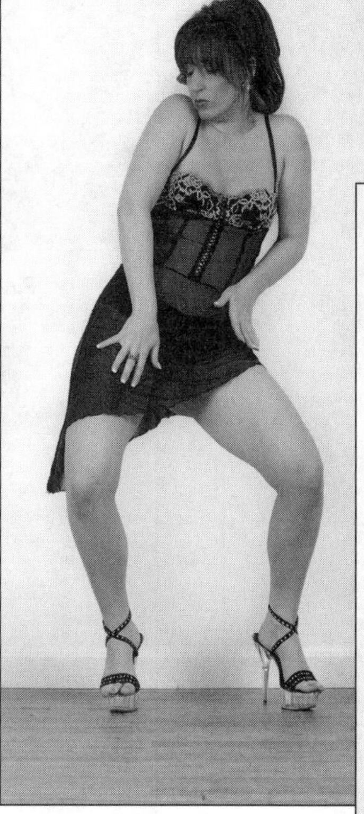

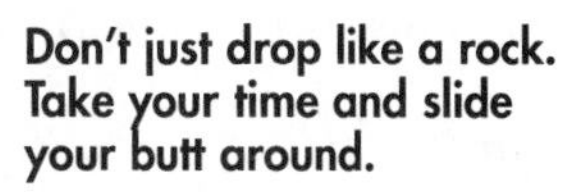

Don't just drop like a rock. Take your time and slide your butt around.

Your legs can either be together or open, depending on what the song tells you to do.

Get Down!

There are several ways to get down on the floor (other than falling), and your music really dictates which move you use to get to the floor.

The most common way to get to the floor is by first putting your hands on your knees and doing a butt circle.

From here, just bend your right knee down to the floor, follow it with your left knee, and there you are.

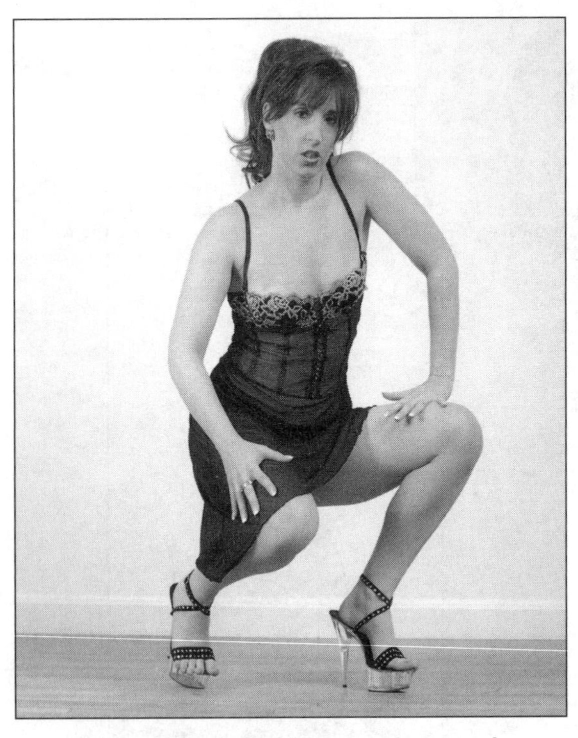

Start with your hands on your knees and squat down.

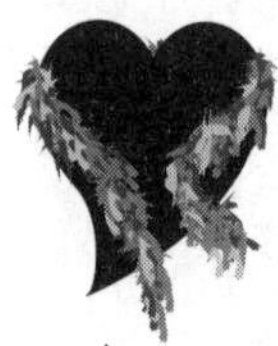

Feelin' the Love

It's nice to see a beautiful and intelligent woman using her body to help other women find self-confidence and the beauty within themselves.

—Peaches, student

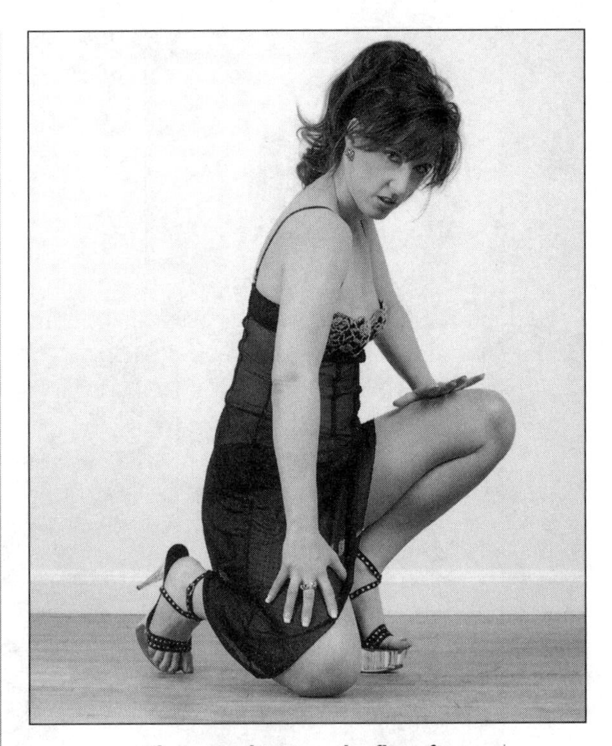

Place one knee on the floor first.

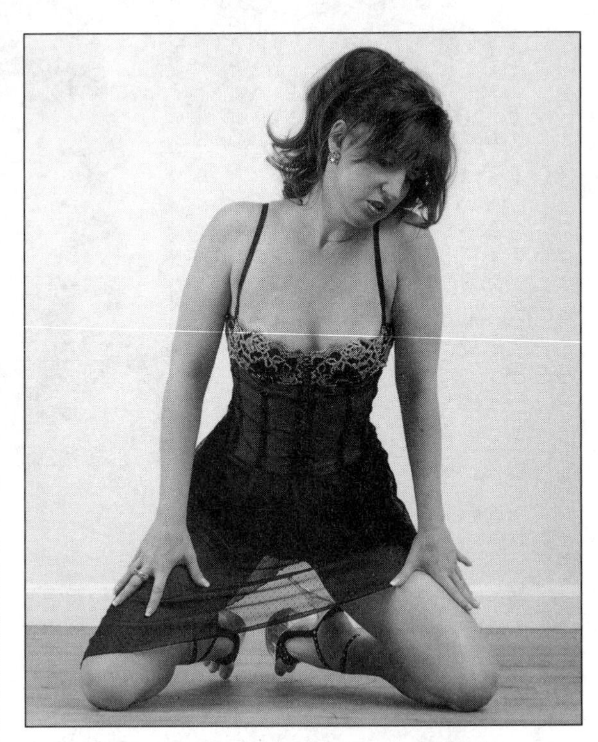

Roll your shoulder as you place your other knee on the floor.

Let It Slide!

A sexier way to go to the floor is to kind of slide forward. Start with your legs about 2 feet apart, place your hands on your thighs with your arms perfectly straight, and then slide your hands down your thighs to a little below your knee.

Then sweep your palms out to the floor and slide them forward while your legs, still straight, sweep around in a wide arc and land back together. From there you can go into a crawl or any other position you want.

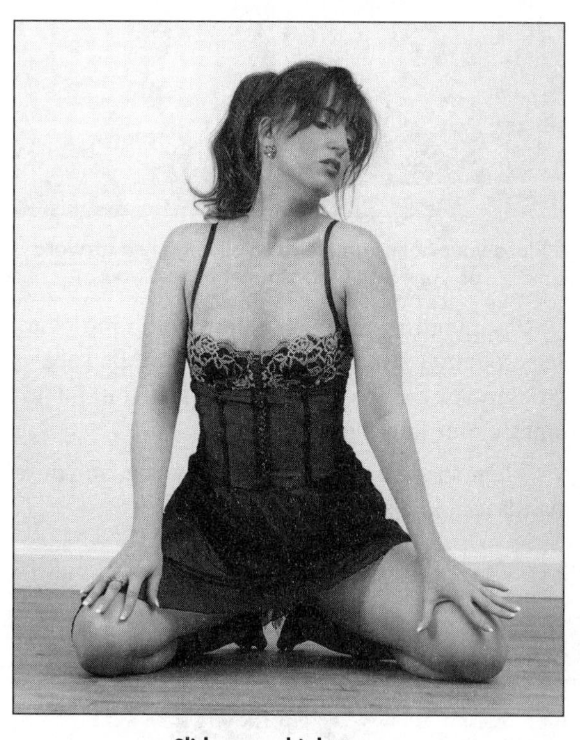

Slide your thighs open.

The Sunset

A flashier version of the slide is what I call the sunset, because your arms form the shape of the sun as they come down to the floor.

Place your feet about 1 foot apart and your arms straight up in the air.

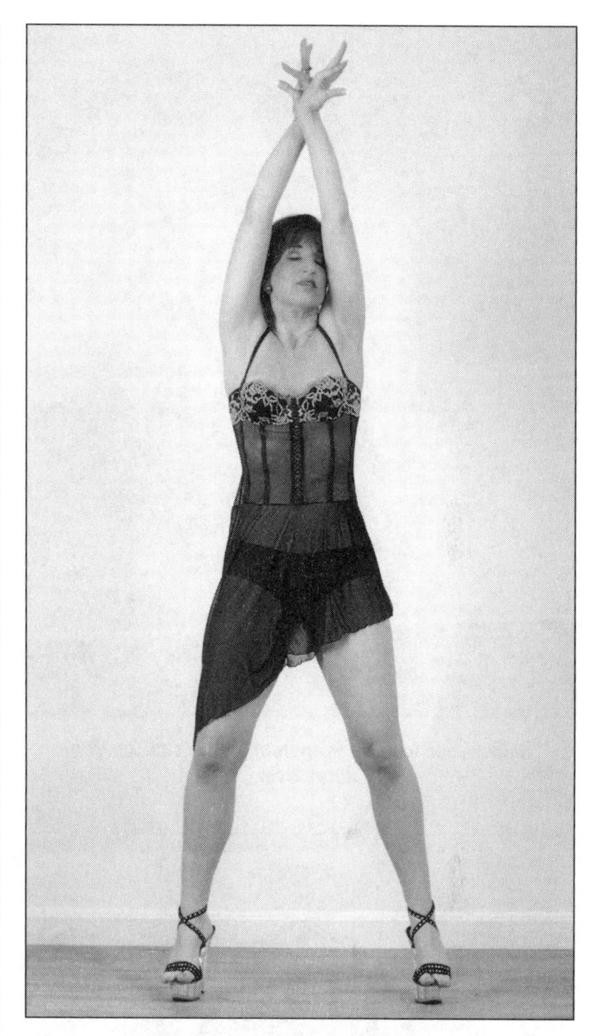

Begin with your arms straight up.

Slide your feet out as your arms come down straight on either side as if you were drawing a giant circle in the air. While you're doing this, lean over from your hips.

Continue bringing your arms down so your palms brush against your shins. This is important because you want to make a complete circle. If your palms don't brush against your shins, you'll be leaning out straight, and that spoils the look of the move.

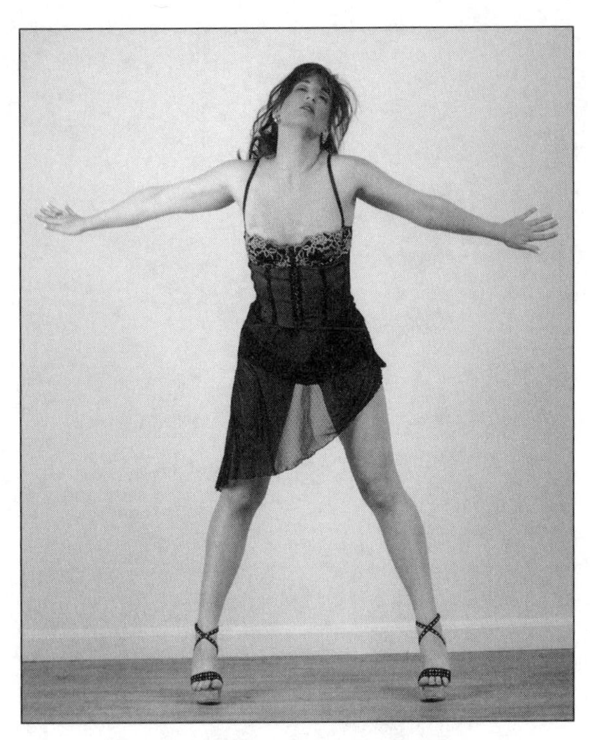

Remember to slide your feet to the side as you lean over.

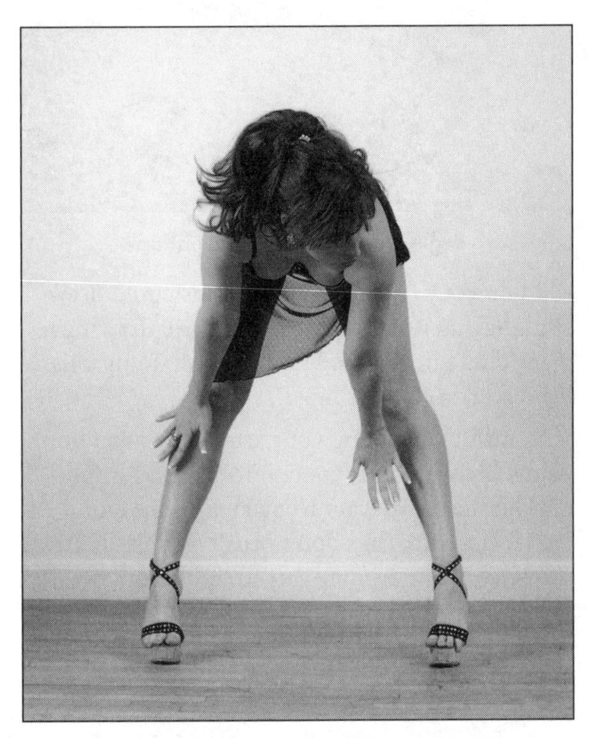

Sweep your palms across your shins to complete the sun circle.

From there, your hands should be about 2 inches from the floor.

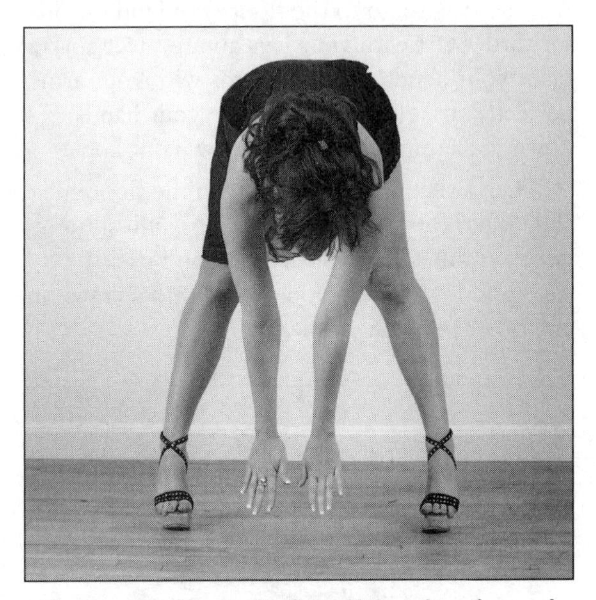

Place your palms on the floor, sliding them forward as your legs snap straight behind you.

Place your palms on the floor and jump your legs together straight out behind you. Be sure to use your toes to brace your fall so you don't smash your knees on the floor!

Then snap your knees up so you are on your hands and knees.

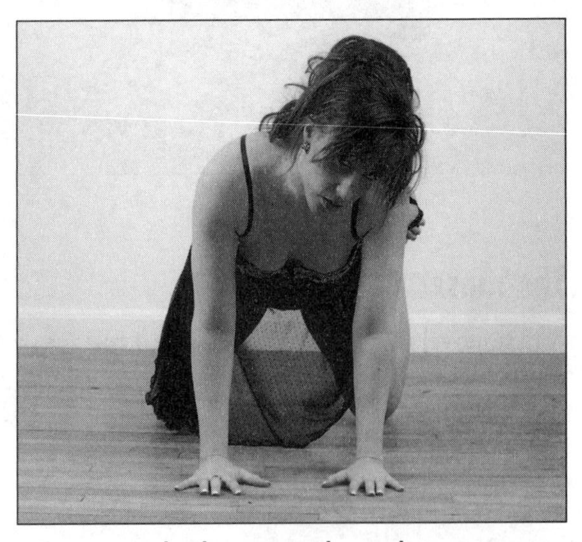

Be sure you land on your palms and your toes, not your knees, when you snap down.

You can also do this move without snapping your legs. When you place your palms on the floor, simply slide both legs out to the sides and around until they are together, again using your toes as the main sliding mechanism.

Snap Down

Harder ways to get down (and by *hard*, I don't mean "difficult"; I mean on more of a beat, like you would do with a traditional tough stripper song as opposed to a soft, slow feminine song) use more of a jump than a slide motion.

First put your hands on your knees.

Snap your palms on the floor and then kick your legs out straight and fold your knees in so you're on your hands and knees.

You can also kneel down off a chair, swing around the pole to the floor, or simply fall over. Whatever method you use to get to the floor, just remember that this is yet another detail to your dance that will add up to make the perfect show!

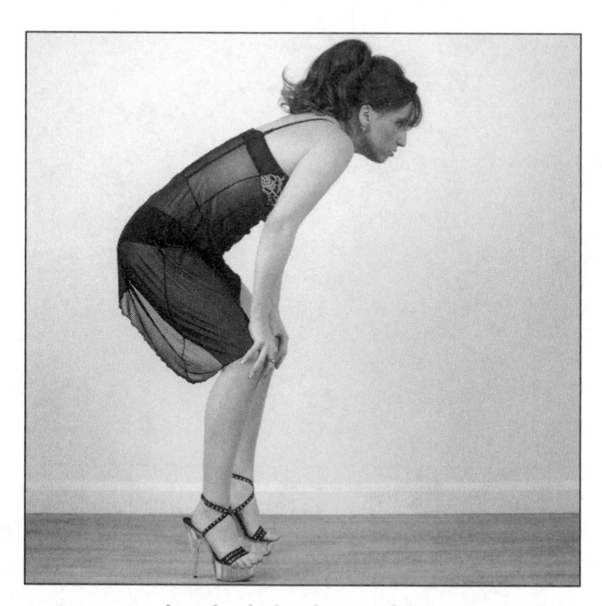

Snap your legs back, but be careful not to smash down on your knees. Your hands and toes are supporting you.

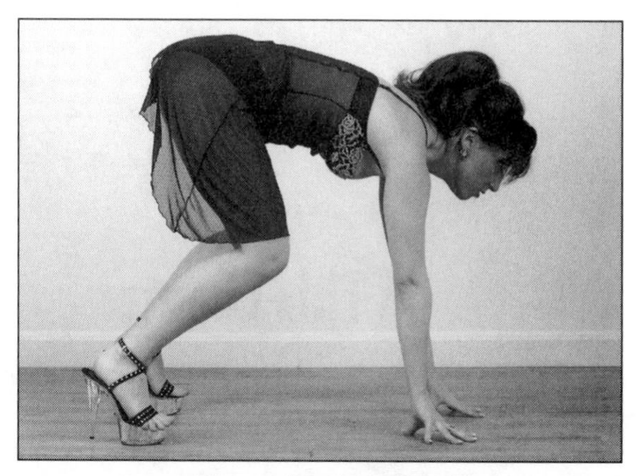

Start with your hands on your knees.

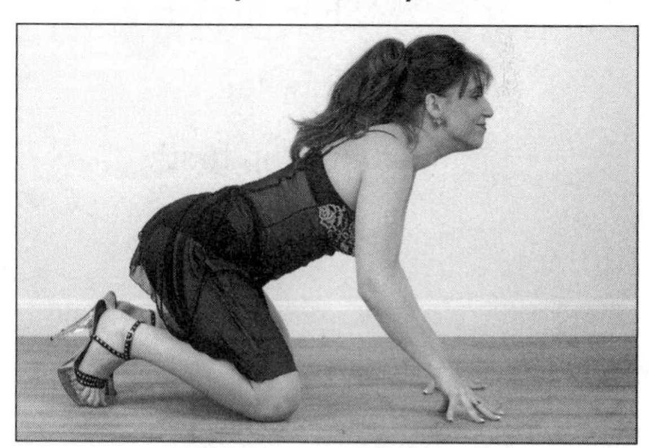

Place your hands on the floor.

The Least You Need to Know

- Don't think about what you're going to do next; let the music tell your body what to do.
- Let the character of the song determine your walking and wall dancing.
- Get to the floor as smoothly and as simply as you can.
- When doing a shoulder roll or half-turn, be sure it's just that. Don't try to go all the way around, or you'll trip over your feet.

In This Chapter

- Fun things to do on your knees and your back
- Transitional floor routines
- Shocking and sexy poses
- Crawling
- Butt up first!

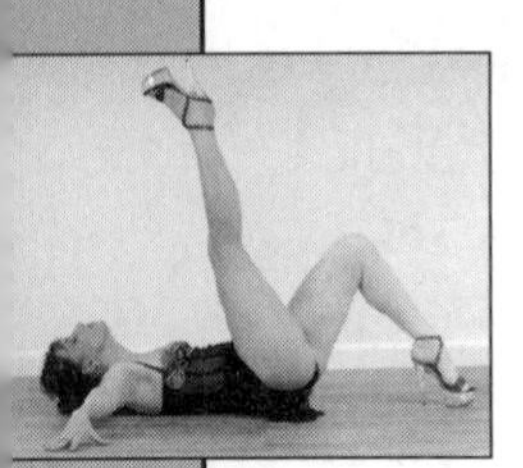
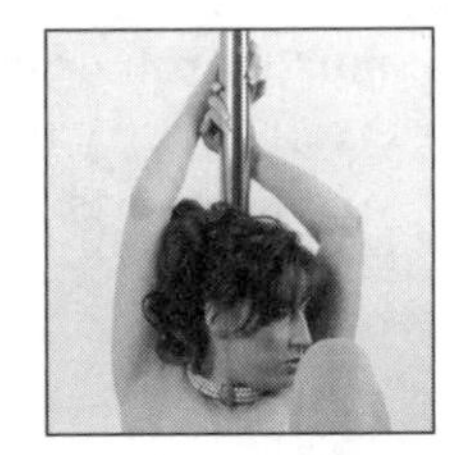
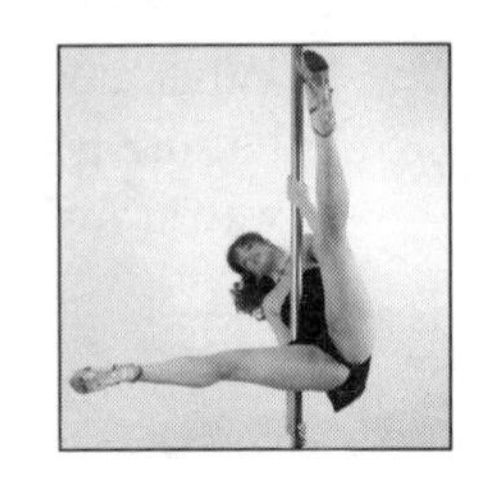
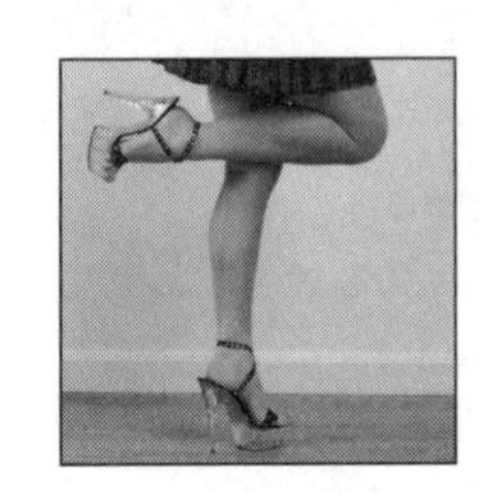
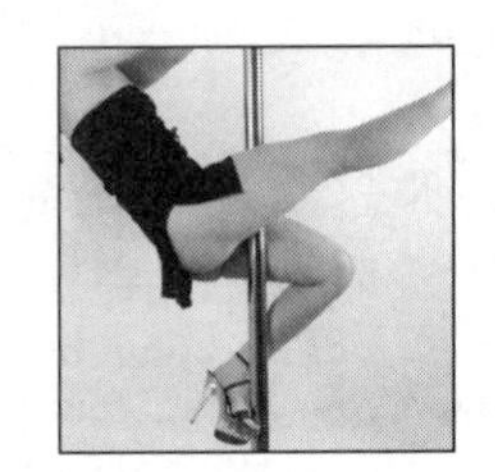
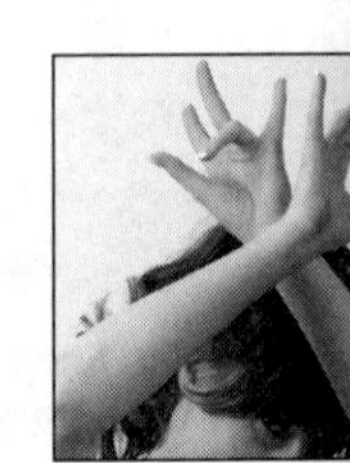

Chapter 7

Seize the Floor

Now that you know what to do when you're standing up, here's what to do when you're lying down. These moves form the backbone of your floor work, and the more you practice these basics, you'll find your floor so clean you'll be able to eat off it!

Thigh Pumper

Now you're on the floor … what do you do? If you come down so you're on your knees, you can begin with the thigh-pumper move, which is a great time-killer and something you can repeat often and with slight differences to make this move look completely different each time.

First—and I shouldn't have to tell you this—spread your thighs and tuck your feet underneath you so you're comfortable.

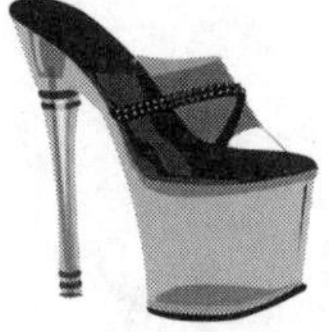

Trippin' Up

The farther forward you sit, the more you'll be on your knees and the more it will hurt, so sit back.

You can do one several things here:

- Lift your thighs up and down. (But remember, you're not doing this just straight up and down as an exercise; you're doing this because that area is sexy and you know it!)
- Swirl your hips around in a hip circle while you're going up and down.
- Pump it up and down with your hands clasped over your head.
- Lean back on your arms and roll your head dramatically.
- Lean all the way back so your head actually rests on the floor while you're continuously pulsing your hips with the undercurrent of the song. Then arc your arms around so you propel yourself back up somewhat quickly.

While you're doing these thigh-pumping moves, your hands are, of course, massaging yourself sensually, or you are using the graceful belly-dance hand arm movements while your neck is rolled back in the passion of that song.

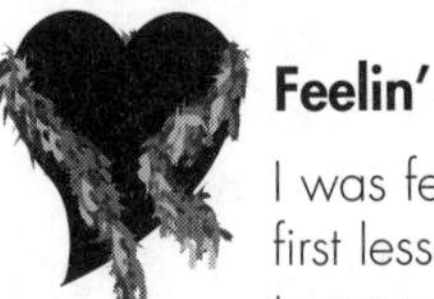

Feelin' the Love

I was feeling different today [after first lesson]. I found myself hip-rolling to any music on commercials … I am so glad I chose to do this and look forward to the day I will become an expert. [Dancing is] the most fun thing I have done in long while. Fun, fun, fun!

—Sage, student

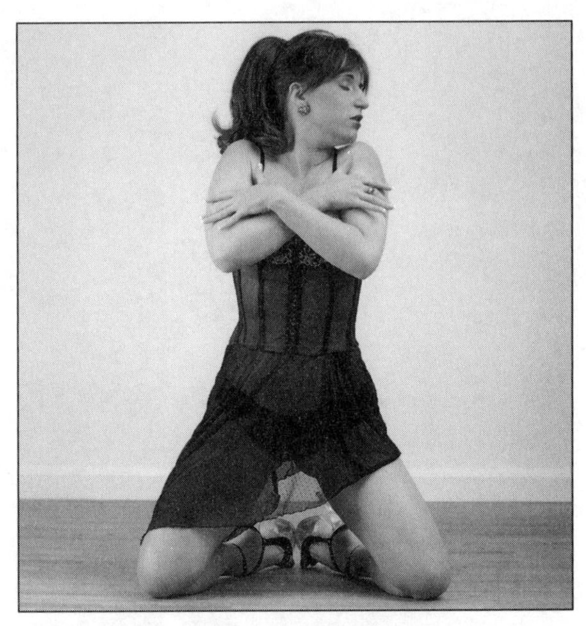

Move your thighs up and down while you're caressing yourself.

The Diva Dive

From here, while still on your knees, you can do a diva dive, a hand movement that starts with your palms up and middle finger pointed up. You then roll your hands back so your middle finger is pointing back at you and then roll your hands over and put one on top of the other as you slide forward with your butt in the air for a butt circle.

Just be careful—you're not diving off a diving board. The movement is in the hands; leave your arms out of this.

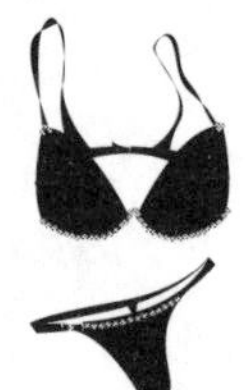

Behind the G-String

Dancing to the undercurrent of a song is so essential to this art that I have often threatened my students with the purchase of an electric cattle prod … *I said no club dancing!*

And now you're in a perfect position for the next move ….

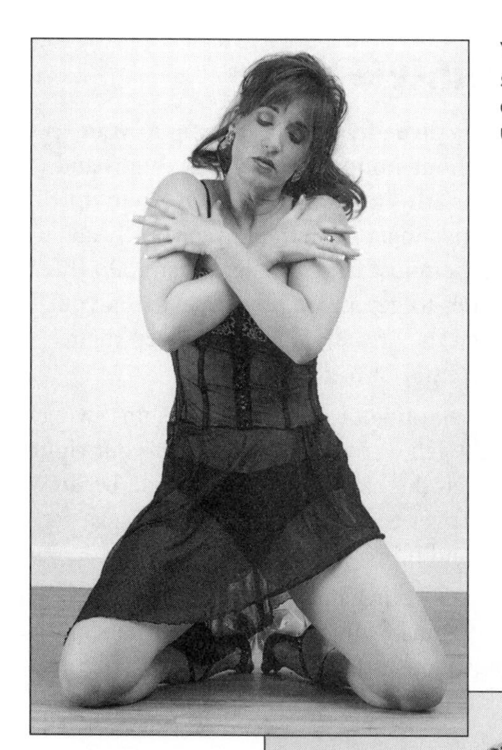

You can also sway your hips as you move up and down.

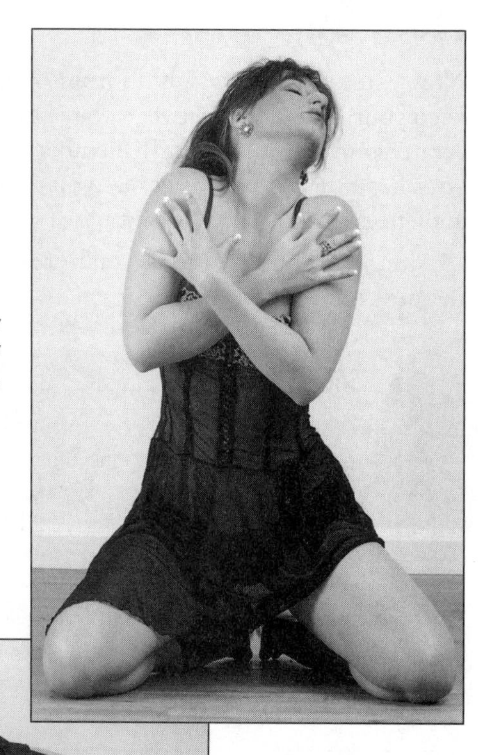

Be sure to stay in the passion by rolling your neck.

You can lean back all the way, or even just lean halfway back on your arms, look up at the ceiling, and rotate or roll your hips.

Keep those fingers moving slowly and deliberately to the undercurrent of the song.

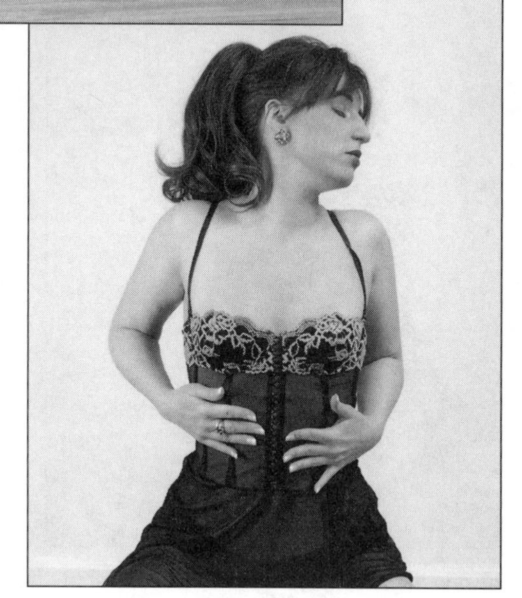

Floor Butt Circles

Now your arms are straight in front of you, so keep your head down between your arms and rotate your butt in the air. Remember to keep your head tucked under because you want the audience to focus on your butt here.

After a few butt rotations, you're ready for the next move: princess pose.

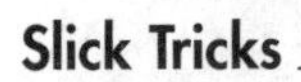

Slick Tricks

While you transition from move to move, pay attention to the music you've got playing. How does the artist sing the words? When do they start the lyrics? And how do they end them? For example, don't just switch moves in the middle of a word. Work with the music and the lyrics, and remember that you want to become one with the song and take on the character of the song.

The Princess Pose

From a diva dive, draw your arms up to your knees. Without stopping, raise your thighs and extend your arms outward, sweeping them up so your hands meet gracefully over your head (don't let them just hang like limp fish). Do this several times to get a nice flow. Don't stop your hands when they reach your knees; keep them flowing up and out to the sides.

Now pivot on your knees so your shins swing as far to the left as possible. Try to get your right foot to touch the back of your left thigh, because the farther over the bottom half of your legs are, the easier and more graceful this will look.

Now cross your hands way over your head with your palms facing down, and dramatically draw your hands down over your face (which is sensually tilted to the right) and then over your chest.

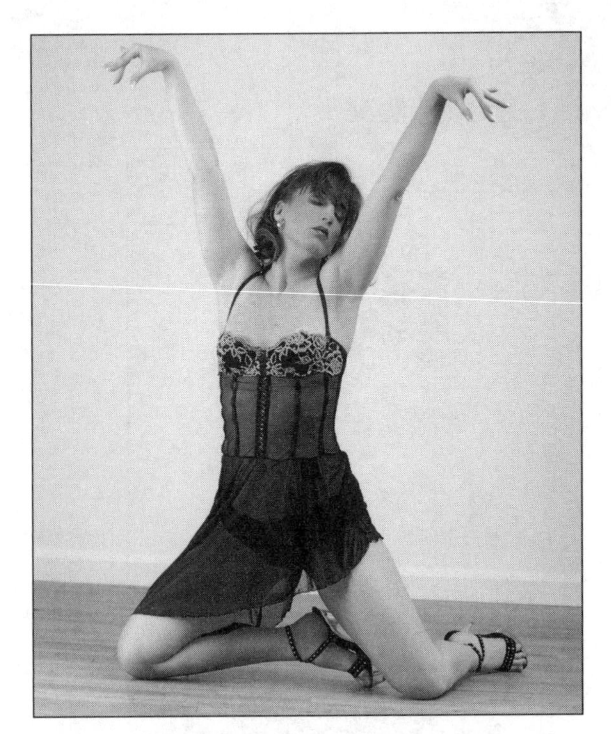

Your arms and thighs rise up together, as your right foot swings as far left as it can.

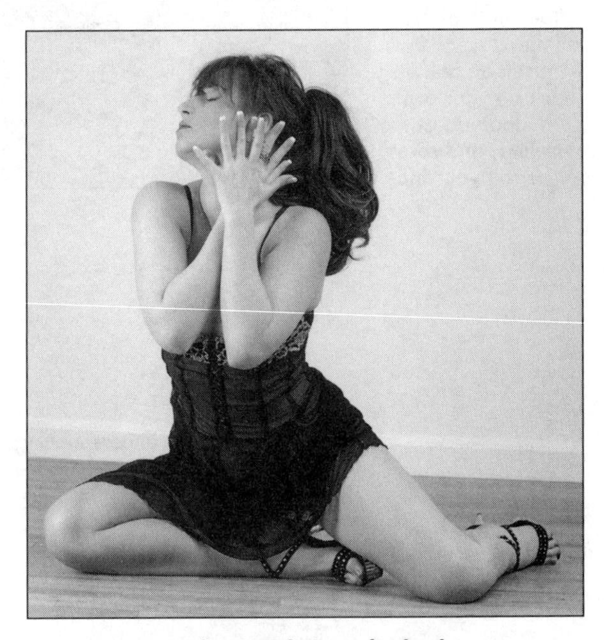

Using muscle control, sit as far back as you can so your butt gently lands on the floor as your hands draw dramatically down the side of your face and neck.

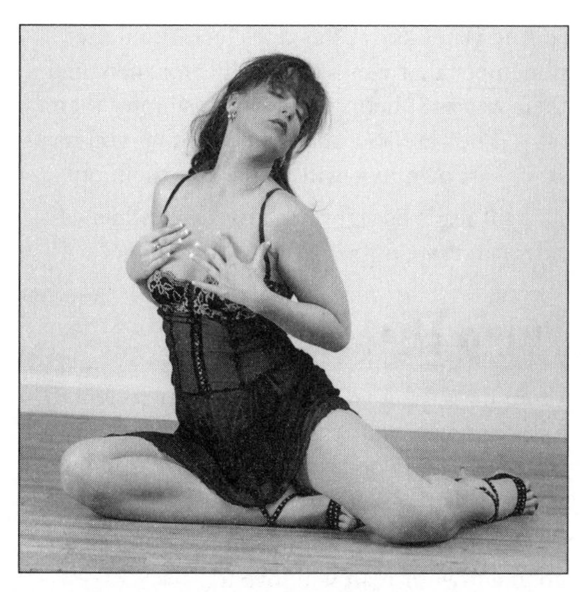

Continue to draw your arms down as you sit with your back properly arched.

As your hands slide down, slowly sit your butt on the floor, ending with your back arched in a very feminine princess pose. If you sat on your feet when your butt came down, your legs weren't over enough to the left and your feet were in the way.

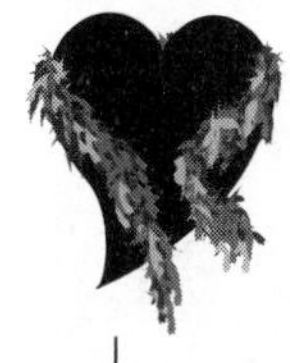

Feelin' the Love

Sometimes, when I'm feeling a little extra confident, I saunter over to the stereo, put some sexy music on, and do a little dance for my boyfriend.

—Jen, student

Love That Leg!

From princess pose, slide your right arm down and behind you, bringing your right side down to the floor. As you rest on your forearm (do not lay completely flat on your side), lift up your left leg straight in the air. Remember, it *has* to be straight, not limp-looking, because this is all about strength and looking strong.

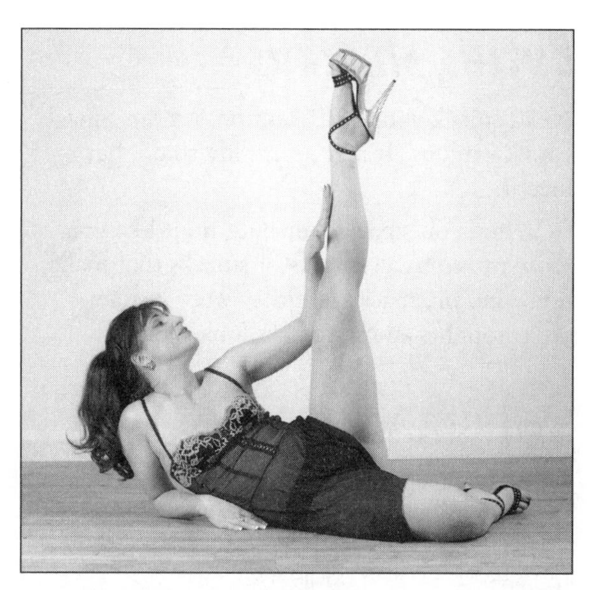

Concentrate only on your finger as you slowly draw it down your leg, ignoring your audience completely.

Place your left middle finger on your raised foot and *slowly*—slower than you think you should—draw that finger down your leg and *stare* at it. Stare at your finger like it's coming down a leg of solid gold and you are in *awe* of your own leg.

When your finger gets to your butt, slowly lower your leg, bending it at the knee so it rests on the other leg. Continue your display of self-confidence by lightly drawing circles on your butt. This is just another way of showing your audience you know you're sexy. Remember, I don't care if you hate your butt or you think it's too big. Act like you love it, and your audience will, too.

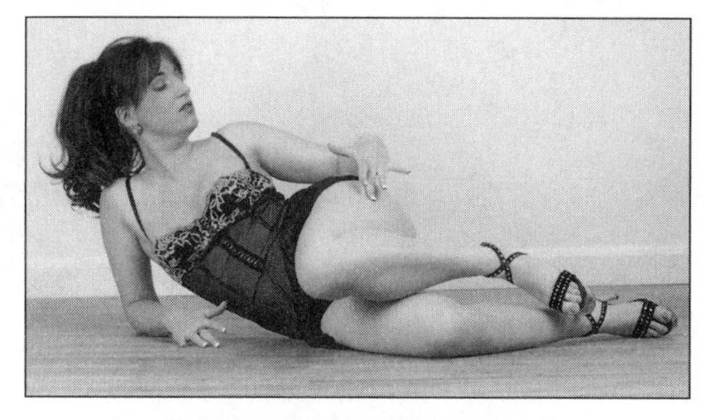

Draw light circles on your butt as you stare longingly at it.

Buttus Smackus

Next, smack your butt. Yes, that's right. Smack your own butt. It may seem silly to do, but men love it.

When you smack your butt, do it like you *mean* it. No weak smacks or smacks that make no sound or smacks as if they were just an afterthought—those smacks looks lame.

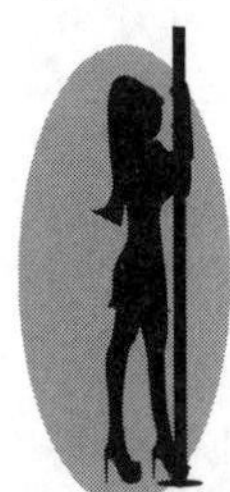

Slick Tricks

When smacking your butt, use a popular dancer trick: cup your hand. This gives you a louder smack, although it does sting a little more.

This Is Your Butt—Love It!

Now massage your butt with the same loving attitude you had for your leg earlier. Don't just rub it—massage it so you can see finger grooves. Act like you *love* your butt, you *want* your butt, it's the best butt you've ever seen and you know it!

And yes, I know, this does feel stupid, but remember that you're doing this for men, and their way of thinking is so much simpler than ours. They are so visual that watching you massage your own butt will really turn them on.

That leads us right back to the confidence rule: *confidence is sexier than any perfect body.*

Pump That Floor

From massaging your butt, roll over so you're lying flat with your tummy on the floor. Extend your arms and your legs out straight, and pump the floor with your pelvis.

As silly as this might feel, it looks very, very good and your man will love it!

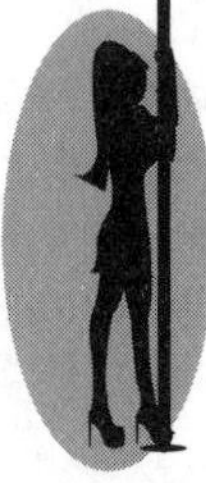

Slick Tricks

If you every don't know what move to do next, just roll over, put the pressure on your fingers, and caress your body while your butt is swirling to the undercurrent of the song.

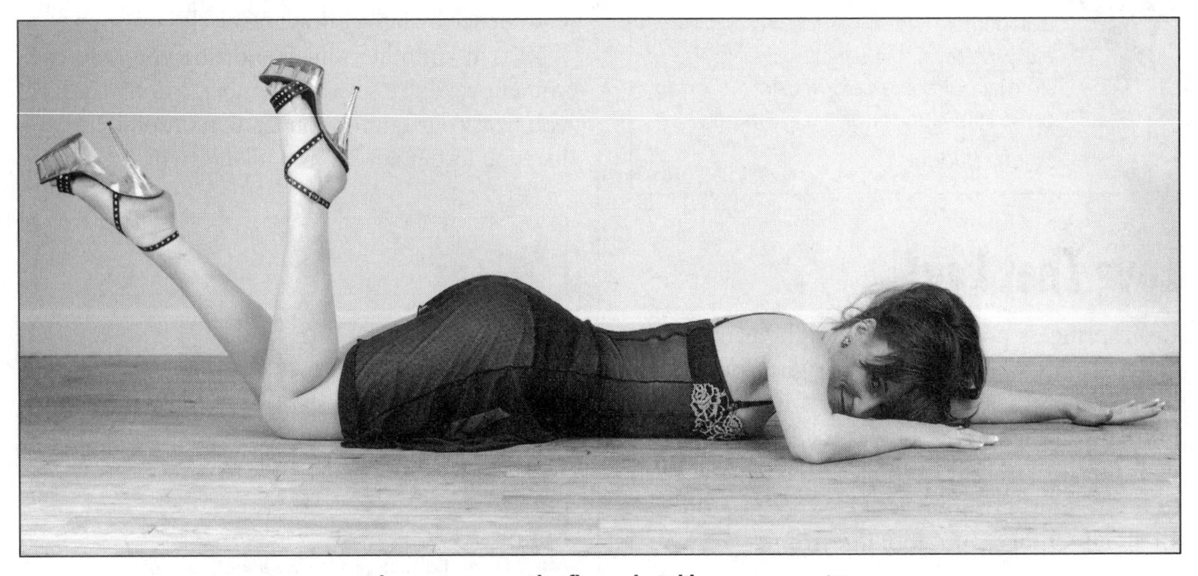

When you pump the floor, do it like you mean it!

Hello! V Legs

The V legs pose is one you'll use often, more for the shock value than anything else. From your position while pumping the floor, simply roll over so you're on your back. Bend your legs at the knee and bring them up together. Straighten your legs and open them slowly so they form the shape of a V.

Be sure to keep your legs perfectly straight. They'll look weak if they're bent, like you can't extend them fully. If you can't extend them fully, that's okay, too, because then you can just bend your knees at a 45-degree angle and keep them open for 3 seconds. As long as you have the sharp, strong angle, the spread legs will look great!

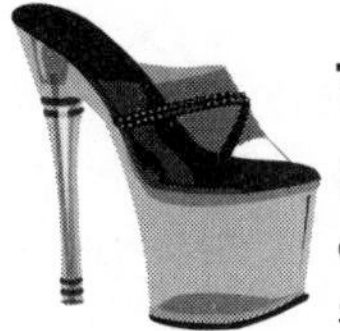

Trippin' Up

It is very, very, very important to always keep your legs open for 3 seconds. If you just open them and shut them, it benefits no one. It's the shock of the position that gets your audience.

While your legs are open, keep your head back and lightly run your middle finger down your legs and then back up. Again, you need to show how much you love your legs and show your audience that your legs are sexy and you *know* it! Then slowly close your legs and ease into your next move.

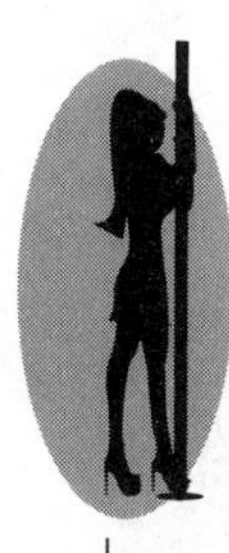

Slick Tricks

Capture the character of the song. In other words, always stay in the drama of your performance through facial expression. The more dramatic you are, the stronger and more believable your performance will be.

Mud Flap Pose

From V legs, you can transition to many moves. One that's popular and very pretty is the mud flap pose, so named because of the instantly recognizable female silhouette on the back of a trucker's mud flaps.

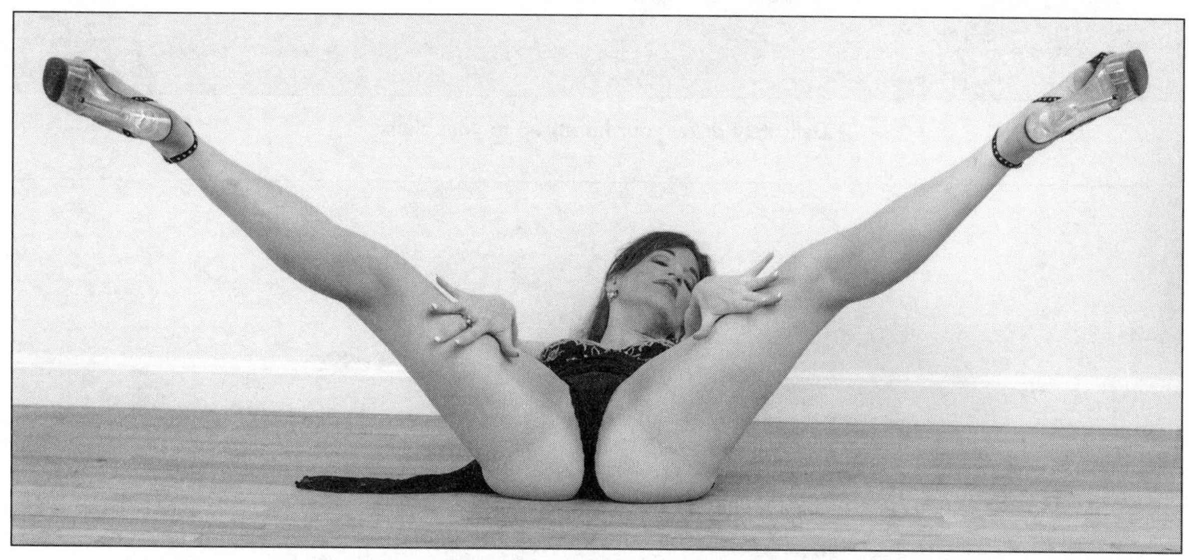

Your legs should be perfectly straight and strong. Hold this position for 3 seconds.

Lying on your back, with both legs together and in the air, gently lower one leg so it's straight on the floor. Bend your other leg at the knee and rest your foot on the floor.

Arch your back as high as you can (the higher the arch. the prettier it looks) and put your head way back so you're looking behind you where the wall meets the floor. Place your hands on your pelvis, and delicately draw them up your tummy and over your chest. (Bring your elbows up as you do this.) Then, extend your arms straight out to the sides.

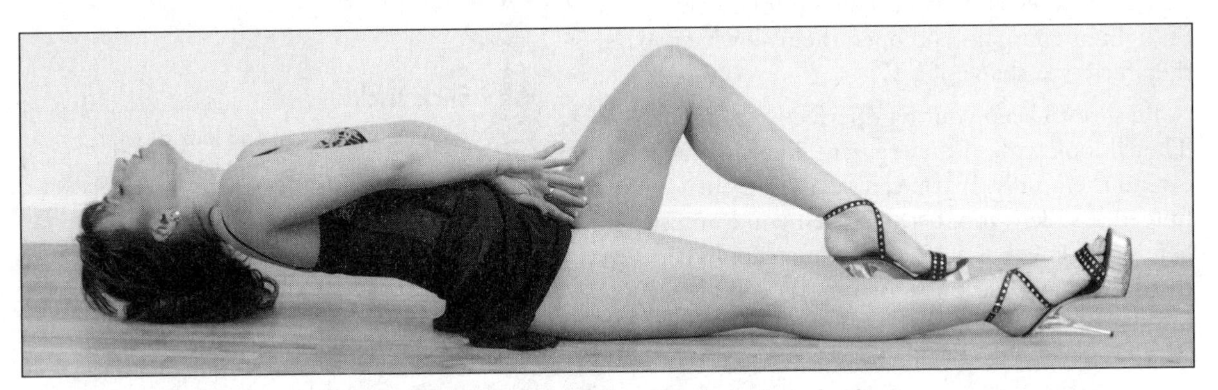

Arch your back, keeping one leg straight and one leg bent.

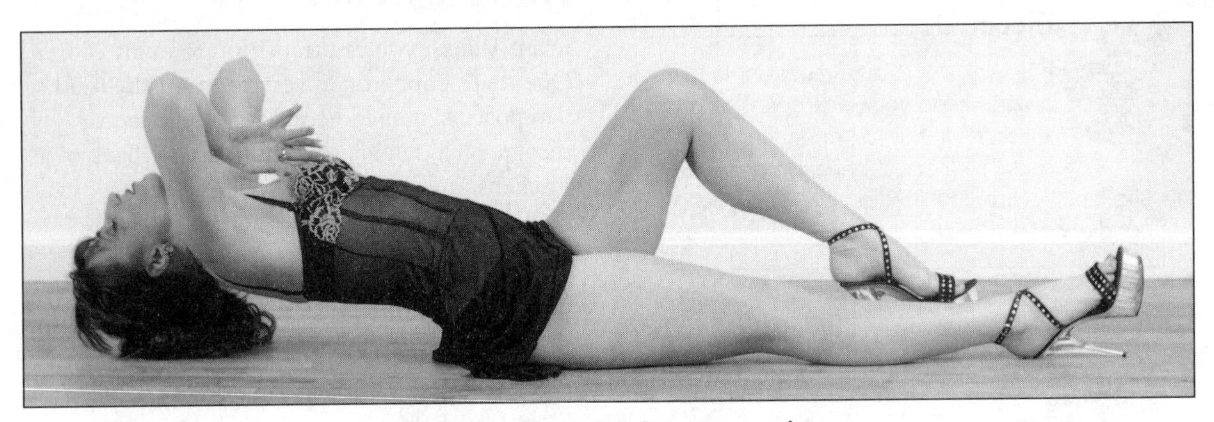

Delicately draw your hands up to your chest.

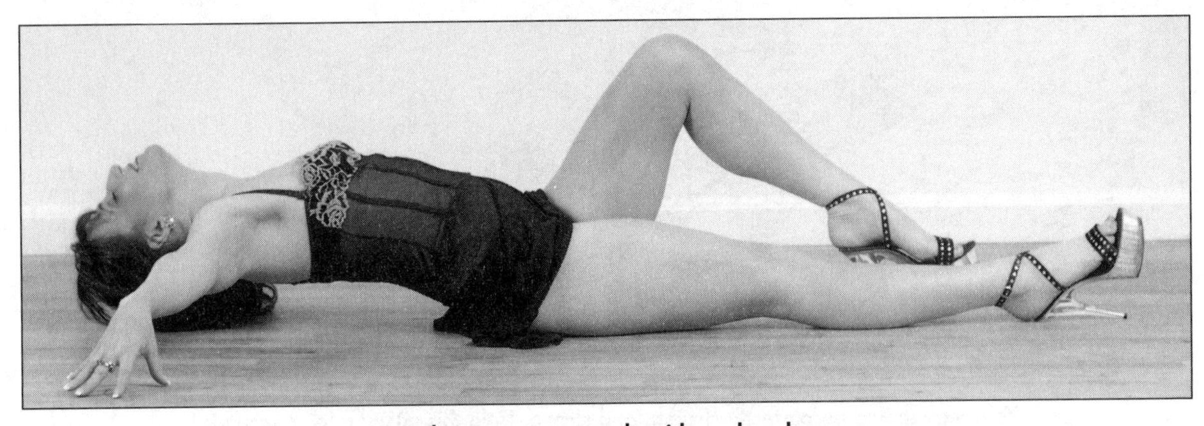

Extend your arms out to the side, palms down.

Relax your back and your head so you're just lying on the floor, and bring your *straight* leg up so your butt is also an inch or 2 off the floor.

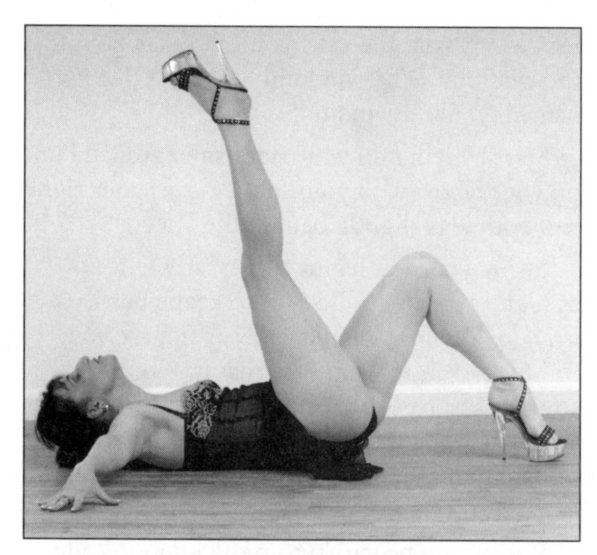

Relax your back completely, and bring your straight leg up.

Use your leg to bring your body into a sitting position as your arms draw up from behind.

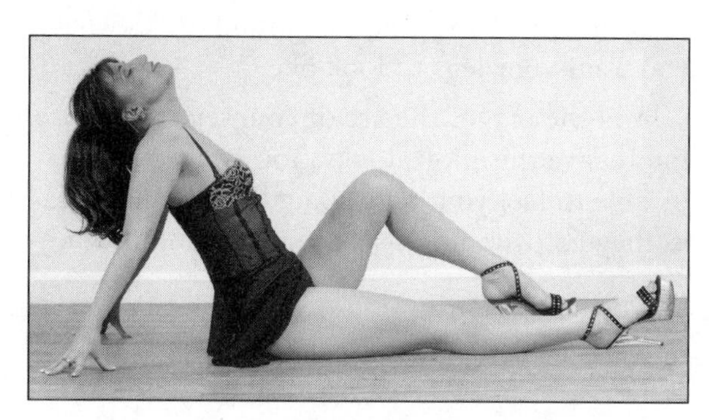

Draw your arms up from behind, keep your head back, and take your time as you come up.

Then, turn your head and look at your audience. Be sure to have a sultry spark in your eye!

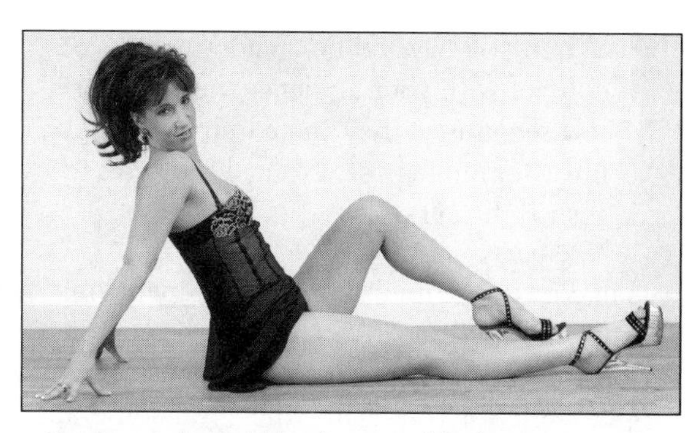

Keep your arms behind you and look at your audience for about 3 seconds so he can admire your feminine pose.

You must follow several rules when doing the mud flap pose to make it really shine:

- Your straight leg must go down and your body come up at the exact same speed.
- When your body comes up, tilt your head *all the way back* and look at the ceiling until you're in your final sitting position and then slowly turn your head to your audience with your sexy look. *Do not come up with your head facing forward.* It will look like you are straining and is not the slightest bit dramatic.
- Come up slowly. Take your sweet time. This is another subliminal message to your audience that this is *your* show, you'll take *your* time, and they'll like it.
- Be sure your hands and arms slide along the floor when your body comes up. Do not lift your arms off the ground and swing them over; that kills the whole move.
- Don't slide your hands too close to your butt. Keep them at a nice angle behind you.
- Do this sideways to your audience. This is an incredible profile shot. (Think of the mud flaps.)

- When you have come up and made eye contact with your audience, hesitate for a few seconds so they can admire your sexy, ultra-feminine pose. No need for you to rush right out of it …

The key to the mud flap pose is repetition, repetition, repetition. Watch yourself in a mirror on the floor if you can so you can see the proper angle for your arms when you come up as well as your speed.

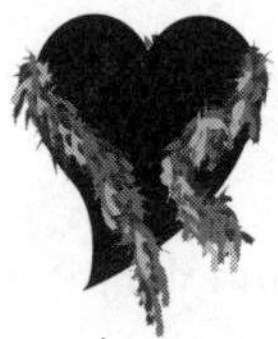

Feelin' the Love

Boys become putty in your hands if you let them think anything is possible. —Suede, student

When done correctly, this is one of the sexiest moves there is. Of course, you can add your own twists and turns to it, like maybe crossing your feet when your legs are in the air and bringing yourself up that way, or even coming up with your legs bent at the knee going over to the side … so many possibilities! Have fun and create your own specialized mud flap pose!

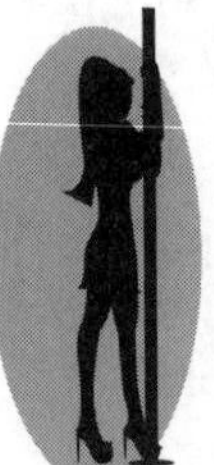

Slick Tricks

Repeat your moves. Your audience is not going to know you're repeating yourself, and he wouldn't dare say anything if he did. Men are simple creatures and will not notice you doing the same move again because their focus is … well, we all know what their focus is …. That's what makes exotic dancing so simple—men are so easily pleased!

The Windmill

If you come out of the mud flap pose with your feet crossed and your knees bent with your legs together at the side, you can easily go into the windmill. The windmill looks just like it's named … like a windmill.

Start by lying on your right side, propped up on your elbow with your left leg over your right leg, both legs slightly bent at the knee.

Swing your left leg over first, arcing it up as high as it can go. Be sure to keep your leg *straight!* When it's about midway up, arc your right leg over, making sure that it, too, is straight and has just as much power going over as your left leg did. (often, the right leg loses momentum as it swings over—both legs must look strong.)

End as you began, but on the opposite side (that is, on your left elbow with your legs bent).

The key to this move is *not* to swing both legs at the same time. They must go over individually, but smoothly—not one *[pause]* and then the other. Imagine a windmill; that's what you want your legs to look like.

And the bigger the arc of your legs, the more impressive this move looks. You really want to be able to feel your legs going in a circular arc as they go over, not just straight up and down.

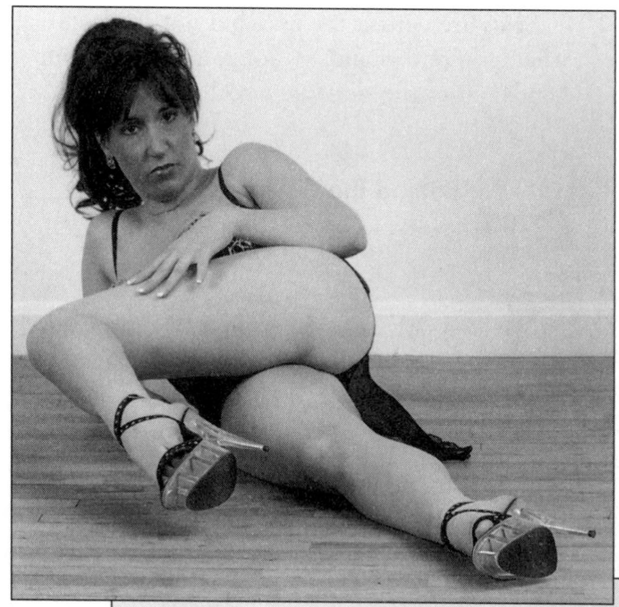

Start completely on your side, not your back.

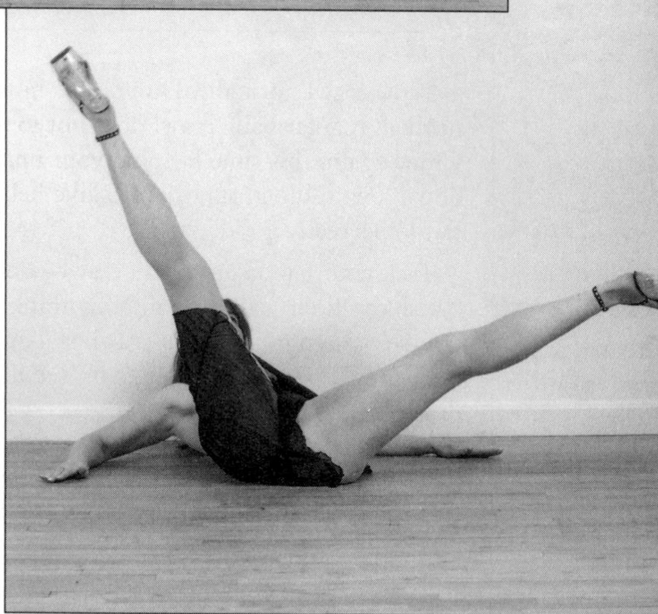

Both legs are straight and strong when they go over one at a time, not together.

Land on your opposite forearm so you're on your side, not your back.

The Crawl

Crawling does not feel sexy; it feels clunky and stupid. But it *looks* sexy, and guys love it. When you crawl, you want to feel like a sexy tiger. Again, it's the mind's-eye thing: picture a tiger crawling, and your body will adjust. That's easier said than done, though, because it hurts like hell, so many of my students will revert to the more comfortable yet dorky-looking crawling with straight arms.

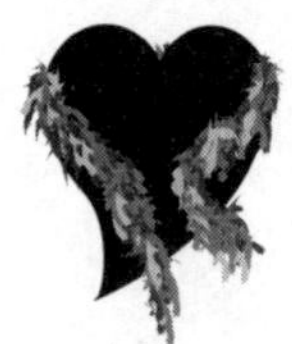

Feelin' the Love

I can tell you that New Year's Eve 2004 was the *best night* of my husband's sexual life! He was in awe of my skills, confidence, and eye contact!

—Maureen, student

It helps if you have a mirror you can place on the floor so that you can watch and see what you do that you think looks sexy—and learn what does *not* look sexy.

For example, proud Americans we all are, it's not necessary to prove it when you crawl, so no "military-under-the-barbed-wire" crawling.

And no Ralphing, either. "Ralphing" is named after my family's dearly departed dog Ralph, who was half Shepherd mix. When he got older, he got hip dysplasia, and his back became paralyzed. To get around, he would drag his back legs around on the floor behind him. This worked for him, but it won't work for you. So no "Ralphing" when you crawl.

Never crawl with your arms straight. Always have at least a slight bend at your elbows.

Nobody wants crabs, and your man is no exception. So don't crawl with your elbows sticking out to the sides like a little crab, either.

Seals are cute at the zoo, but not so much when you're dancing, so don't crawl with your hands out to the side like a seal!

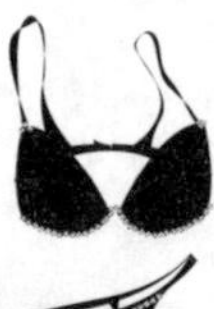

Behind the G-String

When I worked in the exotic dance club, I would crawl up to a guy, staring right into his eyes. He'd stare back into my eyes, we'd be doing this deep, soul-searching thing as our eyes locked as I crawled to him. Then, when I got right up to his face, I'd cross my eyes! Most of the time, the guy would laugh, but some would be taken aback because we had just had a "special" moment, looking deeply into each others' eyes as if we had just discovered that we were soul mates.

Now crawl normally. Do you see how a normal, regular baby crawl does not look sexy? Crawl again, this time keeping your upper back down low to the ground. Hurts like hell, yes, but looks really good.

Pick your hands up as you crawl—don't "wash the floor" with them. Now think of yourself as a tigress as you crawl, stalking your man-prey. If you've got long hair, see if you can drape it down over one eye.

Remember to keep your upper back down, and don't crawl just on your forearms. Repeat this in the mirror to see how you look. And although you may think it looks stupid and feels even more stupid, I'm telling you guys *love* when a woman crawls, and it *does not* look stupid. (Think of Madonna crawling in her "Express Yourself" video. Think she feels good doing that? I bet ya it doesn't feel as good as it looks!)

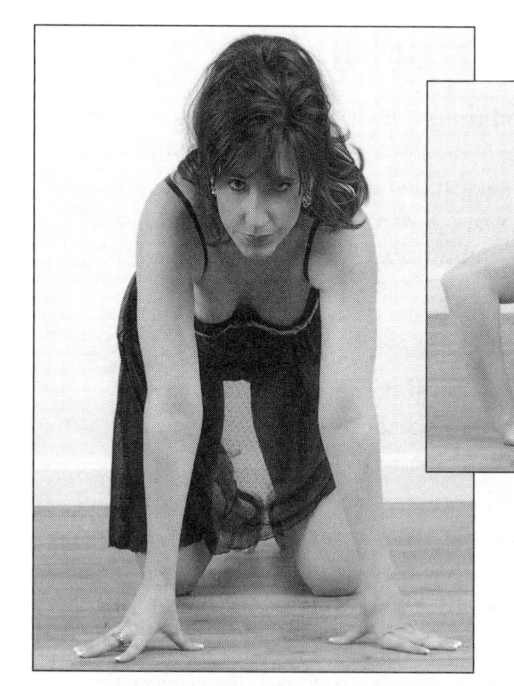

Straight arms are not soft and feminine-looking.

Be sure to keep your elbows bent back, not out to the side, like a crab.

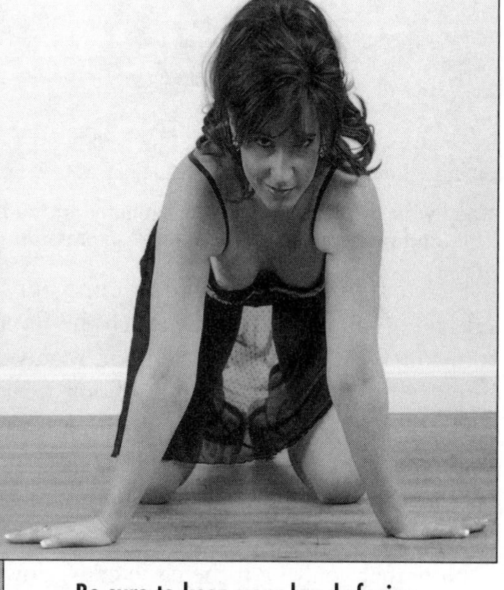

Be sure to keep your hands facing forward and your elbows bent. No seals!

Keep your front end down, your elbows bent, and pick your hands up as you crawl.

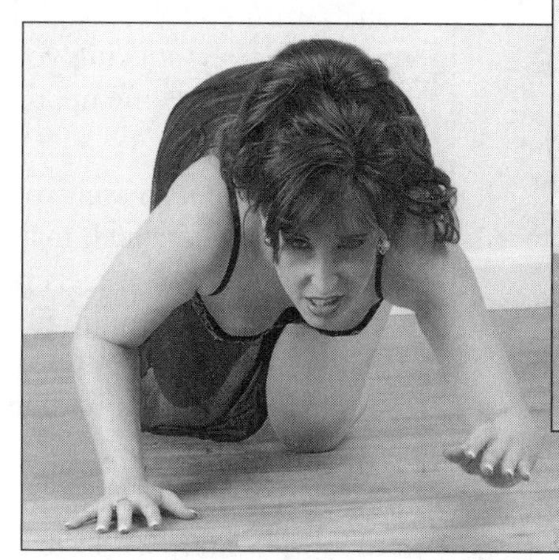

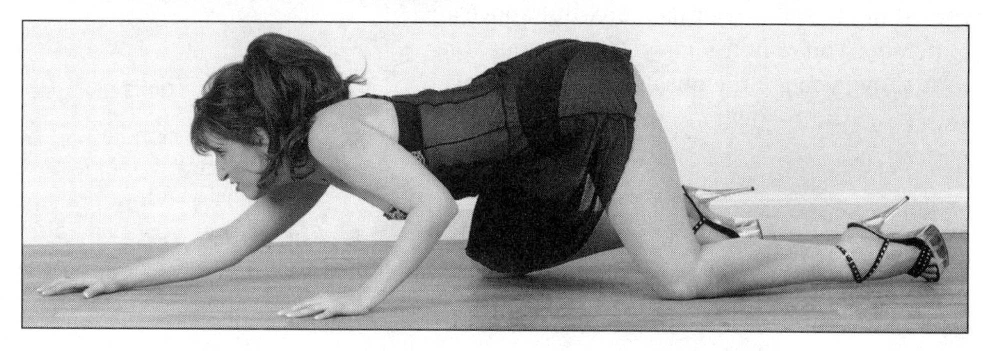

Your crawl is much sexier if you stay low to the ground.

Desperation Pump

This move can also be used as a basic floor move. Lean on your right forearm with your right hand in front of or slight to the right of your face. Slide your right leg back so you're lying on top of your right thigh, with your leg bending at the knee at an angle.

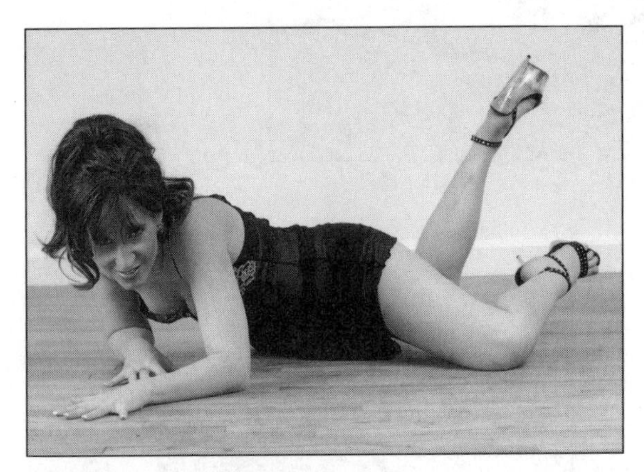

Keep your arms uneven, lift your tummy off the floor, and maintain your "desperate" expression.

Slide out your left arm and rest on your left hand (your arm does not touch the floor). Your inner left thigh is on the floor, with your entire left leg also resting on the floor, bent at the knee. Look up at your mark with a look of desperation on your face, and pump your butt two or three times before continuing with your crawl into your next move.

Now that you've got the basic crawl down, have some fun with it! Stop midway in your crawl and roll your torso up and down, roll your shoulders, flip your hair, etc. But above all, remember you're in no hurry. This is your song, your show; you are the queen and you *will* take your sweet time—he'll *like* it!

Time to Get Up!

All good things must come to an end, and that includes your floor work. But you don't want to just stop and stand up. That breaks the spell you've woven with your dance. Instead, you need to get up sexy.

Butt First

From now until the end of eternity, you will get up butt first—because I will always be there in spirit …

When on your knees, first put up one leg and then the other so you're crouching—do *not* come up yet!—with your feet close to each other. Do not even *think* about standing up until you are completely crouched down first.

Rest your hands on your knees (*never* put your hands on the floor to balance, as that's the sign of an amateur and you're now a professional), turn your feet slightly to the side, and come up slowly, sticking your butt out as far as it can go as you come up, drawing your hands up your thighs.

Be careful not to arch your back. Instead, scoop your back, which makes your butt stick out farther. I know it feels funny to stick out your butt and be proud of it, but remember, when you are dancing, you are the queen, and even if you do have a big butt, *good!*

Also remember the move isn't done until you draw your hands up your thighs, being careful to do it delicately with the middle fingers.

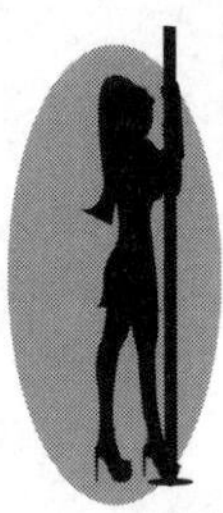

Slick Tricks

When standing up butt first, be sure to keep your feet relatively close together. If they're far apart, you won't be able to get your butt up so it looks nice, and you'll lose your balance.

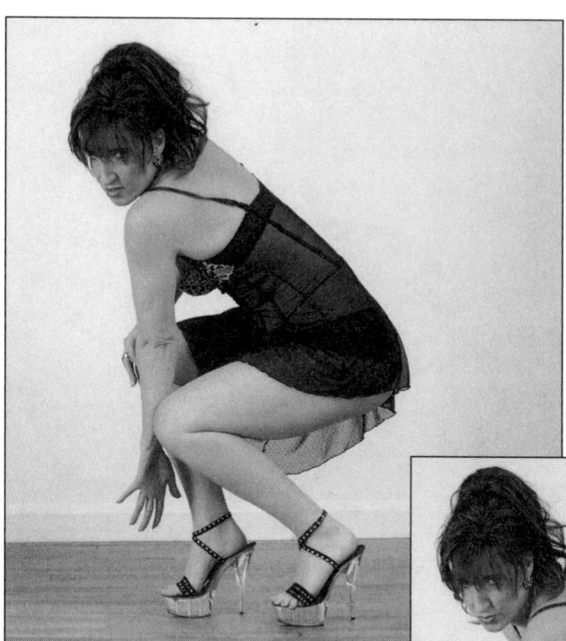

Place your hands on your knees, not the floor, to balance. Keep your feet close together.

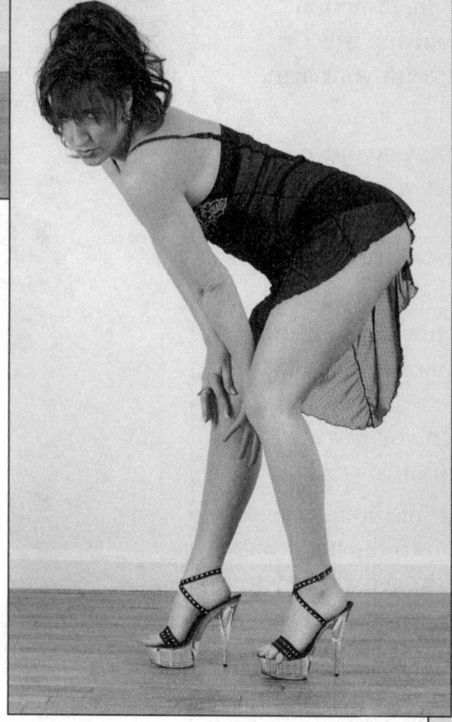

Stick your butt out as far as it can go and come up slowly. Take your sweet time!

The move is not complete until you draw your hands up your thighs. Do it slowly and deliberately.

Snap Up

Another way to stand up like you mean it is to snap up at attention. It's sort of like the snap down position in Chapter 6 but in reverse.

Start on your knees with your hands on the floor.

Snap your feet up so you're in a crouching position with your hands still on the floor.

Then snap up again and step back with your right foot so you're standing sideways yet still facing front. As your right foot comes back, bring your left hand to your hip. (You don't have to bring your hand to your hip if your shoulders look strong enough with your arm down.)

This is just a sampling of routine moves you can do on the floor, so I expect you to master these basics and then add in your own little twists and turns and flourishes to truly personalize your dance.

You can use an infinite number of positions to transition into. Just remember to let your song tell you what to do. Maybe it sounds crazy, but it really will, because when you *feel* the music, your body will move on its own.

These can also be used as transitional moves to get you from one position into the next. Just slide on the floor or roll over to get where you want to go. Don't think about it—just do it. And if you think you're doing something wrong when you're dancing, just keep going and try not to overanalyze yourself. The whole purpose of this dance is to show that you know you're sexy, not to show off actual, physical, dance moves. You're just using the medium of dance to communicate how wonderfully sexy you are.

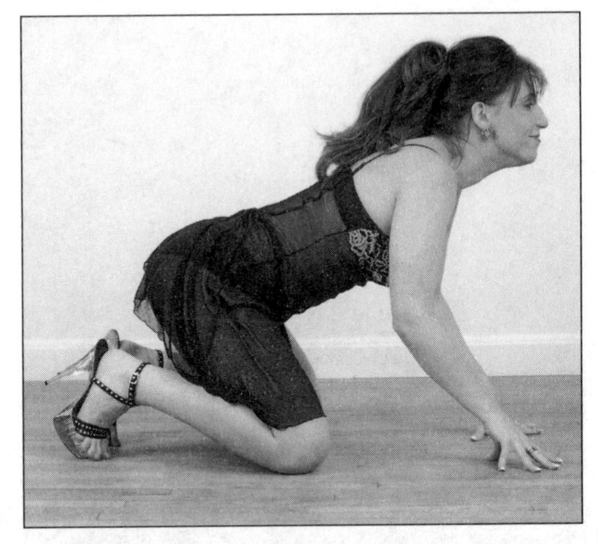

Place your hands and knees on the floor.

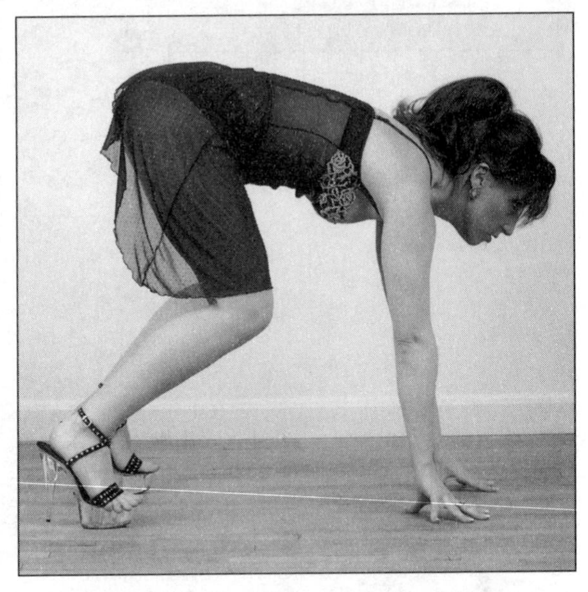

Use a small jump with your legs so you're now in a squatting position, resting on your toes and fingertips.

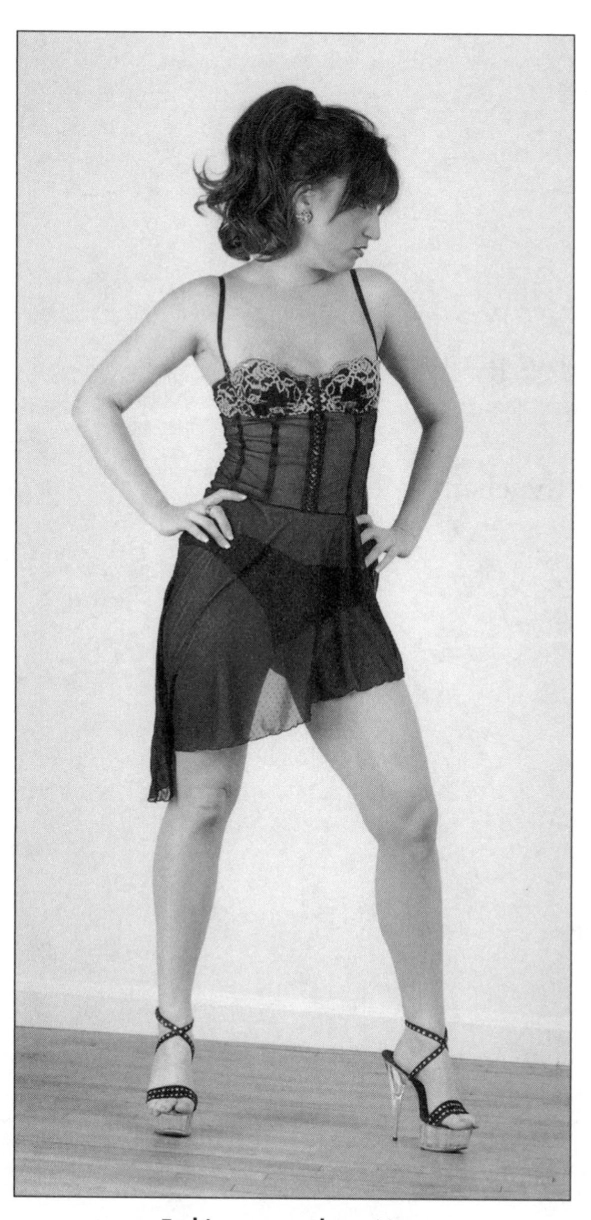

End in a strength position.

The Least You Need to Know

- Your legs should always be straight and strong. Don't let them look weak, 'cause weak isn't sexy!
- Hold all sexy poses for 2 to 3 seconds so your audience can admire your femininity (or recover from shock!).
- Keep your front end down when you crawl. You want your butt sticking up in the air! It doesn't feel sexy, but it looks sexy—trust me!
- Always get up gracefully, either butt up first or snapping up. Keep him under your spell until you're done with him.
- Transitioning from one floor position to another is easy. Simply roll from one position into the next.

In This Chapter

- Using a chair to enhance your performance
- Sexy chair poses
- Transitioning to and from the chair

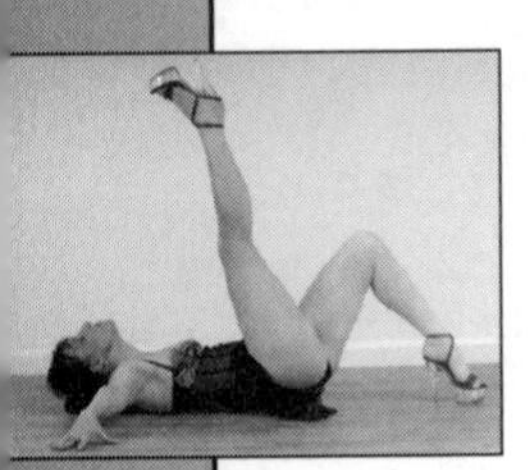
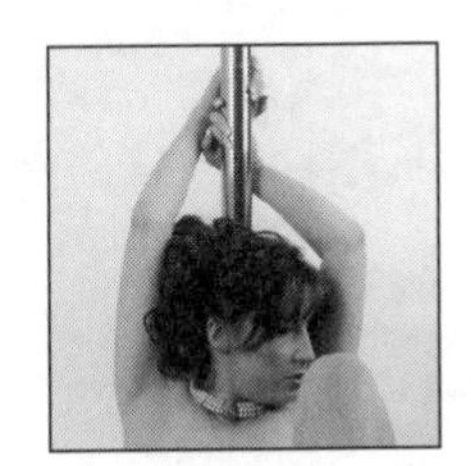
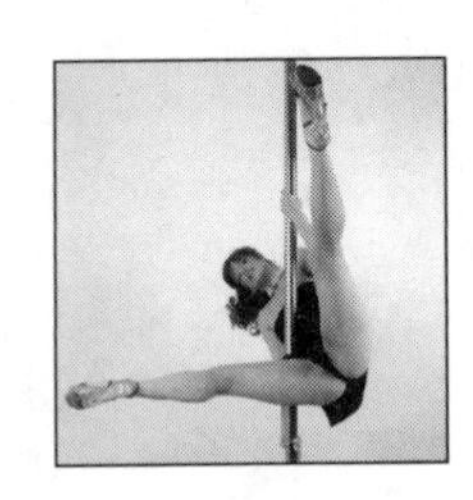
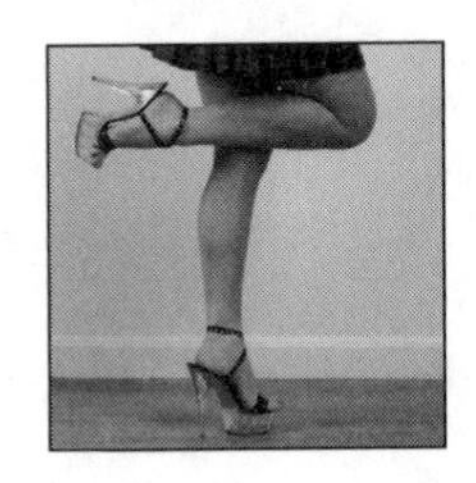
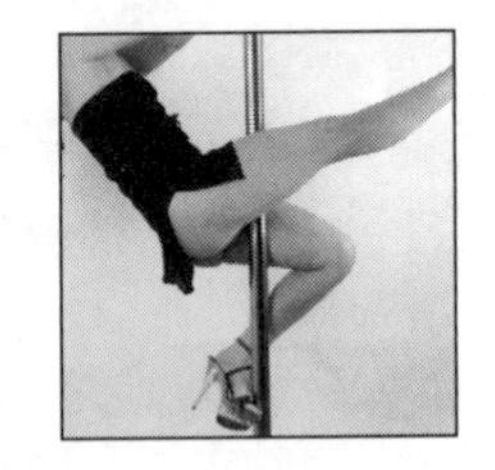
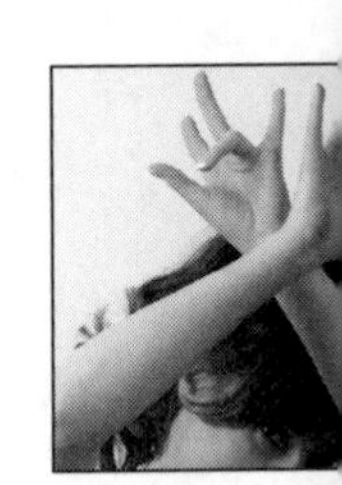

Chapter 8

Chair Flair

You'll never look at a chair the same way again after you learn to see it as a prop to play with. In this chapter, I show you some fun, creative ways to play with a chair that will make your lover jealous!

Kick It Up

First of all, you will never, ever, simply lift your foot up onto a chair again. That is for amateurs. You, as a professional, will snap your leg up onto the chair and push out your butt!

When you snap your leg out, it's just a little snap; you're not kicking anyone high up "where it counts." This is just a fancy way to get your foot up on the chair, because remember, every single thing you do counts, including something as simple as putting your foot up on a chair.

Start by standing to the side of your chair so your left leg can swing out freely in front of it. Now in slow motion, extend your foot forward so it's slightly below the seat of the chair. Then bring your foot up so your toe is on the edge of the chair and, at the same time, push your butt out toward your audience as your left arm lands on your hip. Don't let your arm just hang down blah and boring.

Butt Circles with the Chair

Now do some big butt circles. Remember to go with the undercurrent of the song. Next, bend your knee of the leg that's on the chair down and forward in a swooping motion. (Don't just simply bend your knee—that's boring.) Gently rub your middle finger up and down the length of your thigh—slowly, of course.

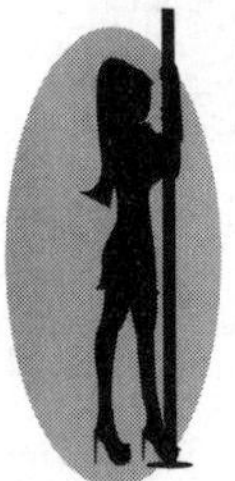

Slick Tricks

Don't feel the need to always be looking at your man. Ignoring him for a move or two in your dance is good for him. It'll remind him this dance is all about *your* sensuality, not performing *for him*. You'll address him when you're good and ready, and he'll like it.

Snap and Rotate

Just as you put your foot up on the chair in a snap, you can take it off in a snap, too.

With your right hand still on the chair back, kick your left foot off the chair and step back around the chair, switching your hands so that now your left hand is holding on where the right hand was.

Now pivot on your right foot, turning your body counterclockwise as you come around to the back of the chair (placing your right hand on the other end of the chair back as you do so).

You are now directly behind the chair. Take a long step with your right foot and slide your left leg way over, sticking your butt way out so you're in profile.

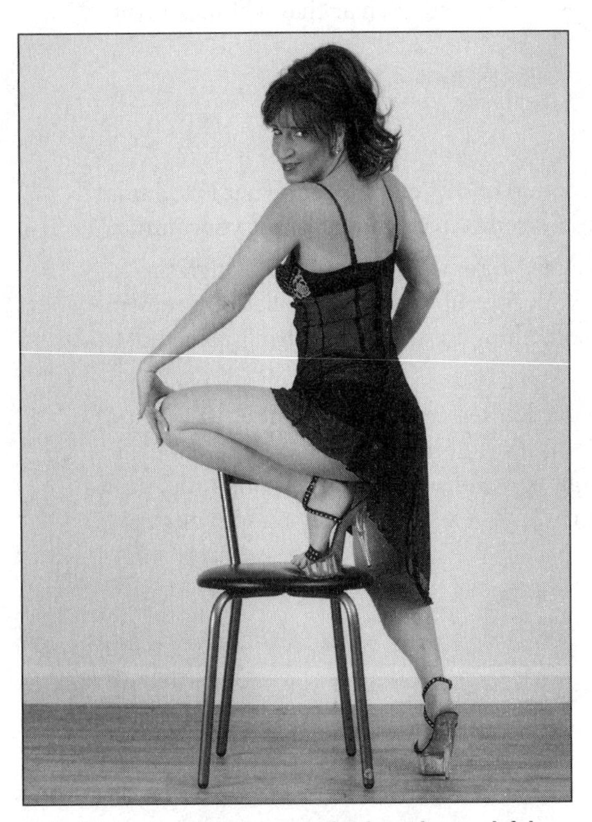

Be sure you're squatting completely with your left leg.

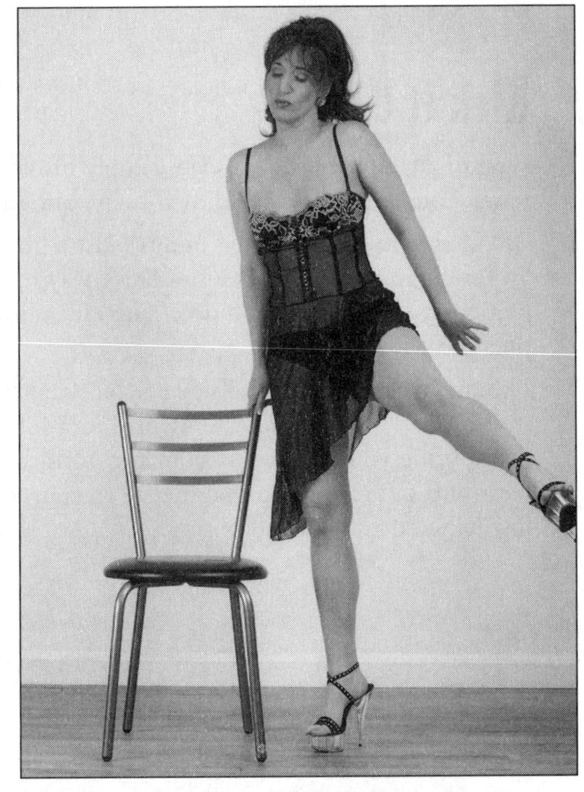

Use the momentum from your left leg kick-off to pivot you around on your right toes.

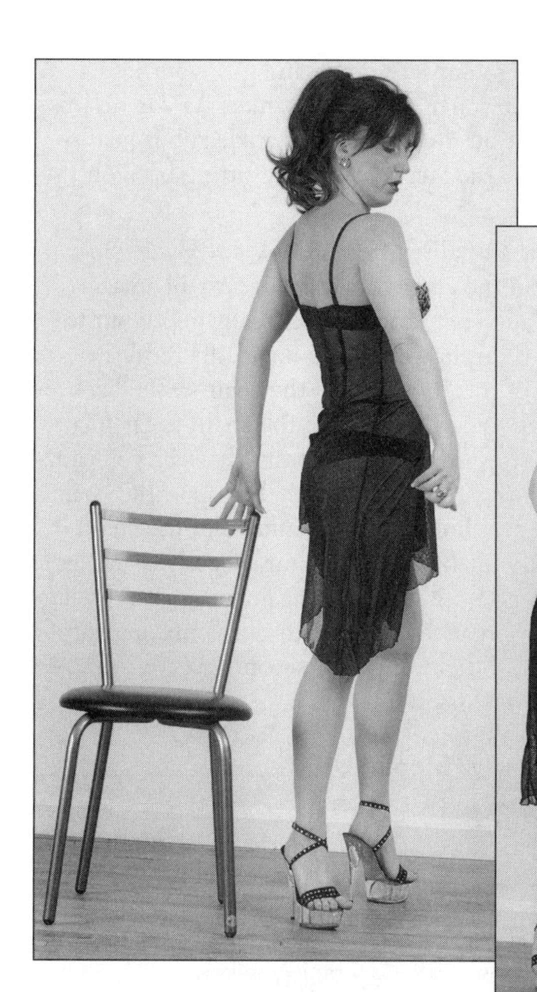

Balance yourself by holding on to the back of your chair with your left hand.

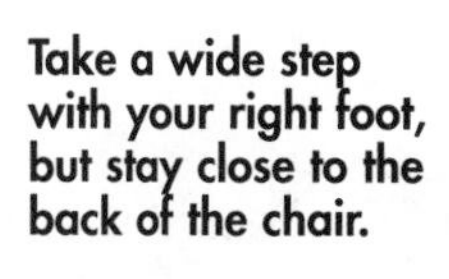

Take a wide step with your right foot, but stay close to the back of the chair.

Slide your left foot to your right foot, taking care to keep your butt out to the side as much as possible.

Back Your Chair

When you're behind the chair, you can do all kinds of things. One thing you can do is to crouch down in back of the chair, play with the sides of the chair delicately, and look through the chair (if it's got bars, horizontally or vertically) like you're playing peek-a-boo. Now turn to the side while crouching, and come up butt first.

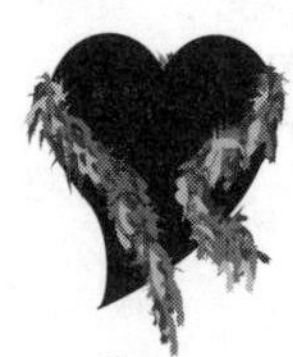

Feelin' the Love

I actually went home, got all dressed up, threw on some music, and sat my husband down to show him all the sexy stuff I learned. It felt great for me and well … y'know his reaction! He liked the chair and floor bounce move the best!

—Tracey, student

Chair V Legs

Here's another shocker for your audience, sure to get a reaction! This is the real "money-maker" shot!

Sit on the chair, and scoot your butt forward, almost to the edge. Lift up your legs, grab your ankles, and spread your legs out straight so they're in a V position.

Now just like with the floor version of this move (see Chapter 7), you want to hold your legs for 3 seconds. What to do during this time? Try rolling your neck around or looking daringly at your audience.

Bring your legs down and give your legs a sexy rub starting from the ankle. As you do this, sit back on the chair. (This ankle rub is just to disguise the fact that you are sitting back on the chair.)

For a totally different look, try V legs sitting on the chair backward! This will amaze your audience, and it looks really good, but to do it right, however, you must adhere to the rules of this move. Turn the chair so the back is facing you. Now sit on the chair, as far forward (toward the front of the chair) as you can. Put both your legs up over the top of the chair while you hold on in the middle of the chair. Scoot your butt forward immediately, as far as it can go, so it's right up against the chair back. Then spread your legs into the V, making sure you hold them out for 3 seconds.

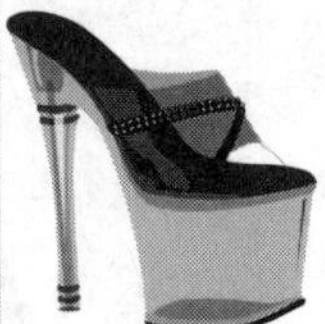

Trippin' Up

If you don't scoot your butt forward, your weight will be on the back of the chair and you could fall backward and bruise your tailbone. This has happened to two of my students, so please take this warning seriously!

The easiest way I find to get out of this position is to swing your right leg over the back of the chair so you're on your *back*, not your butt. If you're trying to balance on your butt, you will fall over backward, so you *must* be on your back.

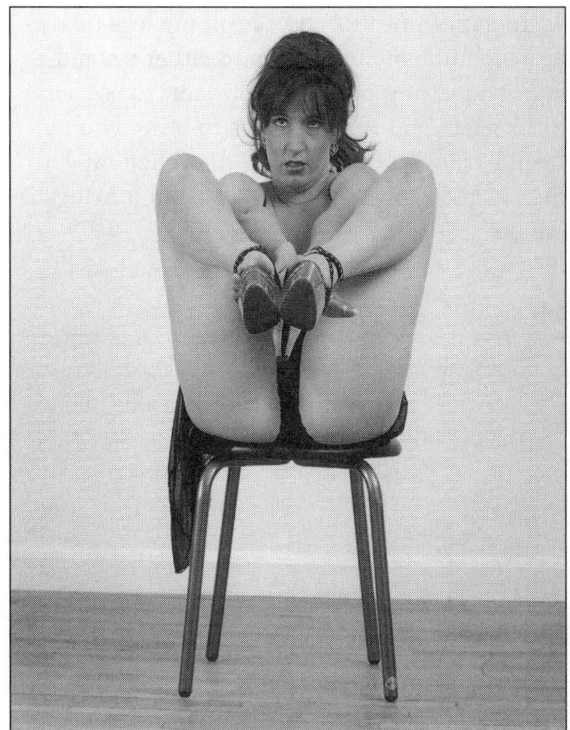

Anyone can do this, as long as your butt is as far to the front of the seat as possible so you're leaning back.

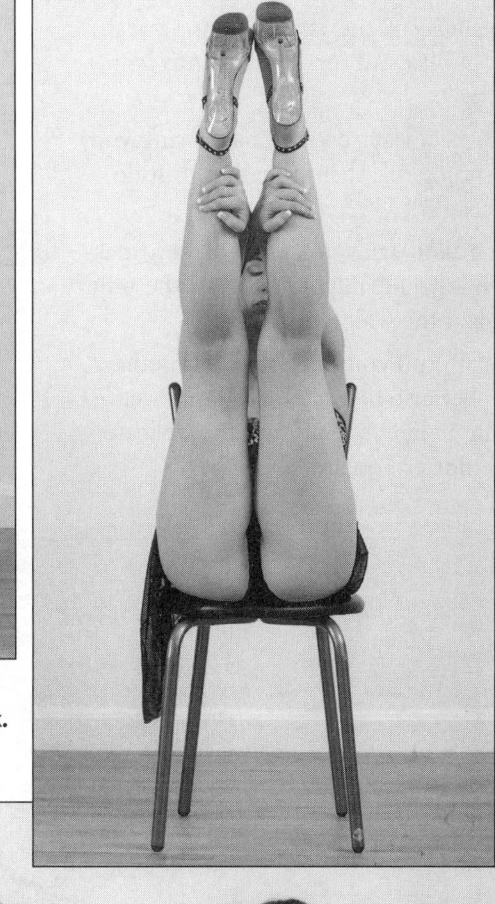

Bring your legs up together.

Slowly spread them, and keep it for 3 seconds.

Prettiest Pose Ever

As the name suggests, this is a pose, not a real dance move, but it's still fun to work into your chair moves.

While lying sideways on the chair, bring your legs up and simply rub them together. But do not do a bicycle!

Then bring both arms up and delicately massage them while you lean your head all the way back and look at the wall behind you.

Remember to rub your legs slowly together, if even at all, because like the mud flap pose, you want your audience to admire the delicate and feminine flower you are.

To get out of this pose, I roll my legs out of it, which lifts my body up into either a standing or squatting position. You want to use some force when you roll your legs to bring you up. I roll hard with my right leg first, then my left, then as the right begins to roll again it brings me up.

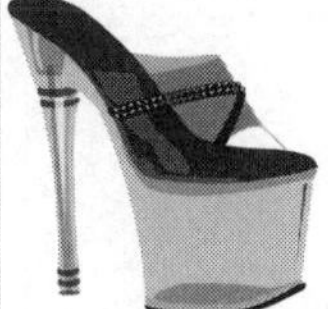

Trippin' Up

A lot of girls want to lift their heads up and look at their legs when they do this pose. Resist the temptation to lift your head, because if you do, you will ruin the beautiful feminine pose you have when you keep your head back.

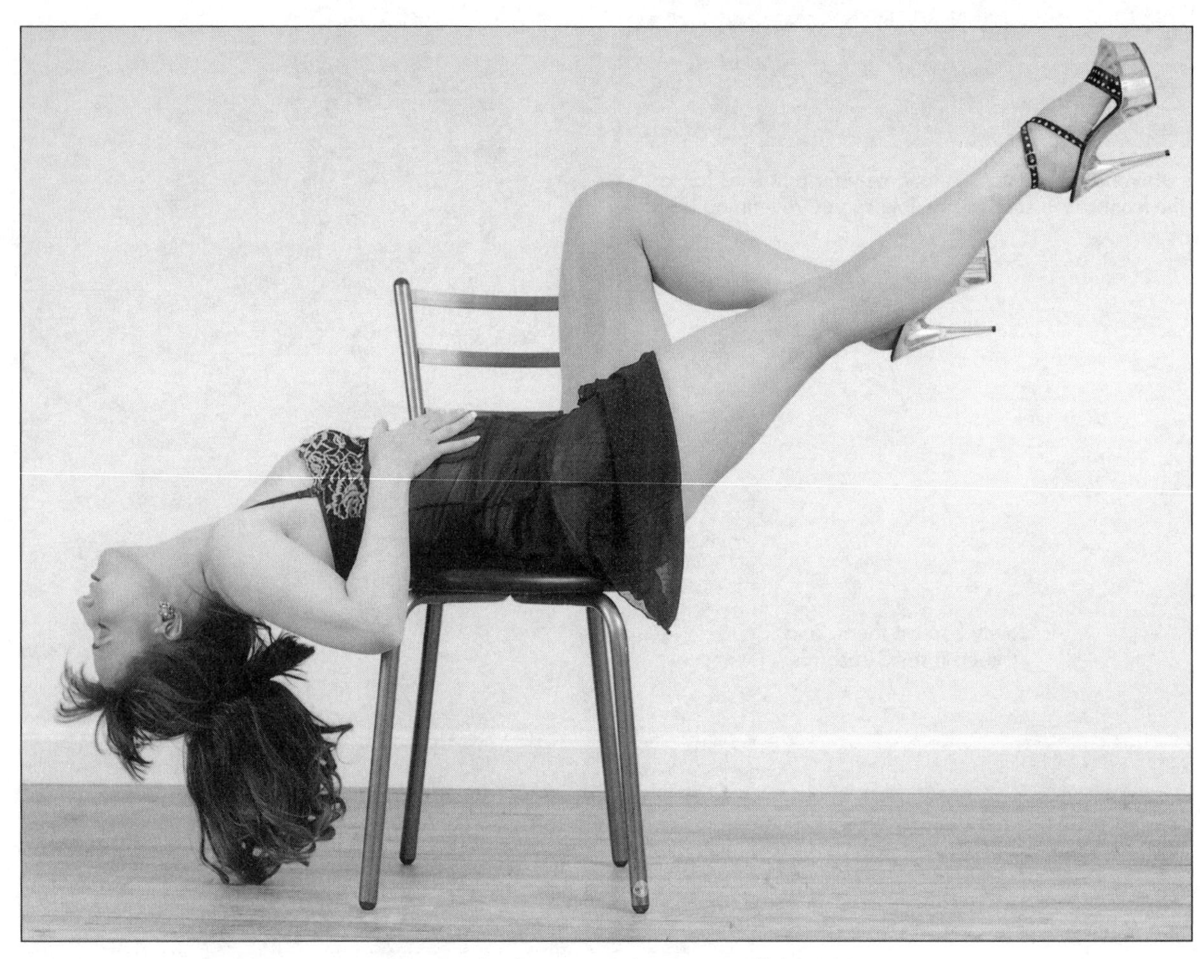

Lay on your back, not your butt, or you'll tip over.

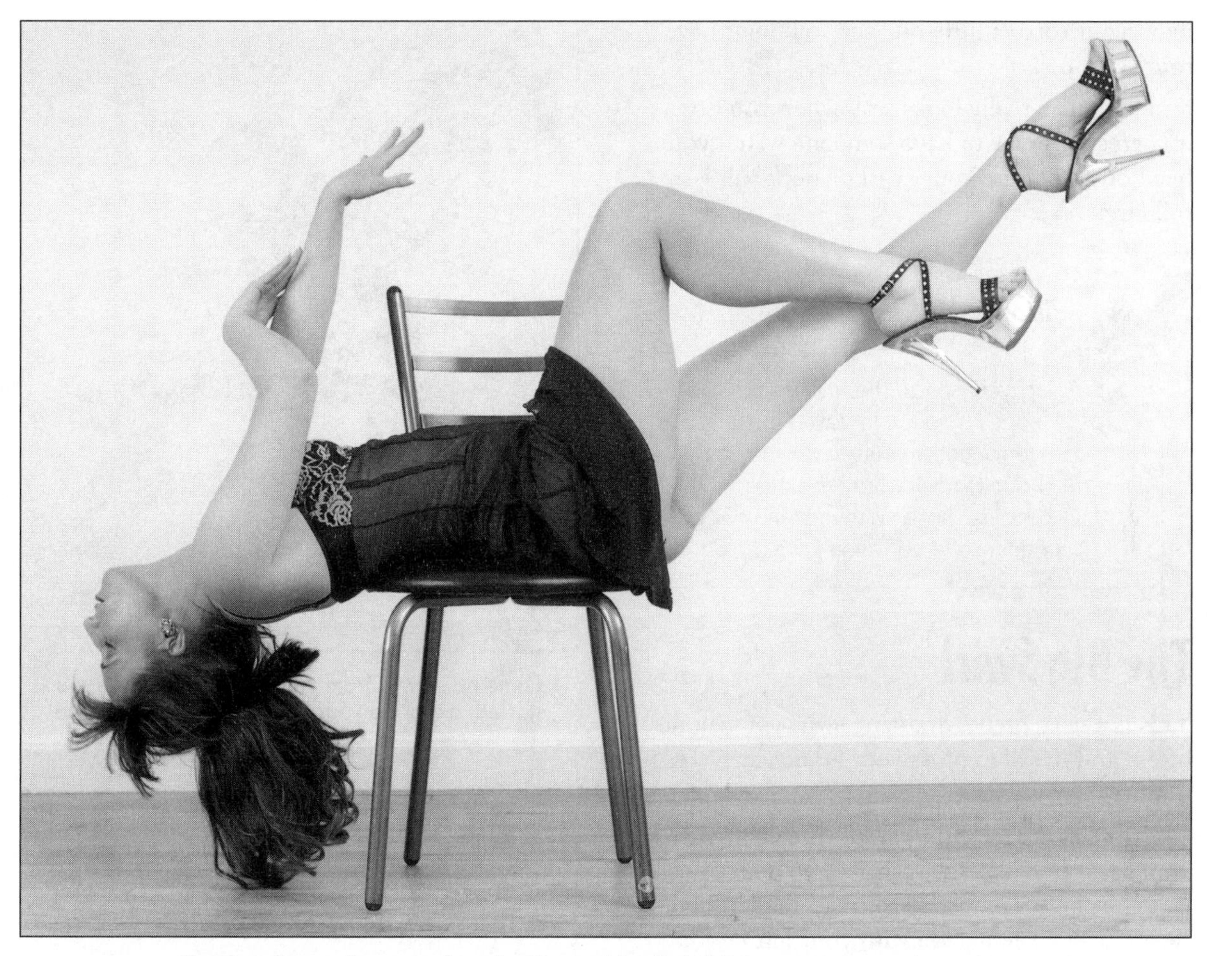

Simply rub your legs together slowly—no bicycles! This is a pose, not a dance move.

Swirl That Hair!

This next move is all about the hair, so if you have long hair, you really want to use it now. And if you don't, that's okay, too! A nice full neck roll is just as sexy!

You can come into this move any way you want. I usually start on back of the chair, facing right with my left fingers delicately on the back of the chair. Starting with the right foot (otherwise it will mess up your footing), take three steps, right-left-right, keeping your body close to the chair as you go around. You must remember to drag your fingers with you as you come around, then let go of the chair when you begin to sit. If you don't bring your left hand with you, you'll end up with your elbow pointing out when you sit. (That looks very clunky and is actually painful.)

You step right-left-right, and then as you go to step left, sit in the chair. Remember not to swing your left leg all the way around the chair to the other side because that looks overexaggerated and not natural, and, of course, this is how you sit in a chair every day.

Sit with your legs spread and place your hands on your knees. Now swirl your hair all the way around. Be careful not to just go forward and back—that's not a swirl. You want to make a full circle with your head, which is basically nothing more than a neck roll. You can bend your torso a little bit, but you don't have to overdo it.

This move really looks sexy when you do it correctly, so try to have someone watch you head on to be sure your swirl or neck roll is a full circle.

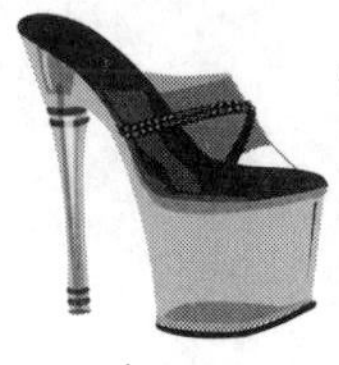

Trippin' Up

Do not come out of character during your song! That means no little "oops I made a mistake" faces, or eye rolling at yourself as if to say "I don't know what I'm doing," because those will weaken your performance. And I won't stand for it!

The Big Swirl

This is a very pretty, dramatic swirl you can do often, and it will impress your audience every time.

While sitting face forward in the chair with your legs spread and your hands on your knees, roll your body completely over to the left and reach for your left ankle with your left hand, while reaching for your right ankle with your right hand. Be sure your hands slide down your shins, yet on the way back up they slide over to the right side of both legs respectively.

As you're swirling toward the right, reach for your right ankle. As you finish the swirl, be sure to slowly bring your hands up unevenly. Let your left hand come up to the inside of your thigh while your right hand makes it to just about your knee. Don't bring those hands up too fast because after you've done the swirl, there's nothing for your audience to look at except your hands coming up your legs, so make that look as dramatic as possible. You can come up with your hands evenly, but I find it doesn't look as nice as when they're uneven. Think of your hands as coming up through a vat of molasses, nice and slow ….

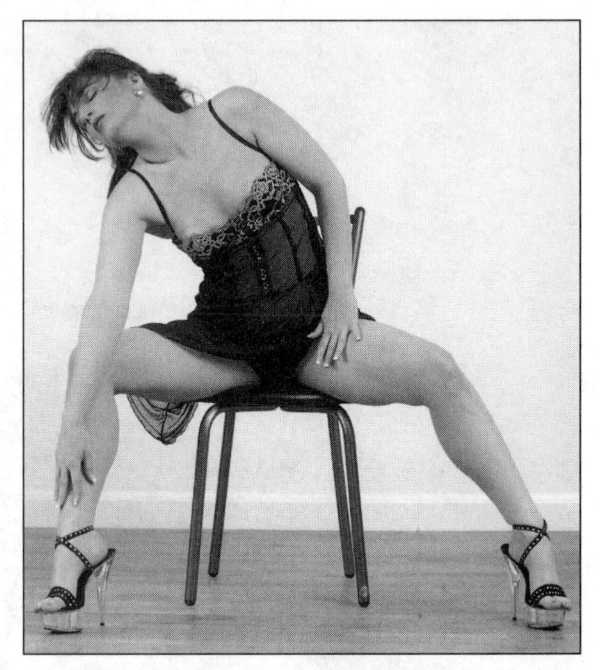

Come up slower from your circle than when you started, exposing your neck as you complete the full circle.

Sit Up Straight!

This move is a classic and is sure to make you look as sweet and innocent as the day you were born.

Sit up straight, with your back off the chair, and cross your leg.

Now reach down to your right ankle with your right hand and delicately bring your middle finger up your leg. If you're wearing a skirt, this is a great time to slowly pull it back just a bit with your middle finger. Be careful not to do that too fast, though!

Now quick as a bunny (as my mother would say) open your legs and stamp the floor with your feet, keeping your hands on your knees. I usually follow this with a big swirl, but you can do whatever you'd like.

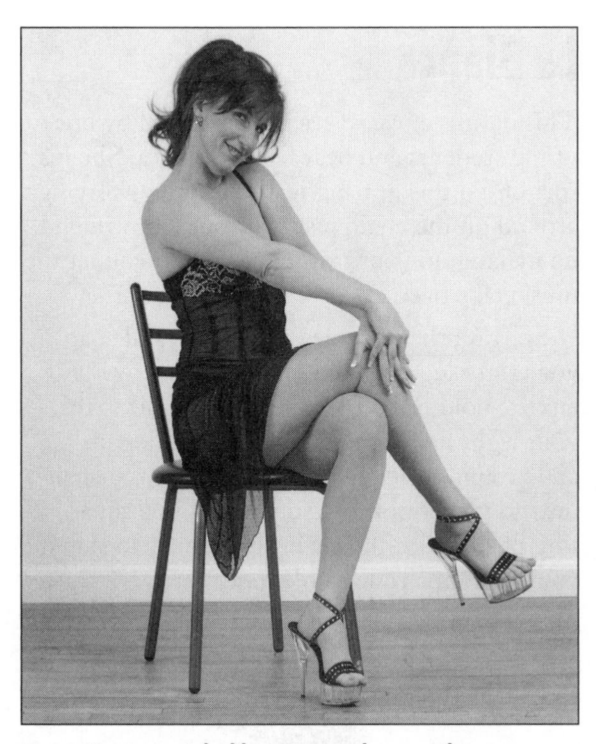

Sit up straight like your mother taught you.

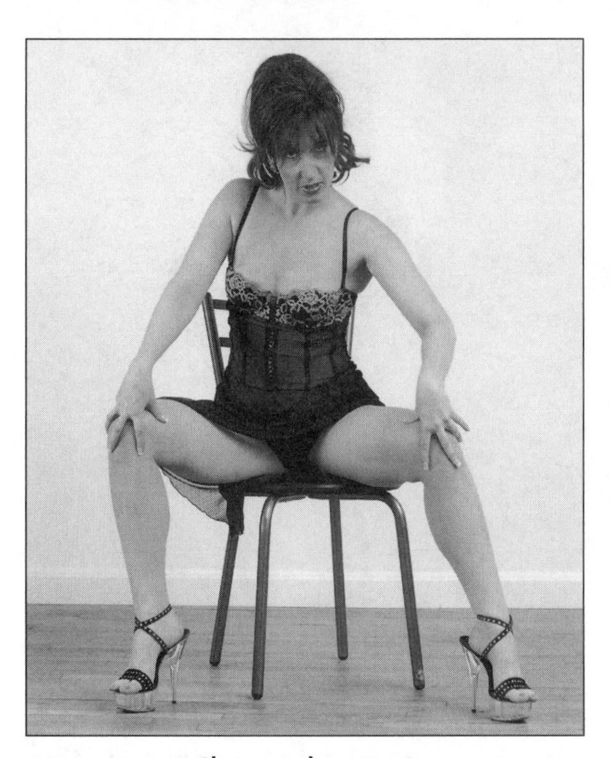

Slam your legs open!

Hip Swirl

The hip swirl is yet another "I'm faking it" move, where the expression on your face and the gyration of your hips make him think you're really getting very, very excited. You should be looking up at the ceiling, not at him, because this is a classic "I'm into myself" move. It's about how you are turning yourself on, not trying to turn him on.

Hold on to the seat pad of the chair and lift up your pelvis. Swirl it around to the music (always going with the undercurrent, of course), with your head rolling back in ecstasy.

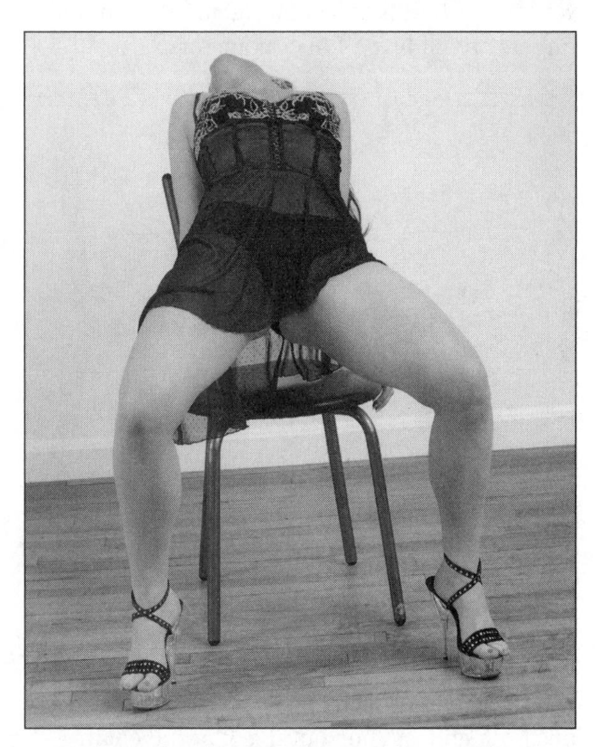

Keep your head back, and envelop yourself in the ecstasy.

Now come down gently until your butt is back on the chair.

Floor/Back Pose

This one can also look incredibly sexy, especially as a result of your facial expressions and your delicate, roving hands. From a sitting position, come down onto your knees in front of the chair, with your back facing the chair. Do a small diva dive down (see Chapter 7), and sport a few butt circles.

Now draw your arms up, flip your hair, and lean your back against the chair (with your legs open, of course), making sure not to lean too hard (otherwise your chair will slide away). Either look up at the ceiling or close your eyes while your butt is still rotating and your middle fingers are gliding all over your torso.

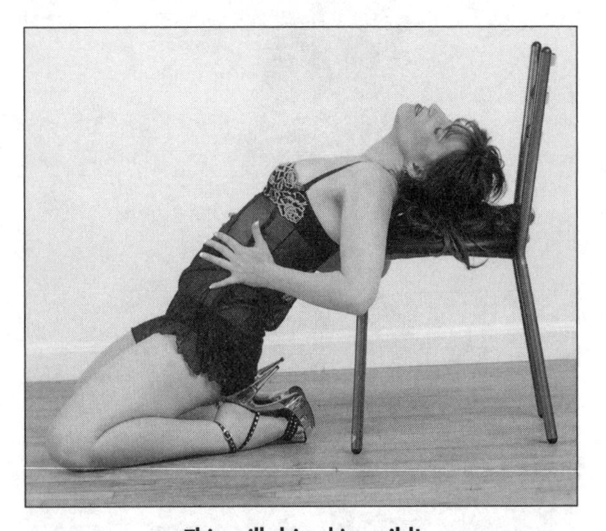

This will drive him wild!

Do this for a few beats and then bring your head up, put both hands between your legs, push off, and sit your butt back in the chair. Flip your hair up and open your legs with a *smack* of your shoes on the floor. Or you can use this opportunity to crawl toward your audience and begin a lap dance or go into another move.

La Bianca

This daring move was actually created by one of my students and dear friend, Bianca. She just sort of did this one night when she was playing around on the chair, just like you, too, will end up making up your own moves when you let the music take over.

Start on the left side of the chair and snap your right leg onto the seat. Toss in a few butt circles, hold on to the back of the chair with your right hand, and swing your left leg up and around, placing your left foot on the chair next to your right foot so you end in a squatting position on the chair. Remember to stay on your toes, not your whole foot.

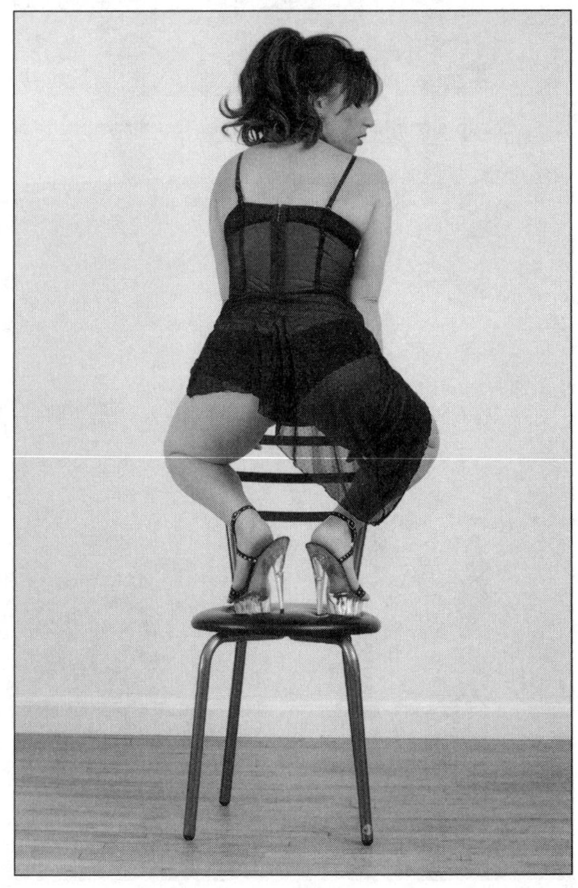

Stay on your toes while holding on to the back of the chair for balance.

Pump your thighs up and down, swish your butt, look over your shoulder—whatever you'd like to do. When you want to dismount, pivot on your toes to your right, kick your right leg out sideways, and use that momentum to twirl your body to the right, all the way around until you need to put your right foot on the floor and step off.

Now you can sit and swirl your hair if you'd like, or pivot on your right foot to turn you around to the back of the chair for a chair slide. With so many possibilities, just let your body go and see what happens!

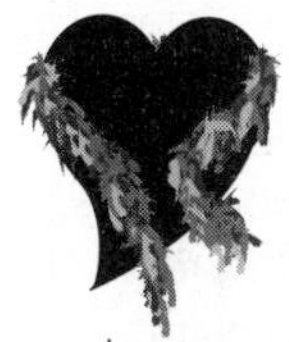

Feelin' the Love

You were absolutely right, I "messed up," but he had no idea whatsoever.
—Appelonia, student

Liberty Legs and the Justice Spread

This sequence was created spontaneously by two of my students whose stage names are Liberty and Justice. (Justice is a law student … how fun is that?)

Lying on your back with the chair at your legs, use your feet to grab the chair and bring it to you. Now roll your butt up so that it rests on the edge of the chair seat with your legs out straight.

Do a V leg and then push the chair away hard as you roll up, bringing both legs to one side and resting your forearms on the chair seat.

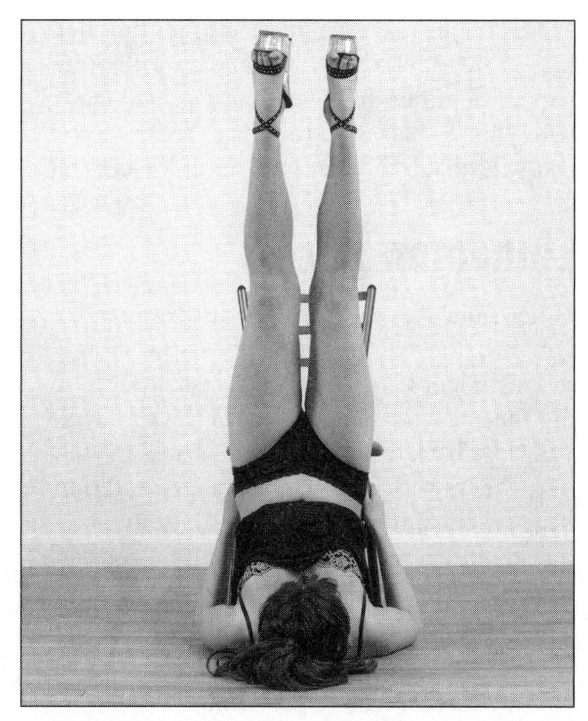

Be sure at least half of your butt is leaning against the edge of the chair pad. This might feel awkward, but it looks great.

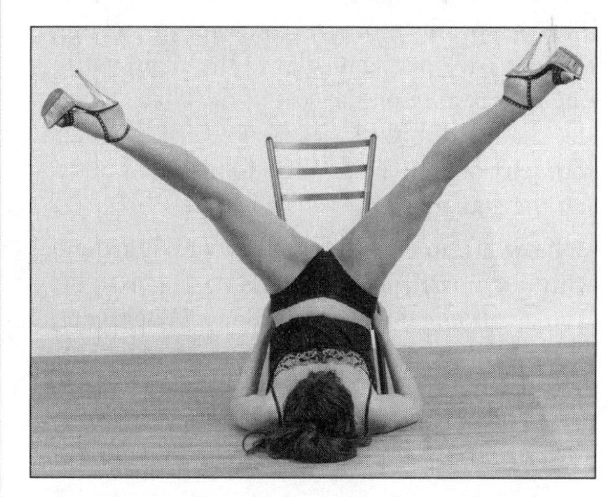

Now spread 'em! Take care to keep your toes pointed, because remember, we want "sexy," not "stirrups"!

For the justice twist, instead of putting both legs to the side, when you come up with your legs straight out, roll over your legs and land with your forearms on the chair. You have to be *really* flexible to do that one, but it looks great!

Cinnamon Spice

When your legs are up in the justice spread, you can, do what my very enthusiastic suburban mom student Cinnamon does: instead of pushing the chair forward and out of the way, roll your legs back over your head (smacking your butt cheeks with your hands is a nice addition here), then continue to roll back, slowly or quickly into a somersault, yet land on your side.

When done correctly, this looks very skillful, so take your time and practice this one, because you don't want to look like you're about to snap your neck when you're performing!

The Swirl and Slide

This is a profile move, so you want to be lying on your back perpendicular to the chair, with one foot resting on the seat of the chair. Place the chair pad in the space between the heel and foot part of your shoe. (This foot should be facing the audience.)

Now lift up your pelvis and rotate it around with the music while your middle finger is, of course, gliding all over your body. When you're ready, lift both legs up straight (with your butt coming slightly off the floor) and place both arms out straight in back of your head.

Swing both legs over to the front of the chair and delicately bend them at the knee as you dramatically tuck your head under and slide your arm up (with your other arm placed on your leg). Now roll your head up so your neck is exposed and keep the pose for a beat. Remember to tuck your head in as you roll it up, and don't come up to fast! Take your time!

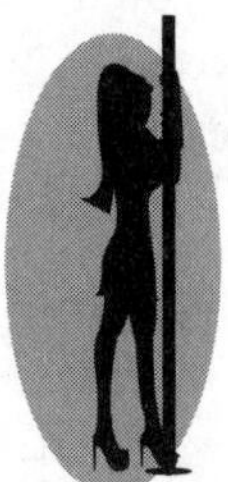

Slick Tricks

I'm not musically inclined, but I do know that when you dance you want to move with your music. Never, ever, ever just do moves to do them! Do a move for a few beats and then transition into another move. Try not to do the same move for more than an 8-count, because then your audience will get bored waiting for the next wonderful thing you're going to do.

Pump and Slide

This sequence of moves works very well when you do it right to the beats of the music.

First, position yourself on your knees, facing the chair, with your hands gripping the sides of the seat.

Then, in one movement, snap your legs up and straight out to the back, landing on your toes.

Pump with the beats of the music and then, with your arms still extended, slide your legs in an arc so that your feet are together and then slide your feet out to the side with your knees bent as if you are sitting. Now slide the chair back between your legs so you're sitting with your back to the audience.

From here you can pump your butt up and down, look back at the audience over your shoulder while you lower your bra strap, and run your middle finger over your bare shoulder … whatever you'd like.

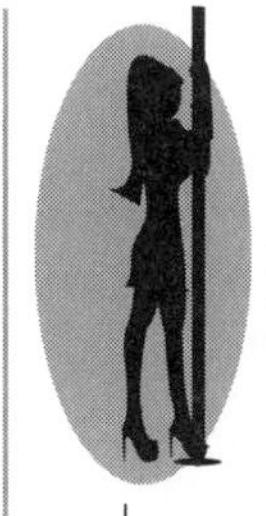

Slick Tricks

Always pulsate to the undercurrent of your song, no matter what position you're in. Whether you're sliding down the wall, finishing a pole move, or sitting on the chair, be sure your body never stops moving.

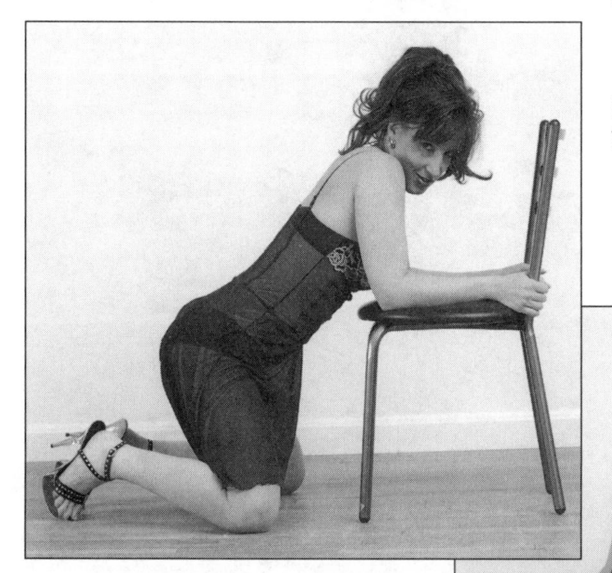

Keep your butt pulsating as your hands grasp the chair.

Be sure your legs are spread as you pump; otherwise, you'll appear to be doing push-ups.

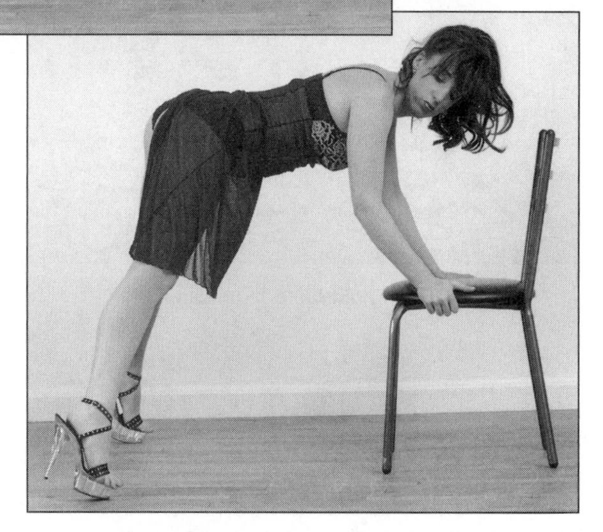

Arc spread your legs out to the side so you can slide your chair between them and sit.

Chair Twirl

This one is really fun because you don't know how you're going to end up! Start by kicking your right foot up onto the chair so your back is facing the audience. Now swirl your butt, but don't actually hold on to the back of the chair, use your hands in the air or massage your thigh.

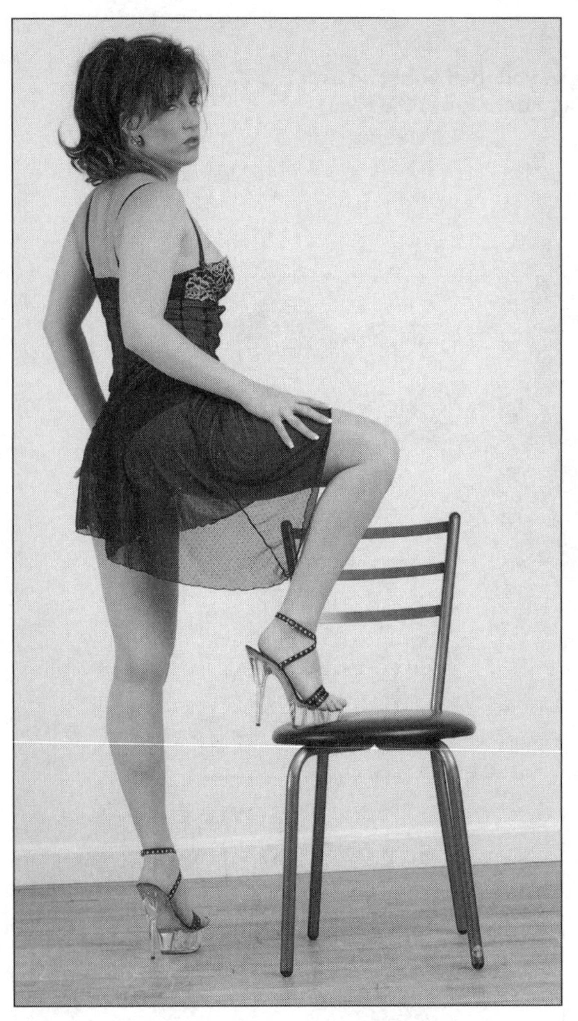

Don't hold on to the chair.

Now kick your right leg up and over the chair with enough force so that it twirls your body around and lands your foot on the floor.

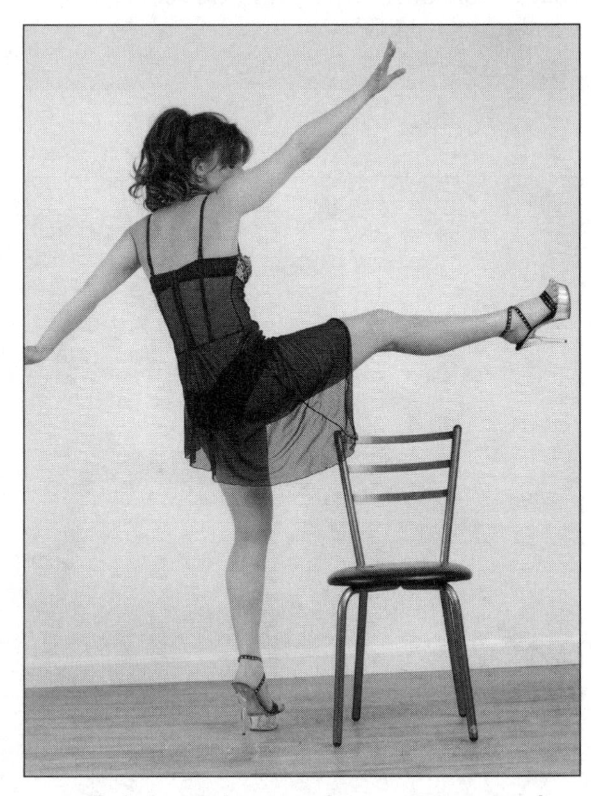

Swiftly kick your leg up and over, using your right arm to balance yourself.

Chances are you're going to lose your balance when you do this, but that's where the fun comes in. When you land, do what you need to do to balance and then follow through. Keep moving so it looks like you planned the whole thing. Sometimes I end up with my hand near my ankles to balance me and then I drag my hands up my legs and it looks like that was my intention all along—when really I was just saving myself from falling flat on my face!

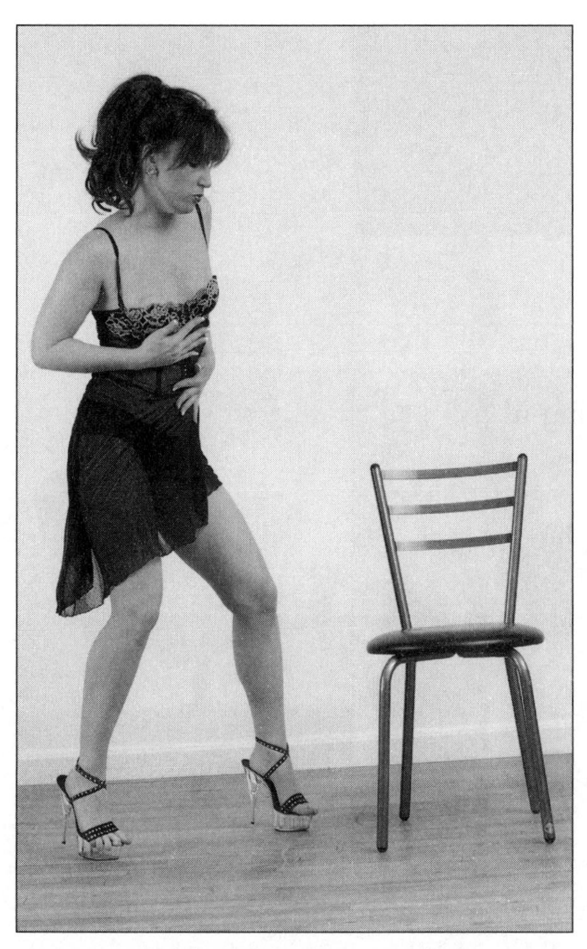

Pivot on your left toe so you turn completely around and follow through, even if you lose your balance.

That's part of dancing and doing these moves—improvising and getting creative. It's more fun that way!

The Least You Need to Know

- Always snap your foot onto the chair like you mean it, because even the little moves make a difference in your overall performance. You make him take notice!
- Always make a full swirl with your head if you've got long hair, or use a simple sultry neck roll if your hair is short and sexy. Whatever the length, make the most of it!
- Always scoot your butt forward as far as it can go when you are sitting backward on the chair doing the V legs. Safety first!

In This Chapter

- Posing on the pole
- Going airborne—and loving it!
- Getting up gracefully
- Transitioning from the pole

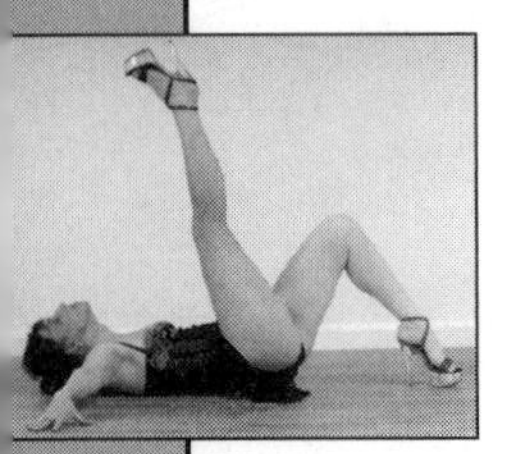
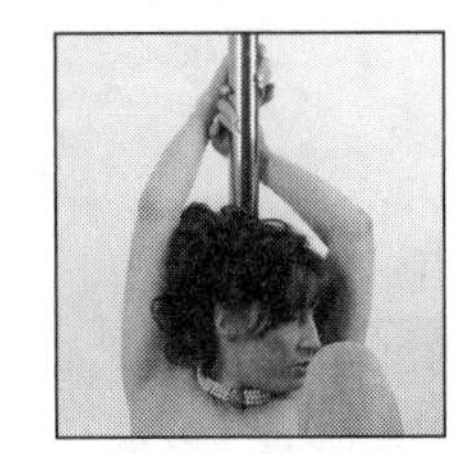
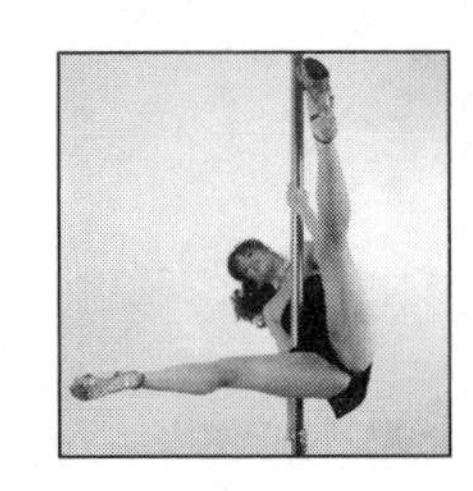
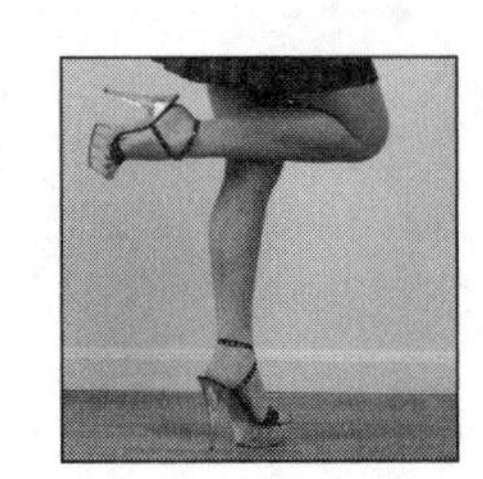
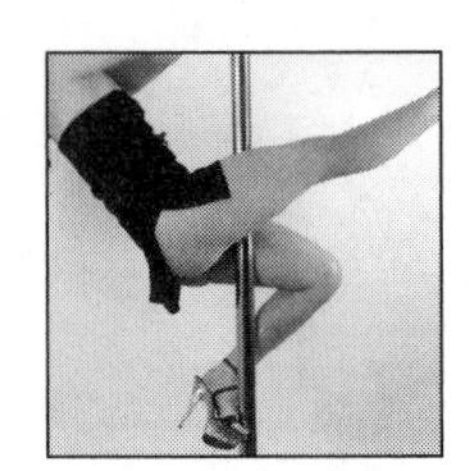
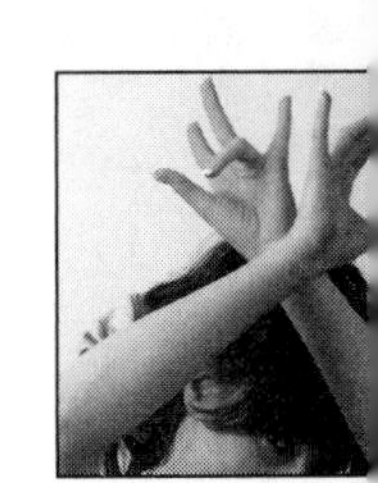

Chapter 9

The Pole Is Your Friend™

This chapter is dedicated to your new friend, the pole. Like all new friends, you must get to know it well before you decide whether you like it or not. And you must give it a chance to get to know you.

New friends can be very helpful, and the pole is no exception. The pole will help you with balance, muscle tone, self-confidence, and of course, the ability to wow your living, breathing friends!

Getting to Know You ...

Rule number one: you must say, out loud, "The pole is my friend." *I said say it!* (Remember the drill sergeant from Chapter 1? She's baaack!) And whenever you get frustrated or feel scared by the pole, you must say it again, out loud.

When meeting your new friend the pole, grab hold of it and walk around it several times to get a feel for it. Hold on to the pole with your stronger hand about 6 to 10 inches above your head. You always want to hold the pole above your head unless otherwise noted because it gives you more control.

Now extend your arm, lock your elbow so your arm stays straight, lean to the side, and walk around the pole several times until you feel at ease with your new friend.

Until your body gets used to how tight it has to hold itself on the pole, you'll probably get pole burn on the inside of your forearm and your wrist. Eventually though, your body will get sick of pole burn and adjust itself as you swing so it doesn't continue to get hurt.

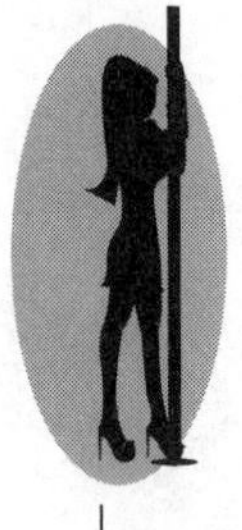

Slick Tricks

Any woman of any height, weight, or age can swing around the pole. Keep in mind that it's the momentum that makes you swing, like an airplane flies. You're not going straight up, you're swinging around.

The Pole's Pet Peeves

Your pole is your friend, and you have to take care of it, cleaning it and being aware of its other pet peeves.

Cleanliness

Your pole has a nasty aversion to hand lotion, baby oil, athlete's chalk, or anything else that will make it slippery. If your pole is slippery, you won't be able to get a good grip, you'll strain your arm muscles, and when you attempt to spin, you will go flying off and *thwap* into the wall, sending your pole into fits of howling yet silent laughter.

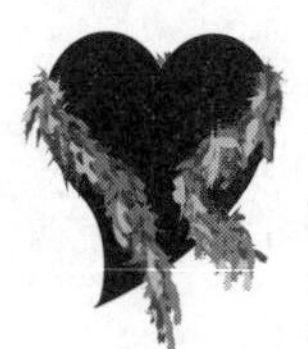

Feelin' the Love

One of the dances I was completely getting into and could not think of another move … I quickly grabbed the pole and banged my entire right leg into the pole, leaving it behind and almost falling to the ground. But I quickly remember my old days of dancing lessons and learned to make it "look" like a cool new move. It made me laugh a little and realize I always have to keep practicing even if no one else notices!

—Chase, student

Use Windex to clean your pole. You'll end up with a clean but sticky pole, which is what you want. When your hands or the pole become sweaty, use Windex and a rag to wipe it down.

The Circle of Death

Like any new friend, you must give your pole its personal space. Most new friends, however, do not have a "circle of death," but your new friend, the pole, has one and enforces it in its own rather amusing way.

In other words, keep your feet out of the 6-inch-diameter circle directly around the bottom of the pole.

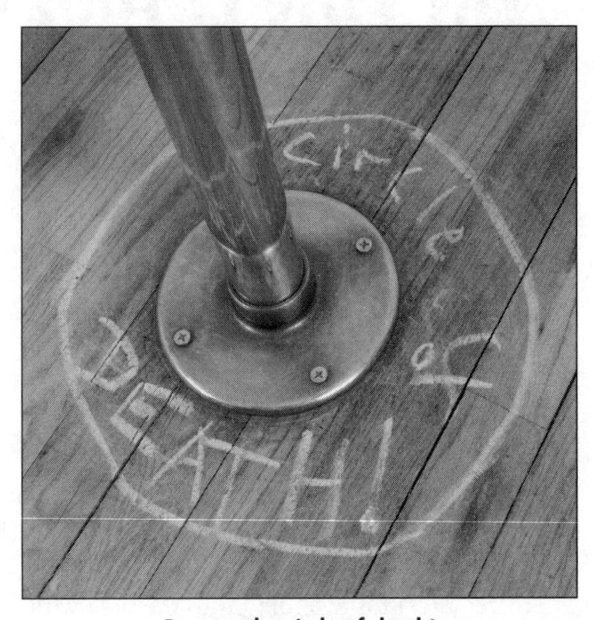

Beware the circle of death!

When you swing around the pole, if you step in this circle, you will get all twisted up in the pole, which can be very painful. Keep in mind that if you are shorter, your circle of death is smaller.

Your pole area is a 3-inch diameter around the pole that extends from the floor to the ceiling—but always outside the circle of death.

Drinking and Dancing

A drink or two might help you loosen up and give you courage for the pole, but do not attempt to swing around the pole when you're drunk, and don't let your friends do it either, no matter how much fun they seem to have. Not only do you risk a lawsuit if someone gets hurt; even worse, you might have to clean up the puke.

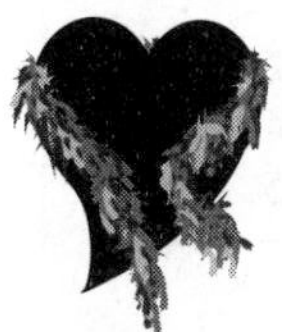

Feelin' the Love

The first night I installed my pole, all my friends got me trashed enough to whip around that pole with no fear or hesitation. I was having a great time … until I lost track of what I was doing and let go of the pole in mid-spin where I threw myself into the wall and knocked the pictures down. When I woke up, my mother was really pissed off, but we laugh about it now.

—Kate V., student

Now, on to the fun stuff—pole work!

Mind Your Wrist

Another one of the pole's pet peeves is when your wrist rests on it. That means you're holding on too tightly and will get pole burn on your forearm. At first, until your body gets used to how tightly it has to hold on so you don't swing off and die, you may get pole burn, but try to never let your wrist touch the pole.

In all the swings I do, my thumb stays with me the whole time I'm going around so that my arm doesn't twist around the pole—no pole burn for me!

Amber P. Poses

Actress, life coach, and my wonderful instructor Amber P. Knight is one of my girls who prefers not to swing around the pole. She's the perfect example of a woman who can really use the pole without having to go airborne. (Yes, I said *airborne.*) You don't feel like you're missing anything during her dances because she doesn't swing around the pole, either. The poses she uses on the pole, along with her other non-swinging movements, make her performances just as strong as those girls who do actually swing.

I've included her sultry sways first so you can practice them and get more familiar with the pole before you go airborne.

The Pole Massage

You can't get much more basic a pole move than this. Essentially, when you're not swinging around it, the pole is your big phallic symbol. You're doing this dance to turn him on, so go ahead and massage the pole. He'll get your meaning.

Stand behind the pole with a slight squat and simply rotate your butt in circles.

Rolling your shoulders, place your hands on the pole and essentially give it a good, sensual rub down … but delicately. Remember to use your middle finger only, and your hands will look ultra feminine.

You can also play a peek-a-boo of sorts with this move: look at your audience and then move your head back and forth slowly to the other side of the pole.

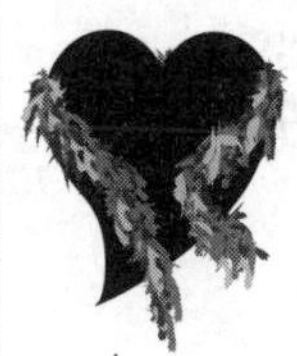

Feelin' the Love

For many years now I know I had this passion to pole dance, and you made it come possible. You saw me go through some spills with the pole … but at least I made you laugh.
—Katie, student

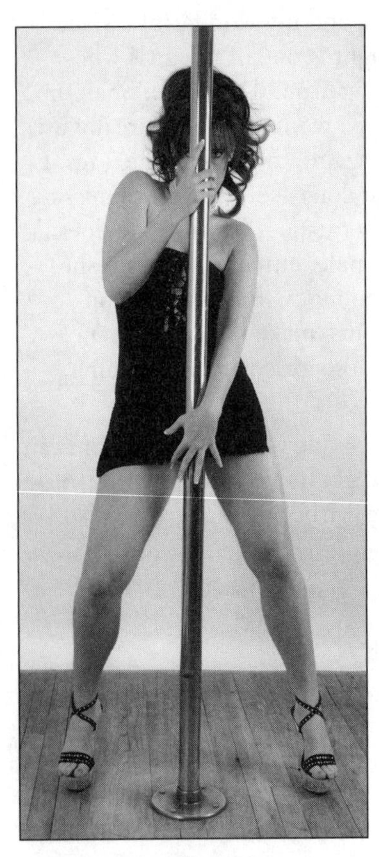

Use your fingertips to massage the pole.

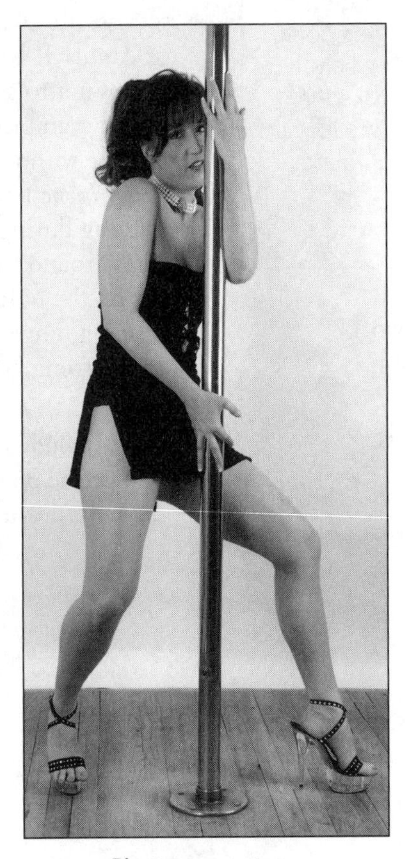

Pivot on your toes.

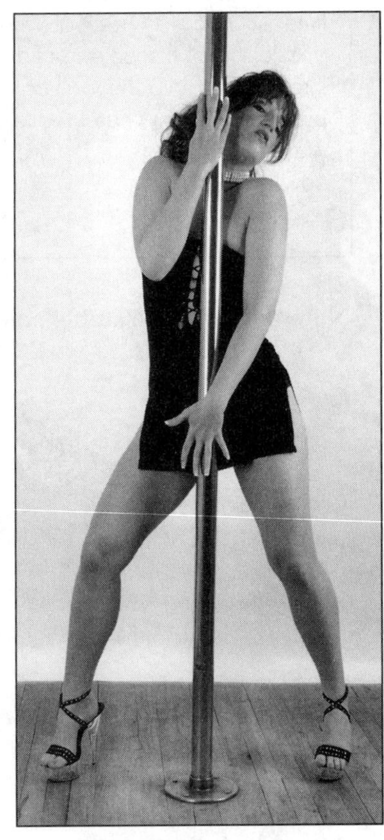

Keep the drama in your expression.

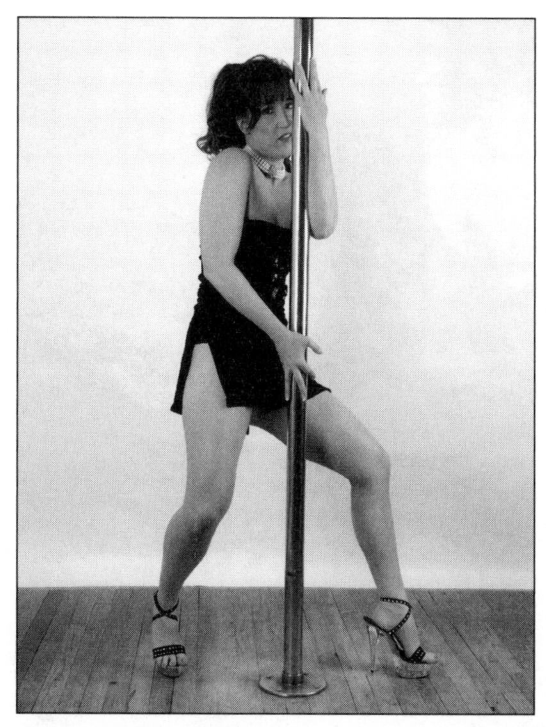

You can also move up and down as you massage.

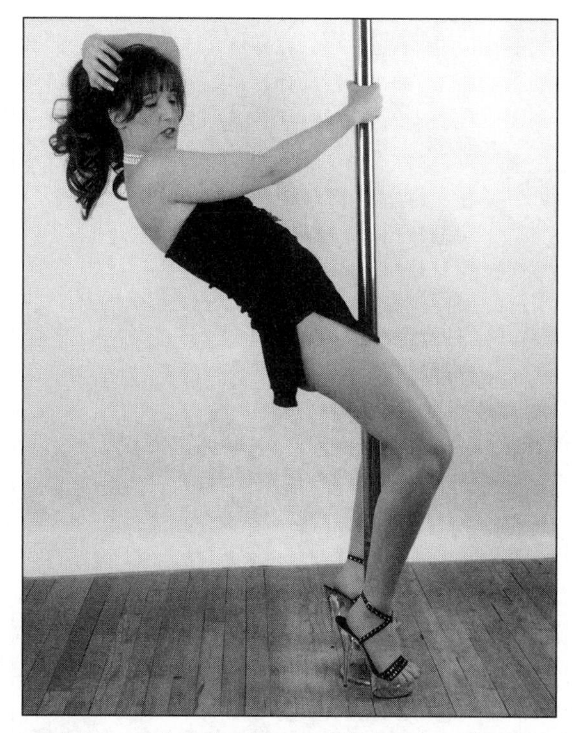

This is one of the few times I'll let you stand in the circle of death.

The Pole Roll

Here's another popular Amber P. pole move. It looks best in profile, so get in position!

Place one foot on either side of the base of the pole. Hold the pole about mid-way down with one arm, and scoop your groin up to the pole and back down. Be sure you use a real "scooping" motion, coming down and then slightly up and back so it looks extra sexy.

Meanwhile, your other hand can be moving all over your body, up over your head—which, of course, is rolling dramatically because you are in the passion of your song.

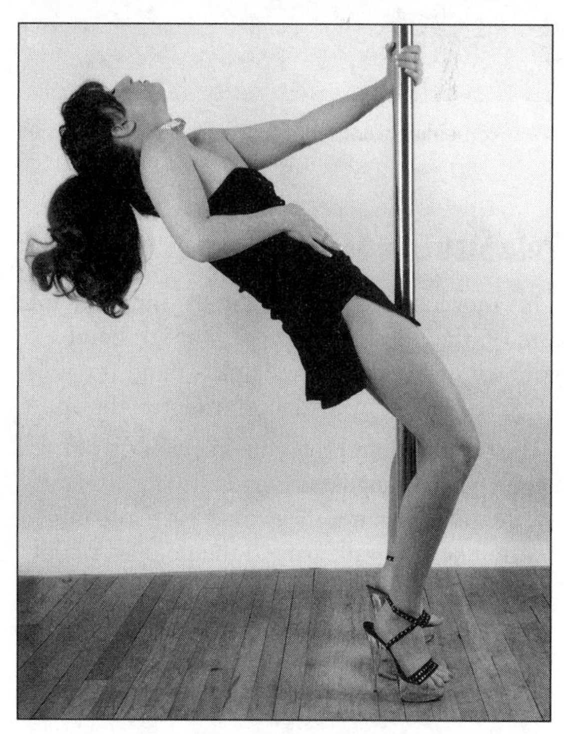

Keep one hand massaging yourself and your expression passionate.

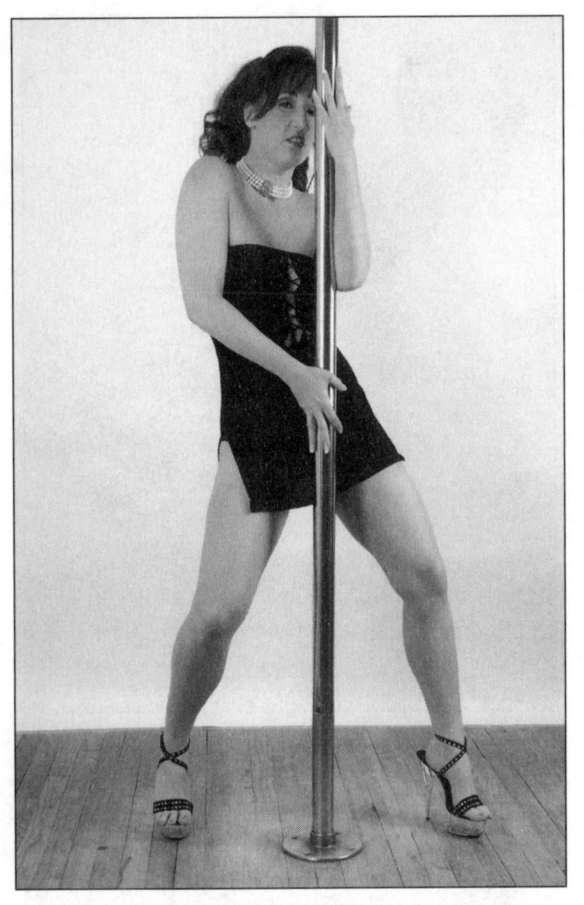

You can either scoop your hips to the pole or rotate them around.

Pole Strut

This move is the one time I'll let you bend your arm on the pole—and you do want to bend your arm when you're walking around the pole because it looks nicer than if it is straight up.

Just walk around the pole like you own it, keep your chin up, and even rest your forearm on the pole as you walk around ever so confidently like you walk around the pole every day.

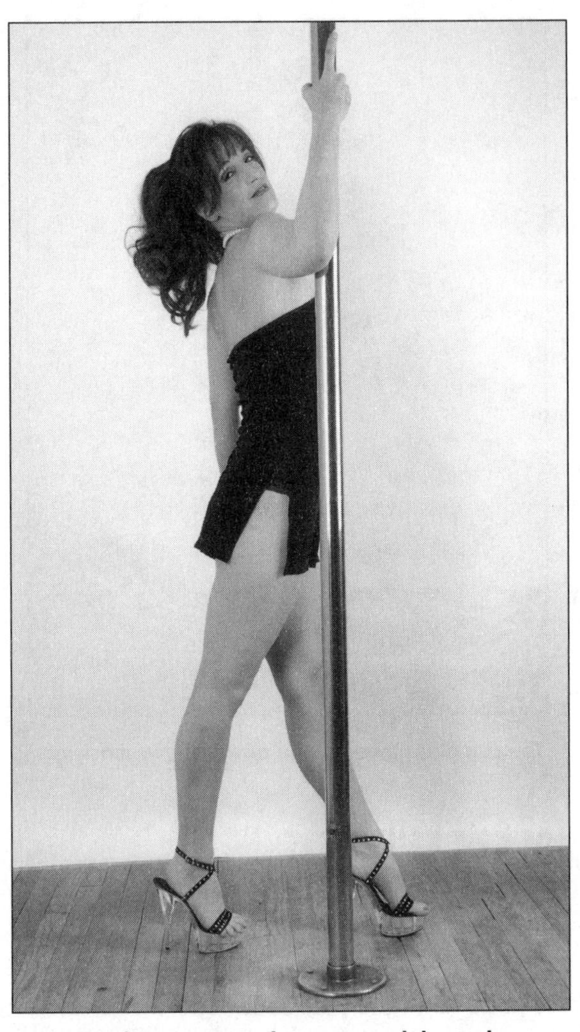

Bend your arm and strut around that pole like you own it!

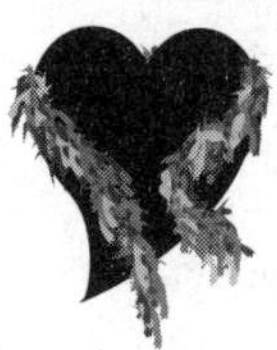

Feelin' the Love

The hardest move to master in pole dancing is walking. It feels strange, like you're pigeon-toed and your chest is all puffed out like a rooster. Once you get it right though, everything falls into place. You posture in general becomes more beautiful.

—Jennifer Solow, author of *The Booster*

Pole Slide

The pole slide is similar to sliding down a wall (see Chapter 6). Stand in front of the pole with your arms up and your hands around the pole.

Bend one knee while keeping the other leg straight, and let yourself slide down the pole as your extended leg stretches out in front of you.

Try to land delicately on your butt, and when you do, scoot it forward and lean back against the pole. The farther forward your butt is, the easier it will be to lift your legs.

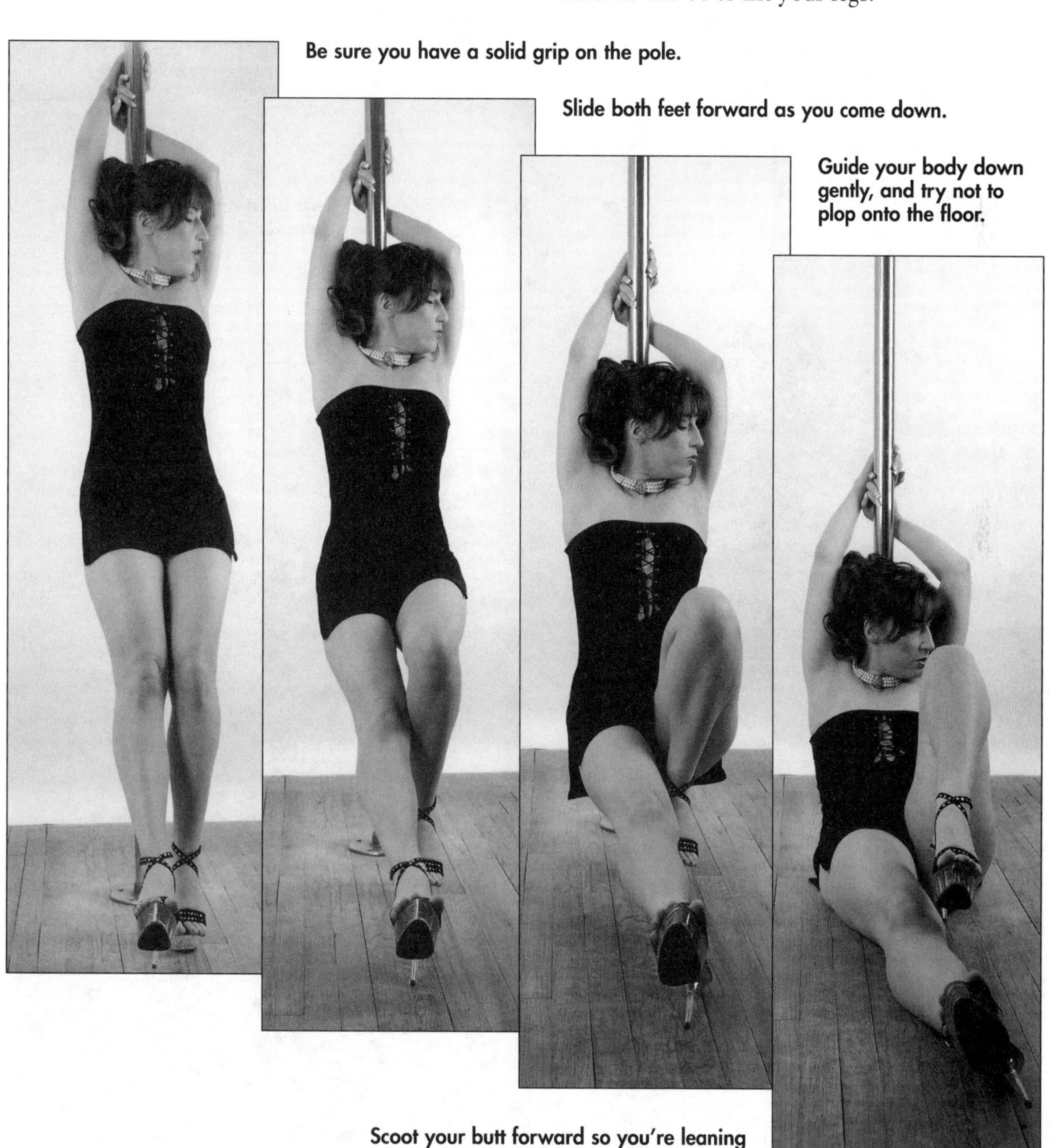

Be sure you have a solid grip on the pole.

Slide both feet forward as you come down.

Guide your body down gently, and try not to plop onto the floor.

Scoot your butt forward so you're leaning your back against the pole.

Now grab both ankles and lift your legs straight up into V legs. Be sure your legs are totally straight and strong, not slightly bent (that would look weak). Keep this position for the count of 3 … because remember, it's the position that shocks the audience.

Then bend your knees down and together on one side, sitting up straight with your neck arched up and your outside arm on your top knee—we are ladies, after all.

Then continue to turn over so you're on your hands and knees.

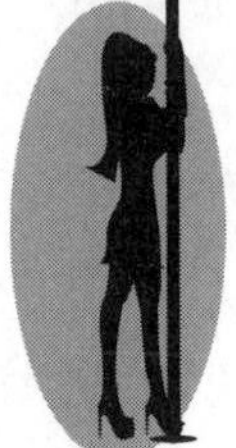

Slick Tricks

If you can't get your legs straight, try scooting your butt out a little farther away from the pole. If you still can't get them to extend, then do a sharp 45-degree angle at the knees.

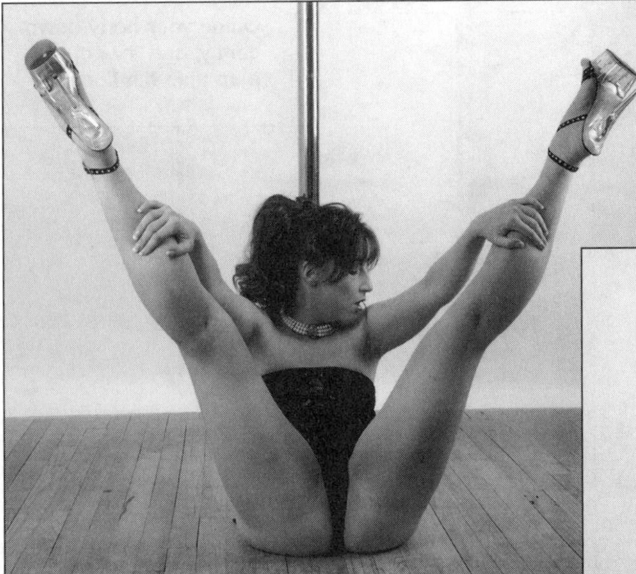

Bring your legs up straight, and keep them there for 3 seconds.

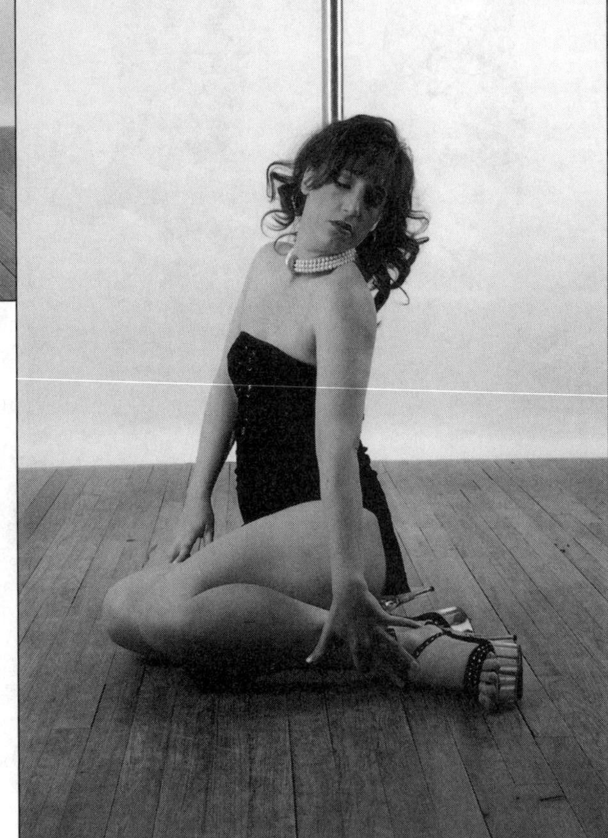

Delicately bring your legs down and together.

Getting Up Gracefully

Most of my pole swings that involve landing on the floor require you to lean back on one elbow (not your full back), let go of the pole, bring your back leg straight up and around the pole, and roll over onto your hands and knees, taking care to stay close to the pole. Now you want to get up with some grace and style. In a kneeling position beside the pole, extend your arms out straight on the floor in front of you.

Then draw your arms up slowly with your head tucked in, and flip your hair up.

Grab the pole with your inside hand and take a step like you're about to stand up.

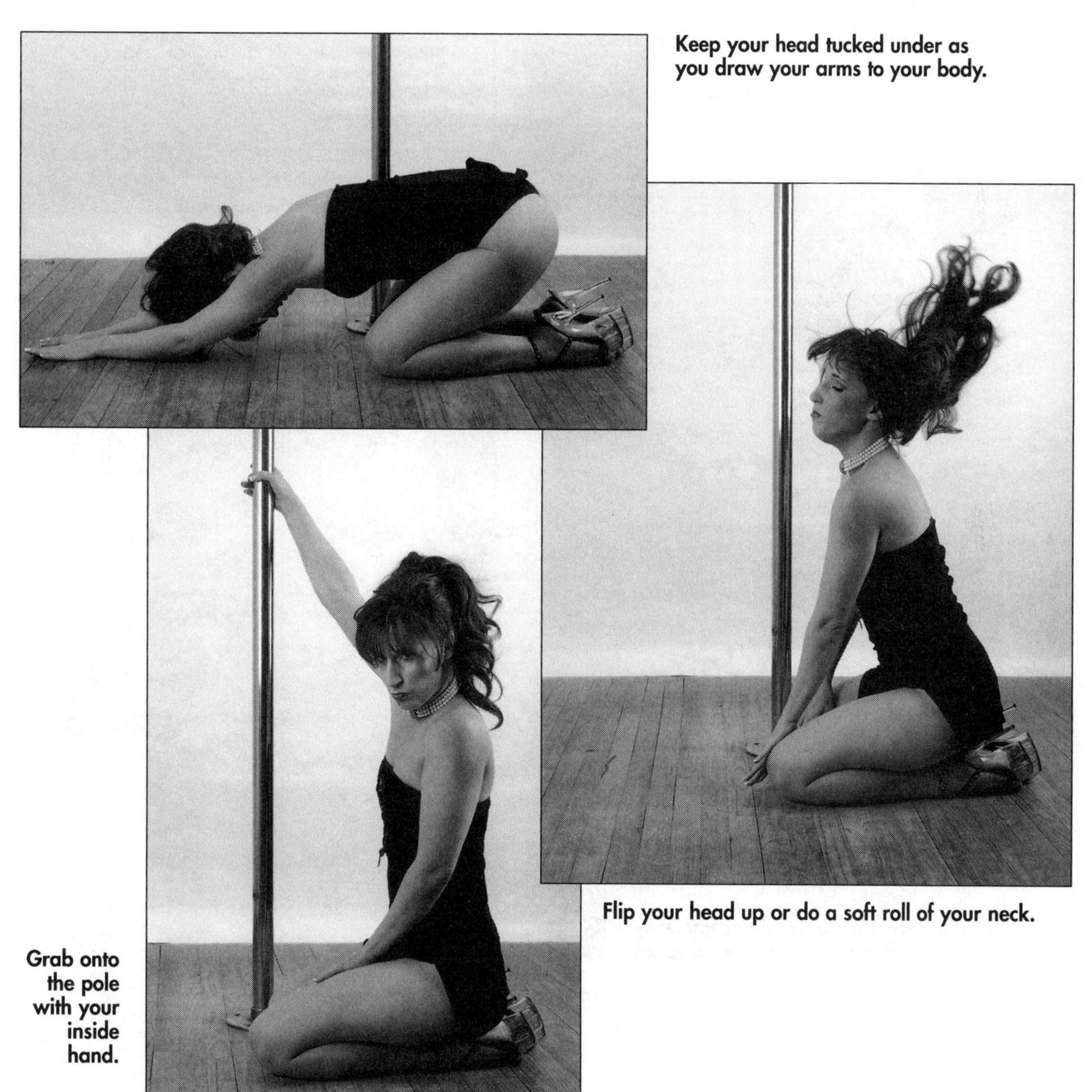

Keep your head tucked under as you draw your arms to your body.

Flip your head up or do a soft roll of your neck.

Grab onto the pole with your inside hand.

Swing around the pole, using your outside leg to propel you around, and grab the pole with your outside hand.

As you're doing this, be sure you pivot on your inside knee (mine is usually an inch off the ground when I pivot so I don't scrape my knee) so your feet end up *together* around the pole. Then stand up butt first.

The key to getting up sexy after you've done a pole swing is to be sure your feet are together, even if you just step into a simple crouch, and bring your butt up slowly, sticking it out as far as you can. Be careful to scoop your back, not arch it.

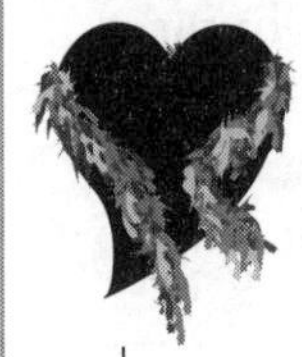

Feelin' the Love

No body type looks bad pole dancing. I have seen people of all shapes and sizes, men and women. A great pole dancer is a thing of beauty.

—Jennifer Solow, author of *The Booster*

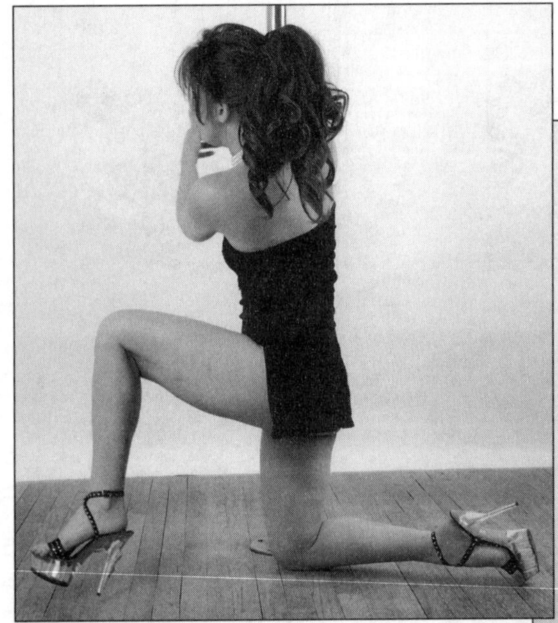

Kick your outside leg around the pole with enough force to bring your body around.

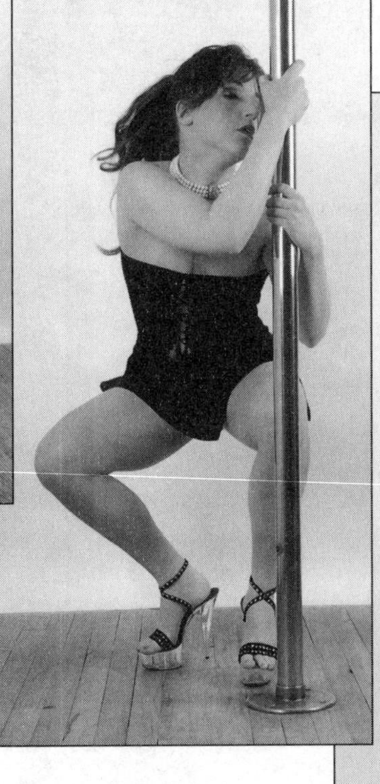

Be sure your feet are together completely before you attempt to stand up.

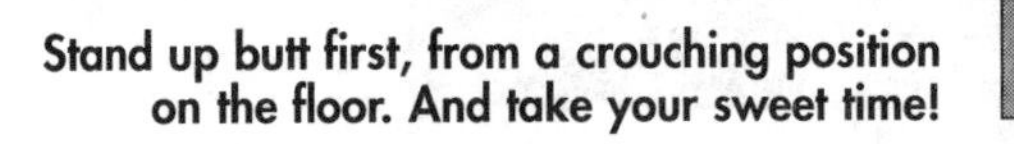

Stand up butt first, from a crouching position on the floor. And take your sweet time!

Honey Jump

This move is fun. To do it, you simply jump up onto the pole. Yes, I said just jump on the pole. One of your legs will instinctively wrap around the pole to help you hold on, while you straighten your other leg in front of you. This pose is best viewed in profile, so be sure you do it sideways to your audience.

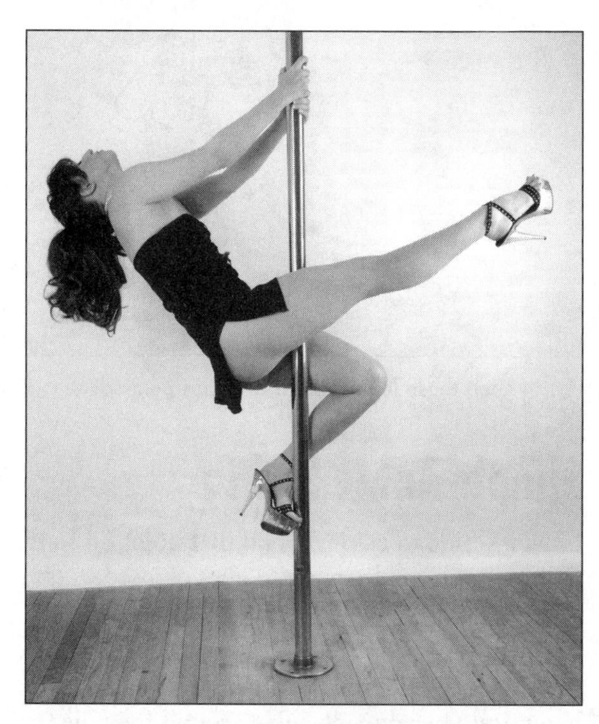

Be sure your leg is perfectly straight and your toe is pointed. Otherwise, this will look weak.

Now slowly lean back and see whether you can hold on with only one arm. The other arm can fall back into a delicate pose as you let yourself slide down the pole.

Honeycomb Slide

This one works well if you're wearing boots; otherwise it tends to hurt the back of your foot. But it sure looks good!

Grabbing the pole up high with both hands, place the back of your foot against the pole while your other leg is out to the back and then slide slowly down to the floor. Again, this is another great profile pose.

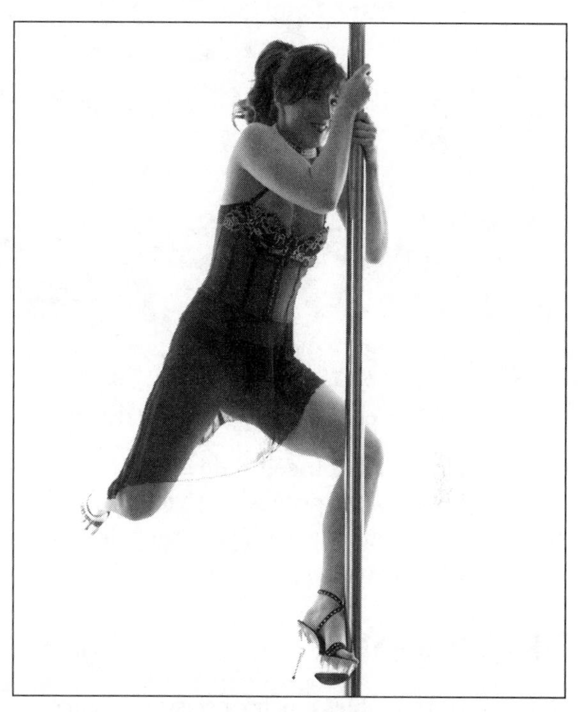

Keep your back leg out straight or at a delicate bend.

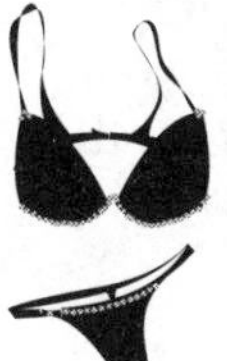

Behind the G-String

Try to maintain your sexy expression on the pole as opposed to the "I'm constipated!" expression, which is very common when you first learn pole.

Pole Spread

This move is almost all leg strength, but boy, does it look great when you can do it.

Using your arms, jump up onto the pole but extend both legs out one to each side, with the pole in the middle. Be careful not to smash your very sensitive area right into the pole!

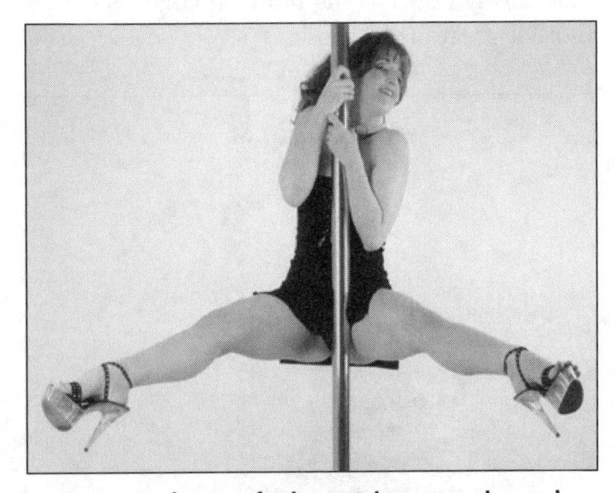

Keep your legs perfectly straight as you descend.

Then slowly let yourself slide down until you reach the floor. This pose is best viewed head on, and if you're really cool, you can roll your neck around as you come down.

The Scissors Slide

This move resembles a pair of scissors, hence the name. To do it, hold the pole with your strong hand so your fingers are pointing to the floor. Extend your other arm and hold on to the pole. Now give a slight jump up with your legs completely extended and slide down to the floor.

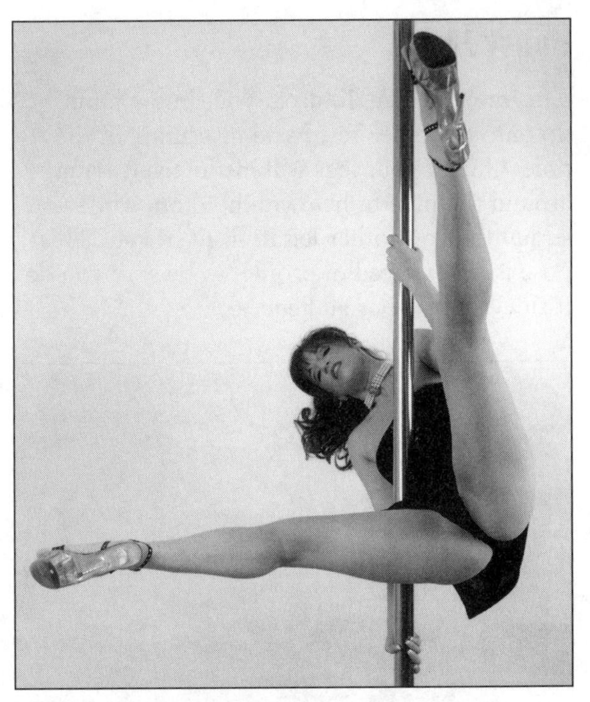

Keep those legs straight and toes pointed!

Simple Ankle Swing

Now it's time to circle 'round that pole! I'll start with a simple ankle swing to get you used to the centrifugal force that will bring you around the pole.

Hold on to the pole with your strongest hand. Put your outside ankle around the pole about 15 inches from the floor and bend your knee. (For example, if you are right-handed, you hold on with your right hand and your *left* ankle is around the pole.) Lean out to the side. (Don't even give a thought to your left arm. You don't use it at all here, so it can do as it pleases.)

Now let yourself fall forward and let the pole slide up your left leg. Then consciously *step away* from the pole, outside the circle of death.

Do not let your foot break your fall! You are in control of that foot, so just slide it down the pole as you come around, and remember to keep your right arm straight. As soon as your body starts moving, that foot is sliding down.

Be sure to step *outside* the circle of death, too, because if you don't step far enough away from the pole, your heel will get caught and the pole and will trip you up. Also, if you step too close to your friend the pole, the pole will get very fresh with you and slide up all the way to … well, all the way up … and that does not feel good!

This is a very gentle move, a very gentle sliding down of the left foot as it goes around the pole. The more you practice it, the more fun you can have. For example, you can lean down into the swing so your body actually dips down. You can use two hands if you want to start out, but it does look nicer with one hand.

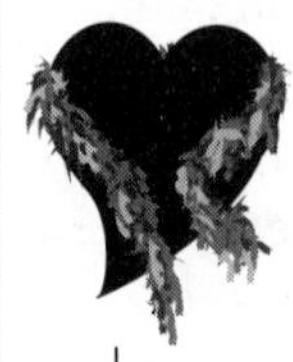

Feelin' the Love

Once I took up pole dancing, no telephone pole, monkey bar, or street light was safe. I swung around everything in my path.

—Jennifer Solow, author of *The Booster*

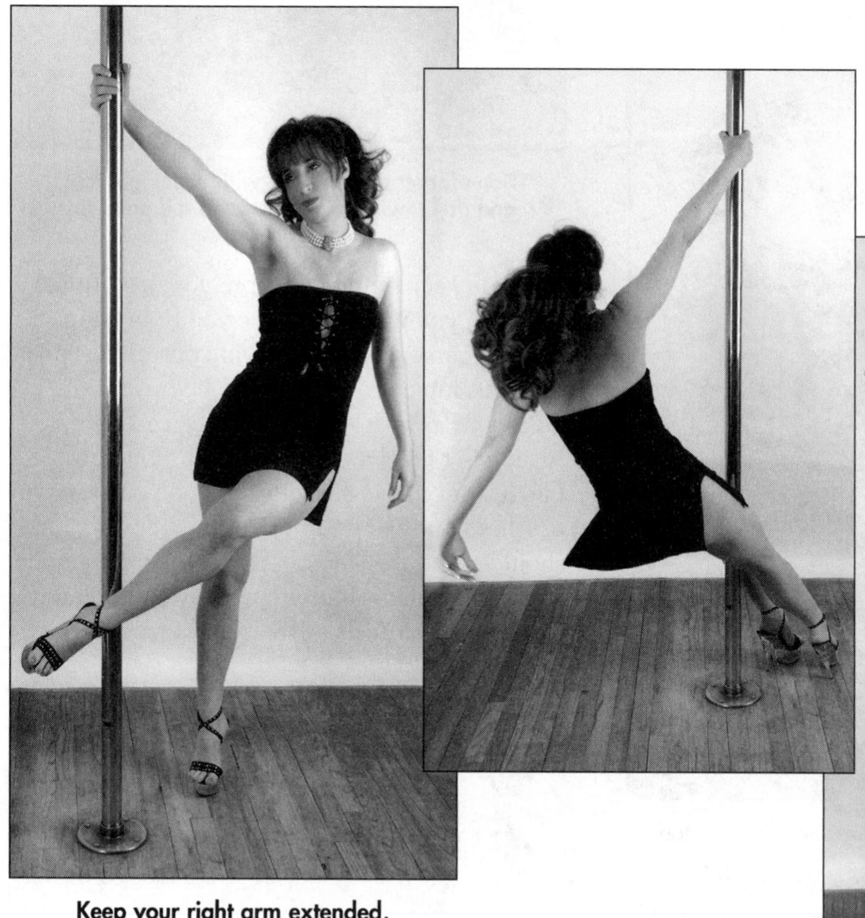

Keep your right arm extended, and lean out to the side.

Dip down as you come around the pole.

Land on your toe so your body can pivot gracefully.

Backbend Finish

This finishing move you can add on to any swing, but it looks particularly nice as an ending to the ankle swing.

Coming out of the ankle swing, as you step on your outside foot (the one you placed on the pole), continue to pivot around on your toe. Switch your arms so now the opposite arm is holding the pole, and *step back* with your other foot (the one that didn't pivot) to brace yourself. (My students always forget to step back, so they're left hanging and looking rather silly as they try to balance with one foot in the air.)

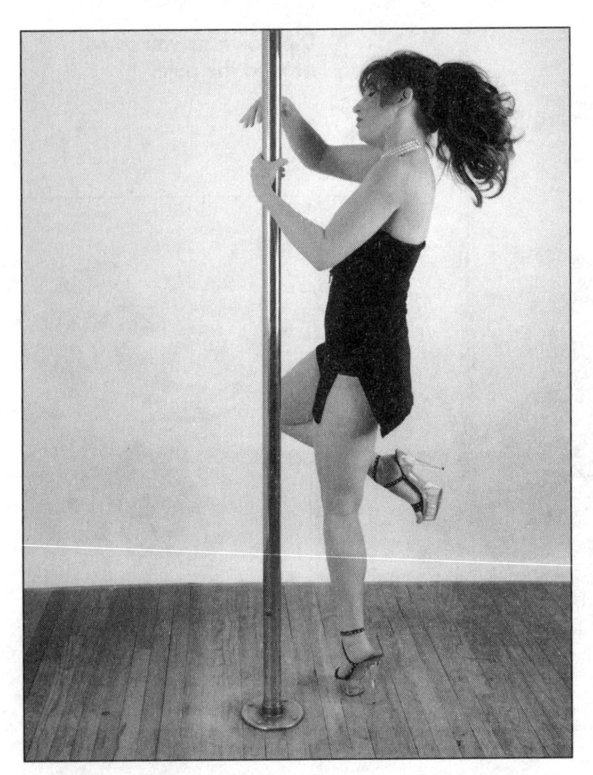

Switch your hands as you're pivoting on your toe.

Arch your back as you use your arm that's not on the pole to sweep over your head, your fingers in the delicate position, your forearm touching your hair as your arm glides over, your hand moving down the back of your head and down over your shoulder.

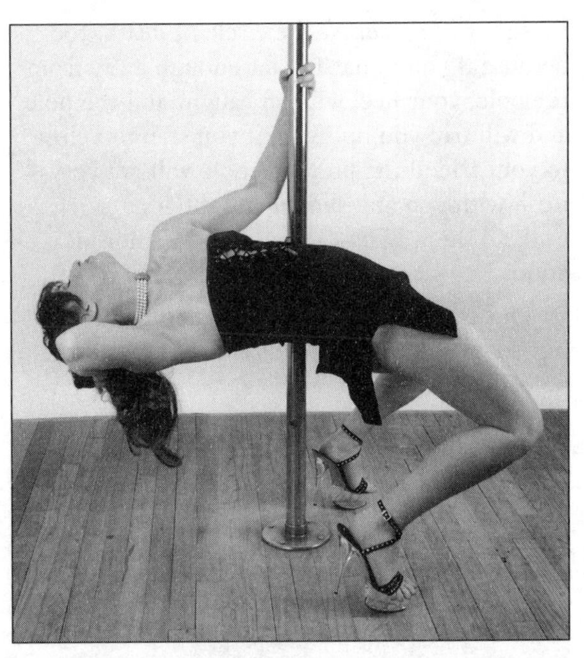

Don't forget to step back with your right foot, and don't twist yourself around the pole. Just go straight back.

If you keep going and wrap yourself around the pole, you won't look like you're in control, and of course you're always in control. Keep your left hip close to the pole, because if you go too far away it won't look nice and tight. Also, don't just let your right arm flop out. Circle your arm over your head so your forearm brushes your hair and then draw it down your shoulder and the side of your body, letting your hand gracefully roll off your body and point at the floor. That feels awkward, but trust me, it looks great!

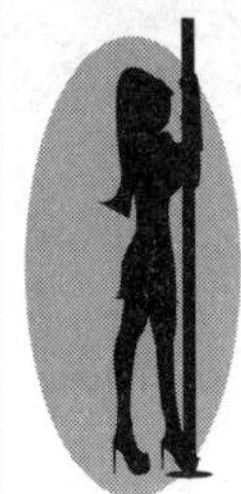

Slick Tricks

If, like me, you can't arch your back, try this trick: bend your knees. It's technically cheating, but it still looks great.

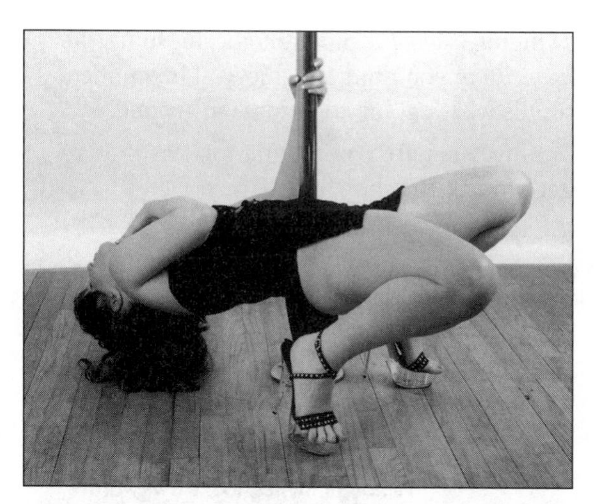

Aim for the floor with the crown of your head, and let your feet slide forward slightly as you slide down.

Keep this pose for a few seconds so your audience can admire it. Then if you're really crazy, you can slide your hand that's holding the pole downward until your back is on the floor and delicately roll away. That takes some practice, but looks really nice. Then you can roll over onto your hands and knees and get up gracefully as described earlier. Or you can just hold onto the pole in a squatting position, pivot your feet so your body turns to the side, and stand up butt first. But remember to accentuate your butt as it comes up. You are in *no* rush!

What goes up must come down, so get up as you did in the "Getting Up Gracefully" section earlier in this chapter. (If you're following along, trying each move in order, you'll already know how to do this!)

Tips for Going Airborne

Now it's time to go airborne! Before you launch yourself into the air, though, you need to keep several very important things in mind:

Do not be afraid. You are holding on with your hands, so you will *not* fall off. Now say, out loud, "The pole is my friend."

When you're airborne, you're holding on with your arms, it is all arm strength. Your legs do *not* give you any support; they simply keep your bottom half around the pole or are just there for ornamentation.

Keep the arm over your head (your main arm) straight. Don't ever bend that elbow. If you bend your elbow, you'll end up stepping in the circle of death and find yourself face to face with your pole, who will be trying very, very hard to keep a straight face.

Always lean out to the side when swinging.

Your outside leg is the source of your momentum, so the more you use your outside leg to swing your body around, the easier the swings will be and the less you will strain your main arm.

When you take your first step before you swing, step *away* from the pole, not *into* it.

To correctly and easily hop onto the pole, pretend like you're kicking a ball. You would wind your leg up first, sweep it down, kick the ball, and your leg would come back up. Although we aren't kicking any balls (unless they're bad tippers), that kicking motion will bring your body up. Pivot on your toe as you do this and then hop onto the pole, wrapping your left leg. And you don't have to try to get your leg as high as it can go—that's not the point. The point is to look graceful.

When you wrap your outside leg, try to do it at the calf. (Leaning to the side and almost pulling on the pole will help with this.) If you grab the pole between your thighs, you'll bruise.

Don't worry if you're heavier or you don't have much arm strength because you're swinging *around* … not straight up, so it's the *momentum* you want to achieve. The momentum is what's going to swing you around.

Now what are you waiting for? It's time to get on with the show!

Step on your toe, not your whole foot, to allow for an easy pivot.

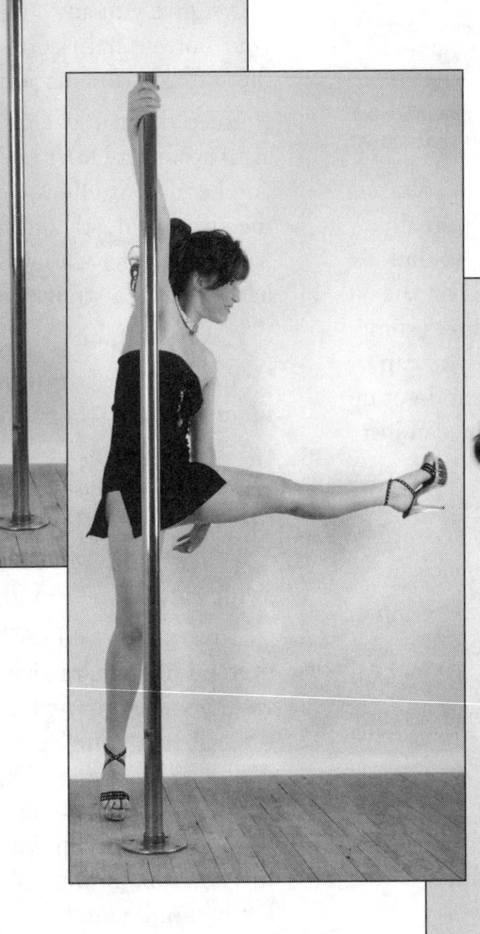

Although my leg looks awkwardly straight in this picture, your outside leg is only out to the side for a second, enough time to wind your leg up for your hop.

Practice wrapping your left leg and getting as many rotations in as possible. Don't worry about your right leg for now. That's just ornament.

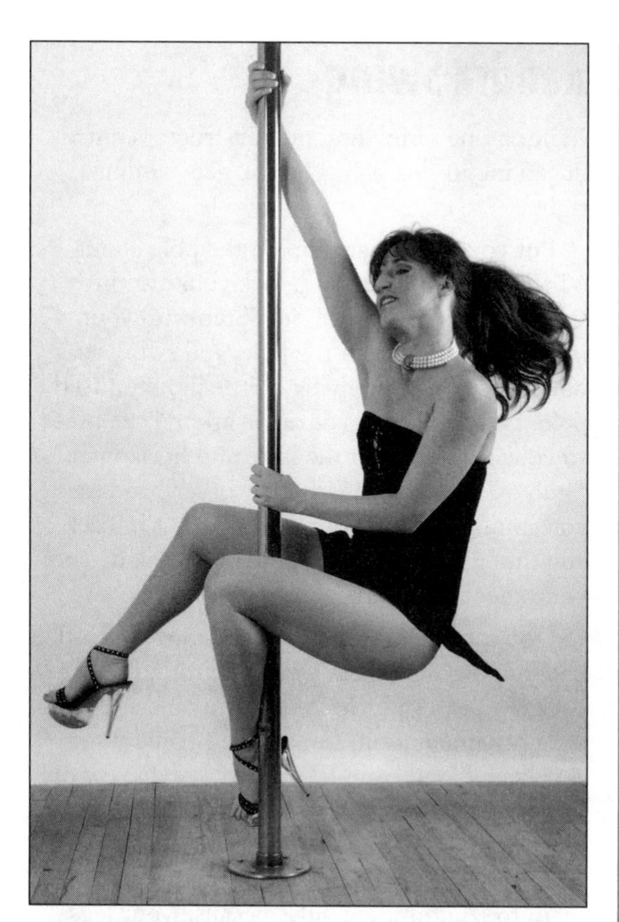

Notice first how far away my body is from the pole because my right arm is straight. Also, see that the pole goes no higher than my calf.

Veronica Swing

Named after one of my first and most diligent instructors, Veronica, this is a great beginner swing to use as a base for others.

Put your strong arm up on the pole about 6 inches above your head, lock your arm in straight, and lean to the side. Step with your inside foot away from the pole, and swing your outside leg around, giving a little jump on to the pole. Wrap your outside leg around the pole and grab on to the pole with your other hand. Place the calf of your inside leg against the pole—don't wrap it around or you'll end up as a pretzel!

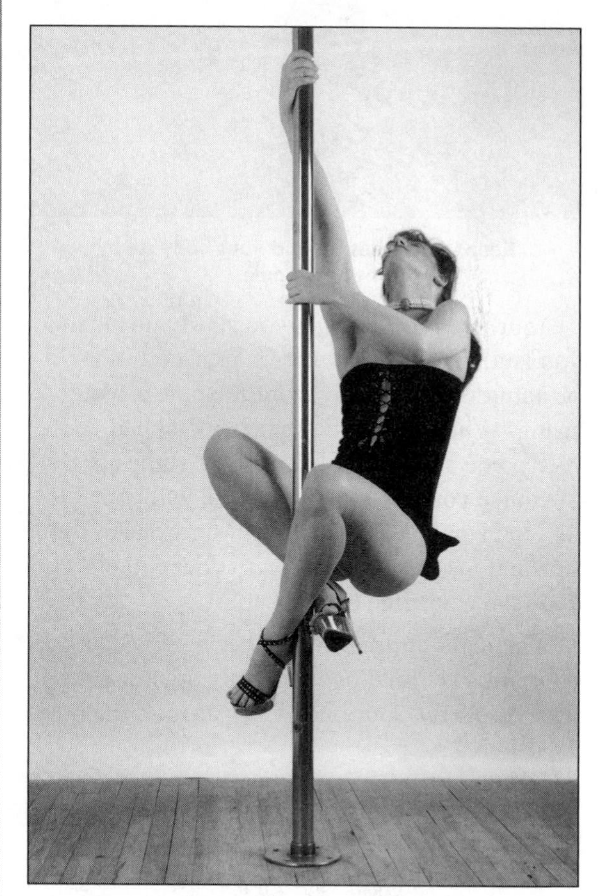

Wrap your left leg first and then gently place your right shin against the pole. Don't try to do both at once.

Feelin' the Love

I was trying out the backward spin move on the pole all night and gave myself a *huge* bruise on my ankle. I had to go out in search of a whole "bruise cover" makeup kit, as I was a bridesmaid in my friend's wedding which was only a week away. The dresses were knee length, and I had a lot of purple spots to cover!

—Kathy, student

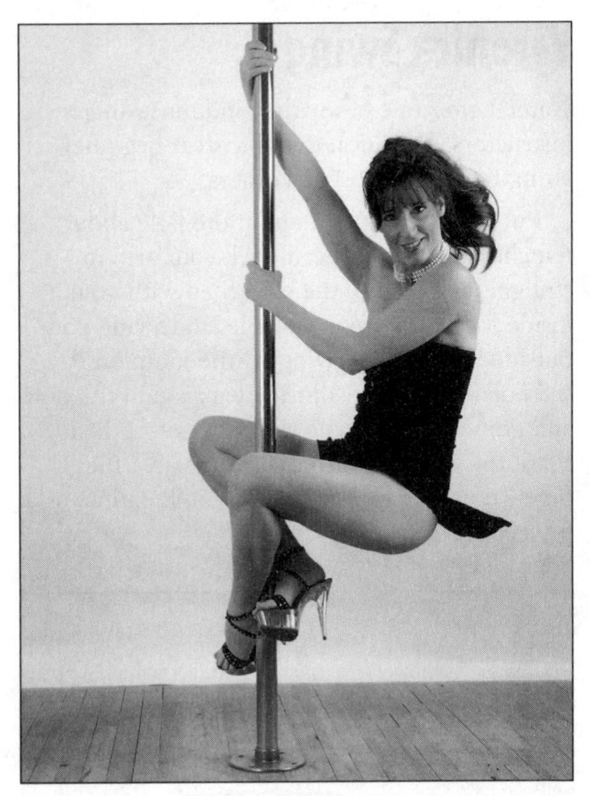

Keep your knees up and your body away from the pole.

Your gravity will bring you slowly down and you land gently on your feet. Your body should be about 6 inches away from the pole as you swing. When you land, if you've wrapped correctly, you should be able to stand right up. But of course you won't just stand up, will you? Oh no, you won't! You'll stick your butt out to the side and massage the pole with your fingers as you take your time coming up.

The main thing to remember here is that your arms are holding your body up, not your legs. Also *wrap* your outside leg around the pole.

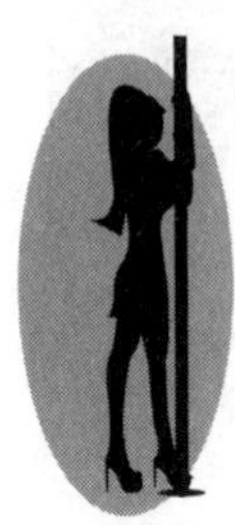

Slick Tricks

You will bruise when you're first learning how to swing on the pole, so use Echinacea to help the bruises heal faster. You can find it in most natural or health food stores.

Xandra Swing

Xandra, one of my first pole instructors, introduced me to this swing, so she gets naming rights.

Put your strong arm up on the pole about 6 inches above your head, lock your arm in straight, and lean to the side. Step with your inside foot away from the pole, and swing your outside leg around, giving a little jump on to the pole. Wrap your outside ankle around the pole so your leg is bent at the knee and horizontal. Grab on to the pole with your other hand as you spin, and place your other leg out in back of you (imagine a male dog piddling), making sure your knee is up to the side, not facing down.

Don't let the knee of your back leg touch the heel of your leg that is wrapped around. That back leg comes nowhere near the pole and is pure ornamentation. Let yourself come down slowly and land completely horizontally, *not* on your feet. You're going to have to fight your feet on this one, because everybody's feet want to land right side up. Don't let them. Force them to land on their sides because your legs need to be horizontal as they come down.

Remember, you're holding yourself up with your arms; your legs do not provide any strength in the swing.

You land in a sitting position, and of course, we want to get up sexily, never just stand right up. Here's one way I do it:

Let go of the pole with both hands and lean back on your outside forearm so you're on your side, *not* your back.

Let go of the pole, and kick your back leg up and around to the front of the pole with the rest of your body.

Roll over on your hands and knees, and continue getting up following the instructions in the earlier "Getting Up Gracefully" section. (But you've been following along and you already know how to get up gracefully, don't you?)

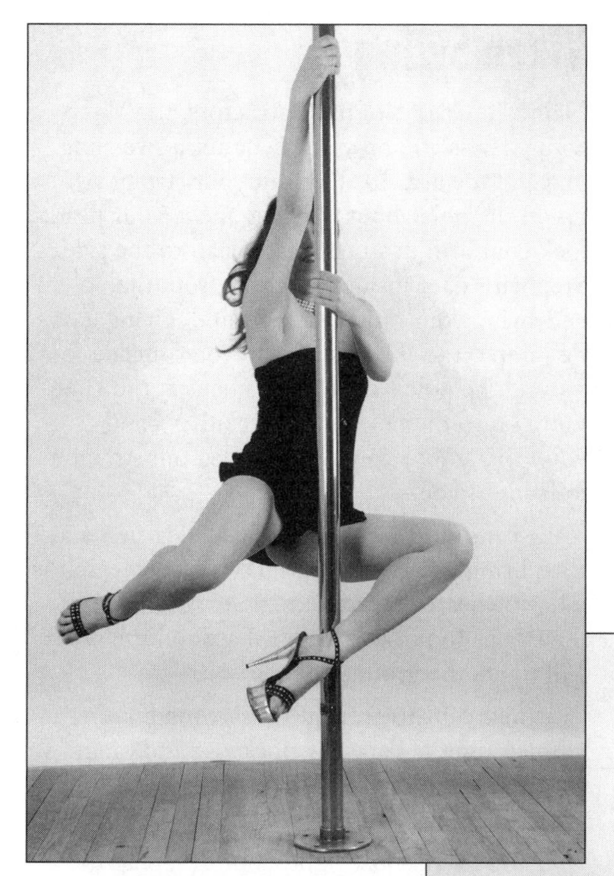

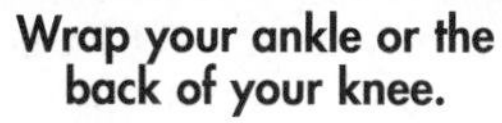

Wrap your ankle or the back of your knee.

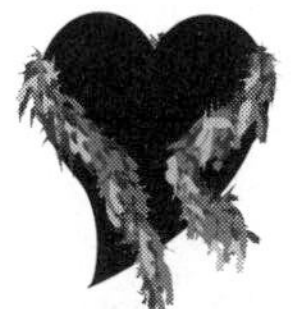

Feelin' the Love

I bought a removable pole for my house because I became so addicted to it that I hated to only have one at the dance studio. Once I put it up, however, the thing became the unofficial property of my seven and nine-year-old. We now all fight over whose turn it is on the pole, and the parents of my kids' friends have to all be reassured that coming over for a "pole dancing play date" is actually more normal than it sounds.

—Jennifer Solow, author of *The Booster*

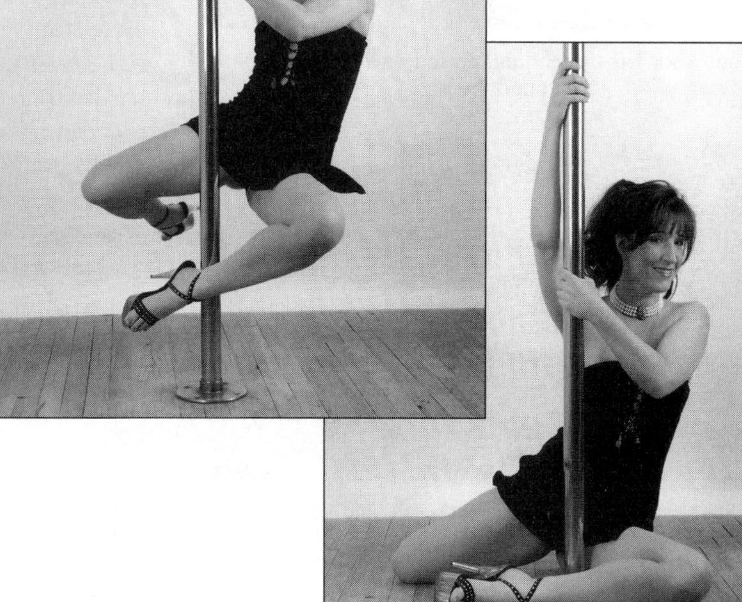

Keep your right leg far out and behind you so it comes nowhere near your other leg or the pole.

Land on the side of your legs, not your knees.

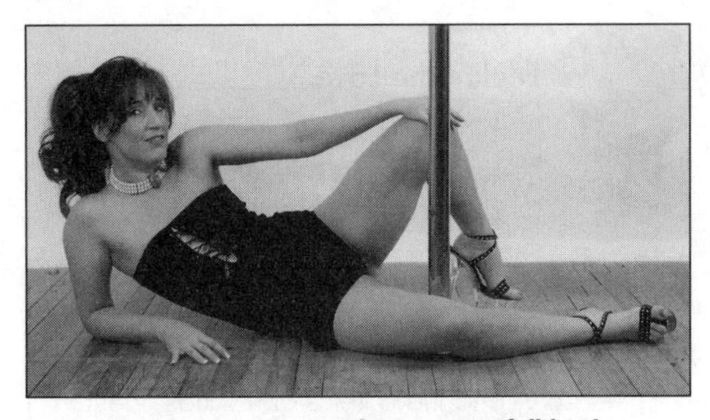

Lean over on one side, not your full back.

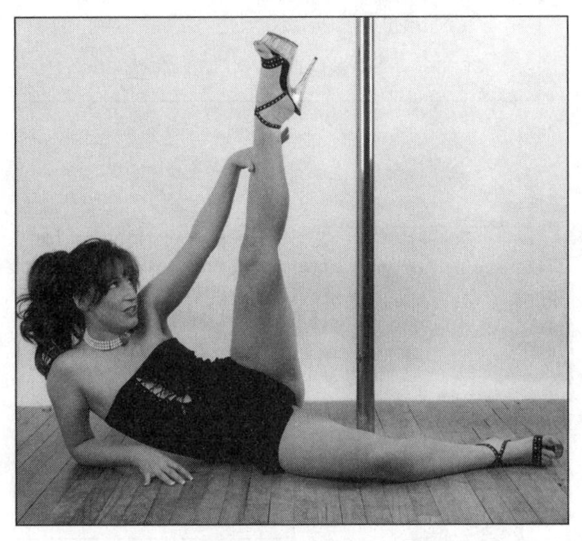

Keep your leg straight and poised as it comes up and around the pole.

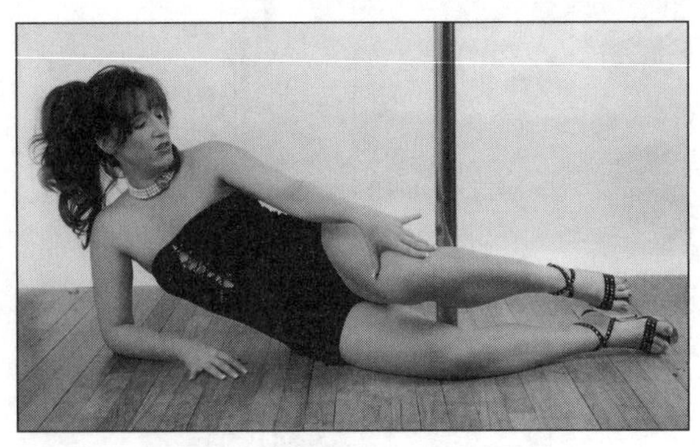

Stay close to the pole when you roll onto your hands and knees.

Vixen Swing

Named after one of my instructors, the Vixen Swing lands you on your feet after a sweeping graceful toe arc. To start, put your strong arm up on the pole about 6 inches above your head, lock your arm in straight, and lean to the side. Step with your inside foot away from the pole, and swing your outside leg around, giving a little jump on to the pole. Wrap your outside foot around the pole so your leg is bent at the knee. Grab on to the pole with your other hand as you spin, and place your other leg out straight in front of you.

Be careful to wrap your outside leg first and then bring your other leg up straight, keeping it a few inches away from the pole. As you come down, the foot that's wrapped around the pole will touch the ground.

When your toe touches the ground, swing your straight leg around clockwise and drag your toe in a large circle as you come back up into a standing position.

If you do this just right, your dragging toe will spin you around until you come to a complete stop, and you'll look incredibly pretty! Just remember not to go down too far, or it will be harder to get up. Use your toe that's touching the ground as your cue for your outside toe to arc around.

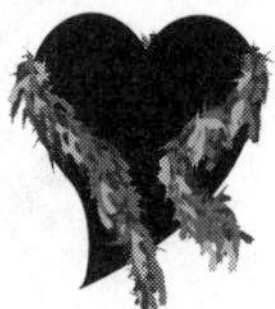

Feelin' the Love

I had taken your class once before, so I thought I was quite the pro and was trying to teach other people how to do the basic swing move with one leg wrapped around the pole and the other straight out. The only person who would actually try it at this bar that had poles was a guy, and he was really good!

—Kathy, student

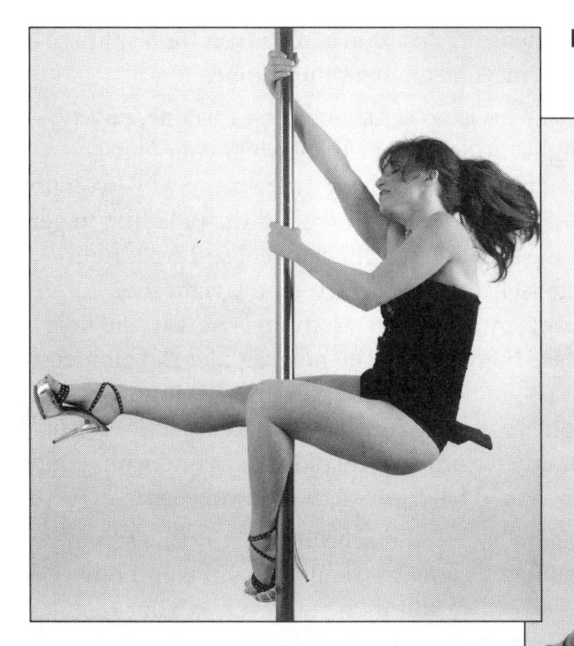

Leg bent: wimpy. Leg straight: strong!

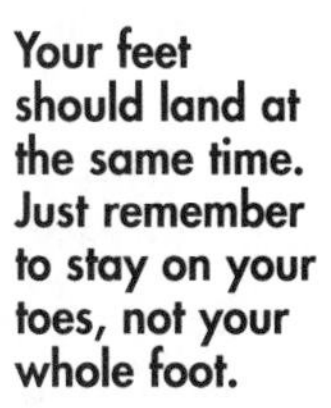

Your feet should land at the same time. Just remember to stay on your toes, not your whole foot.

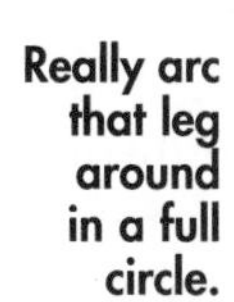

Really arc that leg around in a full circle.

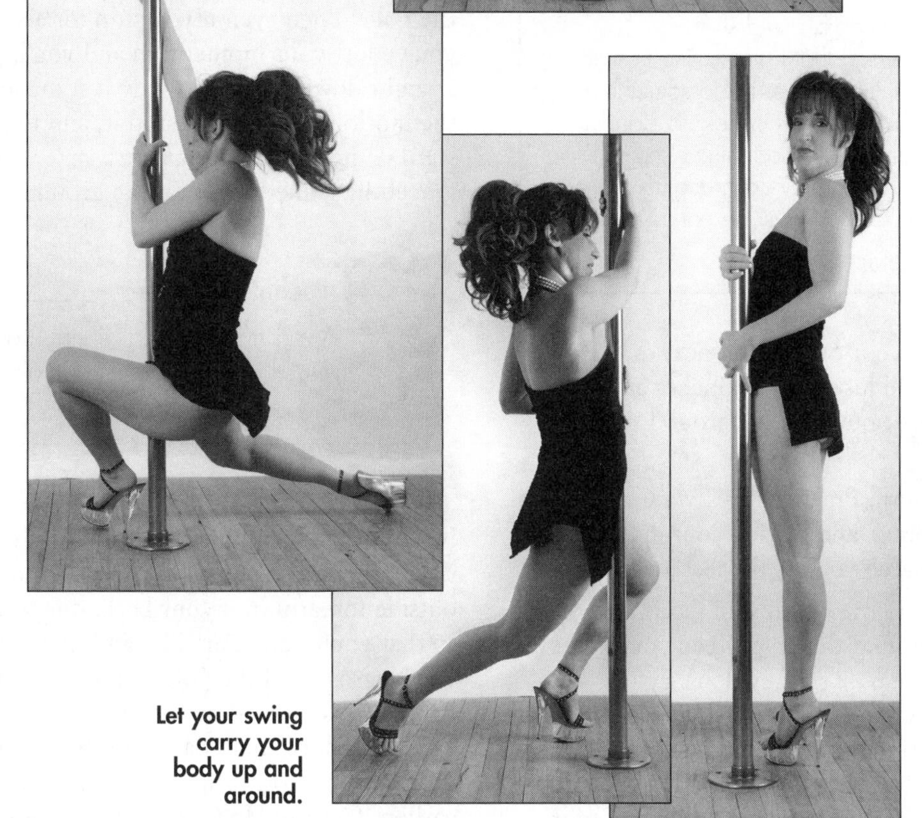

Your body will naturally turn in to the pole, and that is the only time your heels touch the floor.

Let your swing carry your body up and around.

Marilyn Backward Swing

My students claim this is the easiest swing of all, and when you get the concept of the turn and it clicks into your head, you, too, will see that this one is super easy.

The key to this swing is *motion.* You must always be in motion. You can't stop; otherwise, you'll lose your momentum and get all twisted up in the pole or land in a heap.

First you need to practice the actual turn with this move. So holding on to the pole with your strong hand about 6 inches above your head and your arm straight, step on your inside foot so it's about a foot away from the base of the pole. Lift your outside leg, bent at the knee, and turn in to the pole by pivoting on your inside foot.

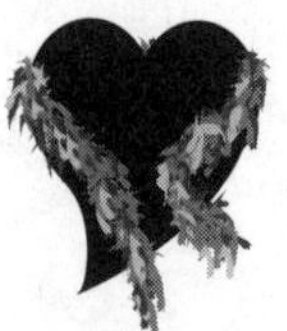

Feelin' the Love

Even my sister said she was impressed that I was doing this and it's motivating her to do something … so all in all learning exotic dancing has been one of the best things I have done … and I still have a grudging respect for the pole … but it will be conquered!

—Calypso, student

This brings your outside leg next to the pole. (Your hip should just be a few inches away from the pole.) Place your bent leg around the front of the pole.

That's the turn. Practice this several times, just stepping, pivoting, and placing your inside leg around the pole so you get the feel for the move.

When you do the actual spin, both legs go up together around the pole. Keep your ankles anchored to the pole so they don't fly off because that doesn't look tight and in control, which, of course, you are when you're swinging. You really want to lean forward as you do this, even take a few steps around the pole for momentum. Just don't stop, even for a split second, or your momentum is gone.

There is no actual jump on this one, just a slight lifting of your body when your legs go around. You must have momentum when you do this, so walk *normally* around the pole first to get some speed. I'm right-handed, so I walk right-left-right; then, as I step on my right foot, I pivot my body so my left hip is next to the pole, place both legs on the pole, and let the momentum spin me around backward. It's almost as if you are waiting for the very last second to turn. In other words, if you didn't turn and wrap your leg, you'd fall forward, flat on your face.

You can even do this using only one step of the foot as long as when you step your body *keeps moving* and then you pivot on your foot and around you go.

Whatever you do, *don't* stop between pivoting on your toe and putting your legs on the pole. Then even if you stop for a second, you've lost your momentum and you'll go straight down. Let your body just move with the motion, don't try to stop it, and then go forward … just let it *flowwwwwwwww* … until you gracefully come to rest on the ground.

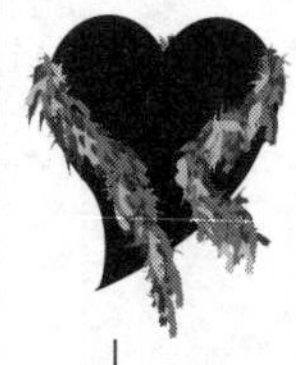

Feelin' the Love

Working the pole like that, I amazed myself.

—Sage, student

When you've landed, you can get up sexily by doing the windmill move. Simply release your grip on the pole and lean back on your outside forearm (not your back, only *one* arm so that you're on your side) and then windmill your legs around the pole, roll over on your hands and knees, come forward with your arms extended, draw them back, and flip your hair up. Continue to get up as you learned in the earlier "Getting Up Gracefully" section.

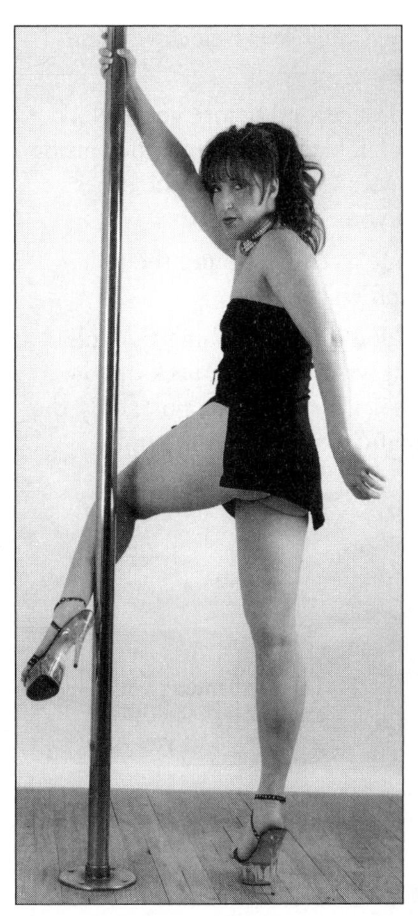

Step on your toe so you can easily pivot all the way around.

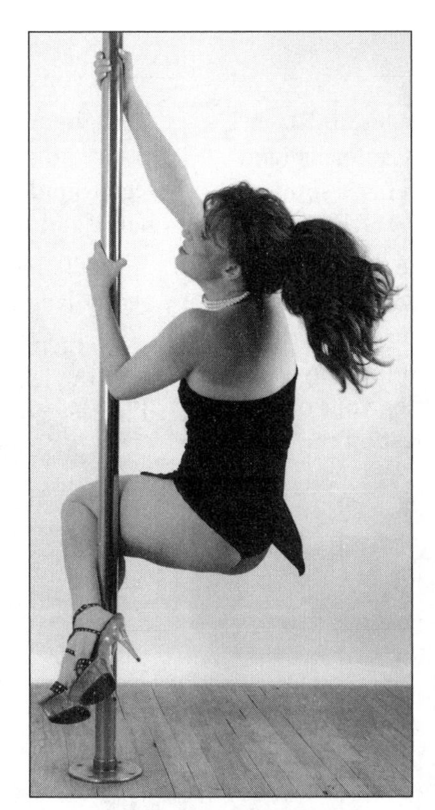

Don't fight the momentum. Let it carry you backward after you pivot.

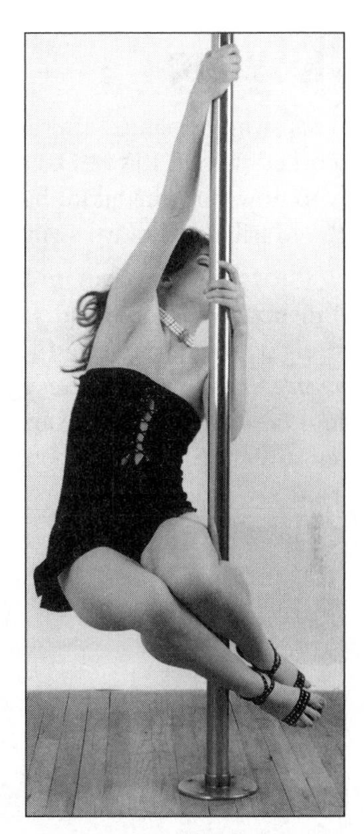

Keep your ankles anchored around the pole by concentrating on them as you spin. Don't let them fly off. Look dramatically down at them if you need to.

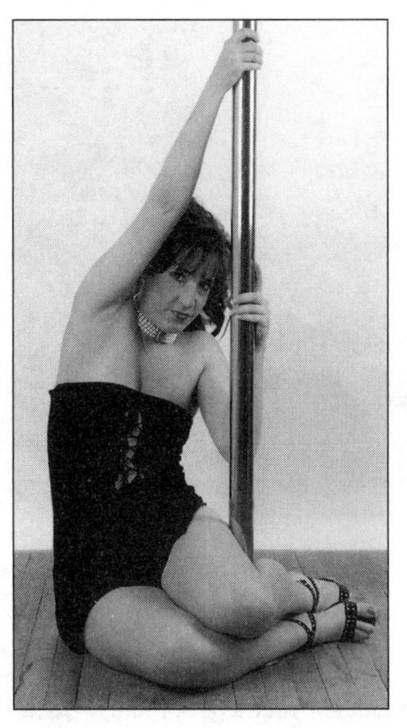

Let your arms come down with you; otherwise, they'll get tangled and you'll have a nasty case of pole burn.

JK Swing

This swing is named after a wonderful dancer I worked with at PJ's in Oxnard, California (and who now runs the bikini bar!). This is similar to the Marilyn backward swing.

Put your strong arm up on the pole about 6 inches above your head, lock your arm in straight, and lean to the side. Now step with your *outside* foot (I'm right-handed, so I use my left foot) away from the pole and bring your other leg straight up in back about 3 feet off the floor.

Let your straight leg swing clockwise and bring you around.

Right at the last second before you feel like you're going to fall backward, wrap your inside leg around the pole, grab on with the other hand, and bend your knees.

You'll continue to come around the pole, gently landing on your knees.

Remember, you're not grabbing the pole with the leg that was straight in back of you. That leg comes *nowhere* near the pole; only the foot you originally step on is on the pole.

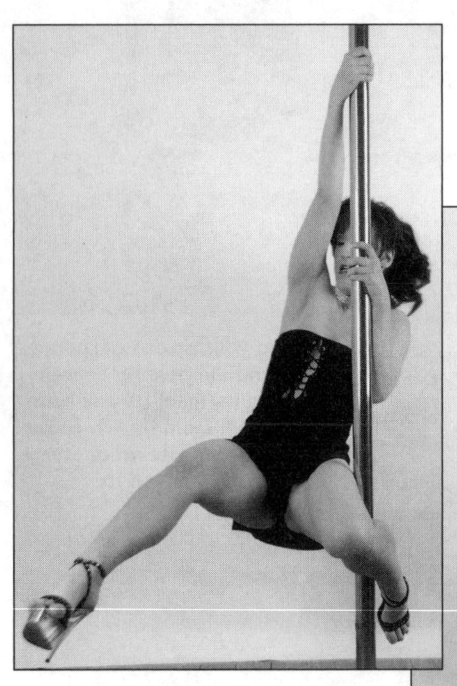

Use your straight leg to bring you around the pole.

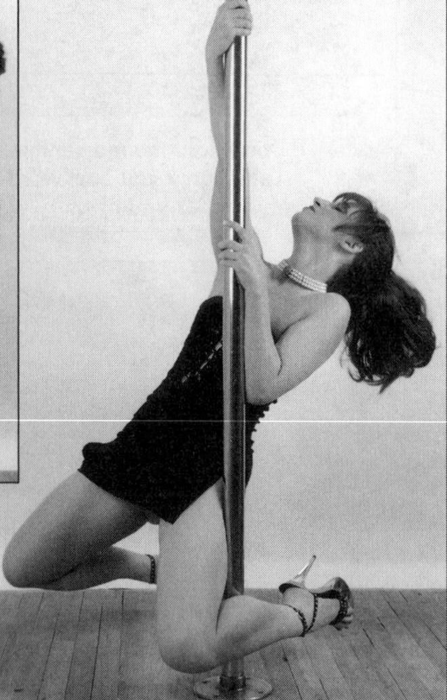

Quickly bending your straight leg increases your speed as you spin.

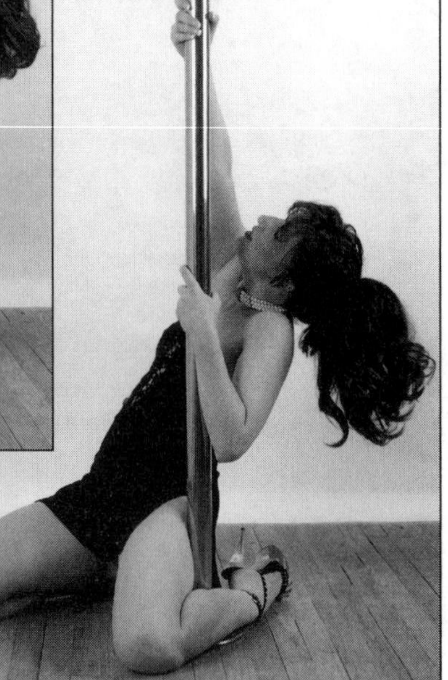

Be sure to keep your legs spread.

Harley Swing

I've named this great-looking sideways swing after my instructor Harley. You'll feel all your weight with this swing, so you might want to practice the other swings first to build up some arm strength.

The easiest way to learn this swing is to start by holding on to the pole with both hands and leaning way out to the side. Now simply fall forward and bring your legs up in a sitting position, as if you were sitting in a chair, and let yourself swing around the pole until you come down.

Be sure your body is about a foot away from the pole as you swing around, and don't hold on so tight that your arms twist around the pole. Try to keep your thumb facing you as you go around so your wrist doesn't rub against the pole.

When you're comfortable doing that and you're swinging away from the pole, try it again but this time bring both your legs up to the side together and let yourself land gently on the sides of your legs, *not* your knees.

As you get better at this swing, you can begin by just lifting your outside leg straight out and letting your body fall forward while putting both legs out to the side as you come down.

You can do this swing backward as well! Swing the same way, but just turn your shoulders slightly clockwise. Your body will magically turn around so you land backward.

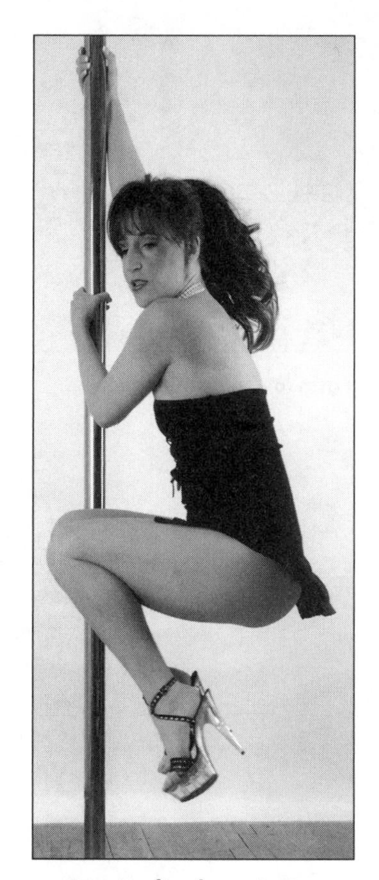

Practice first by swinging in a sitting position.

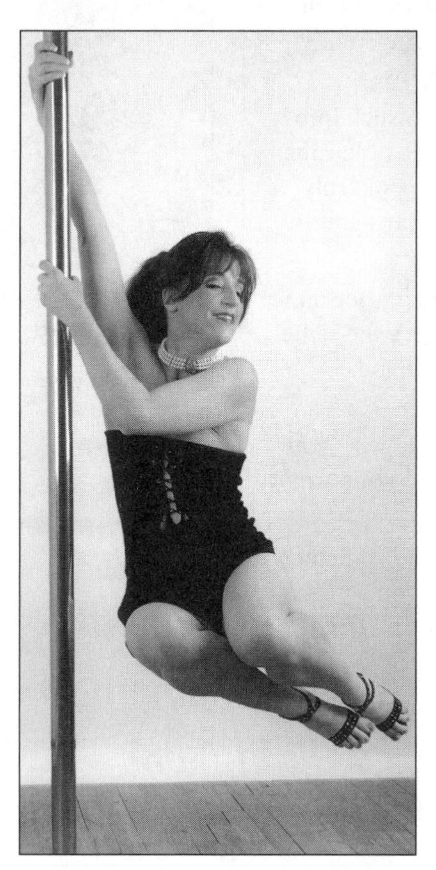

Shift your legs up and to the side.

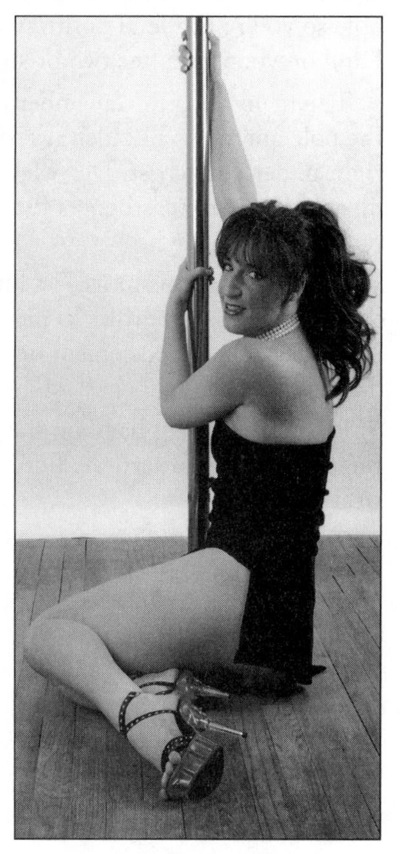

Gently glide around until you're on the floor.

Juliana Swing

You *must* wear something over your tummy for this swing; otherwise, the pole will rub against your tummy—which, let me tell you from experience, hurts like hell!

This is a sideways swing, so the main thought going through your head here should be *sideways sideways sideways.* To get sideways, you have to use your outside leg to swing you into a sideways position.

Hold on to the pole with your strong arm below shoulder height. Step with your inside foot, and swing your outside leg around hard. As you do, grab on to the pole with your outside hand *over* your other hand. Let that leg swing your body around and then suck into the pole so you're in a fetal position as you spin. Land on your feet after two or so spins.

The main thing to remember is to suck into the pole and try to be sideways so the pole rubs right under your chest. Don't let the pole rub up against your breastbone—that means you're not sideways enough.

A variation of this move is a little harder on the arms, but I think it looks nicer. It's the same basic idea, just the placement of the hands differs.

Place your strong hand on the pole with your fingers pointing toward the floor and your arm straight.

Swing your outside leg around, and remember to put your body as sideways as you can while your other hand grabs higher up. Then, land on your feet.

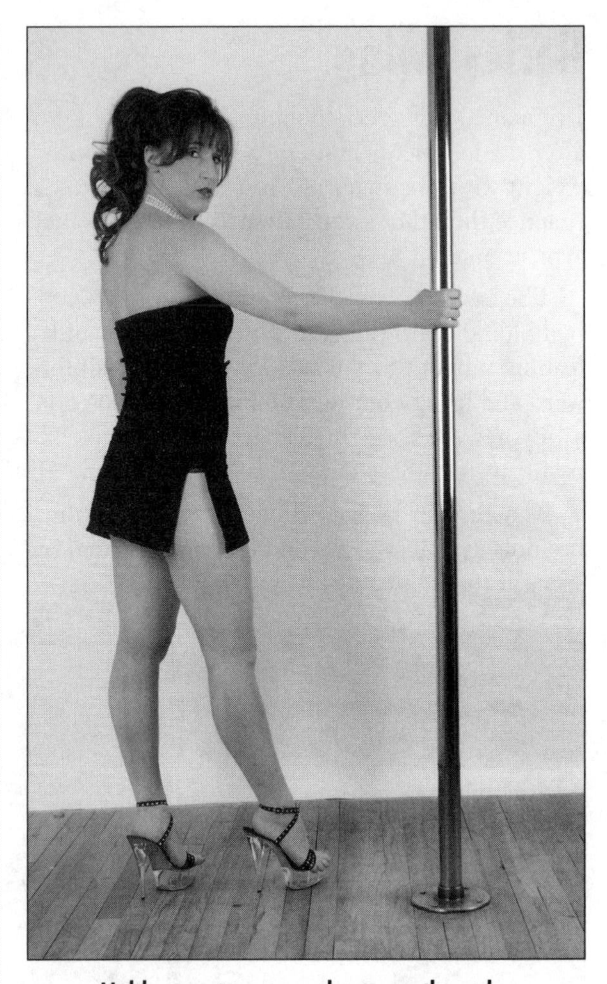

Hold your strong arm lower on the pole.

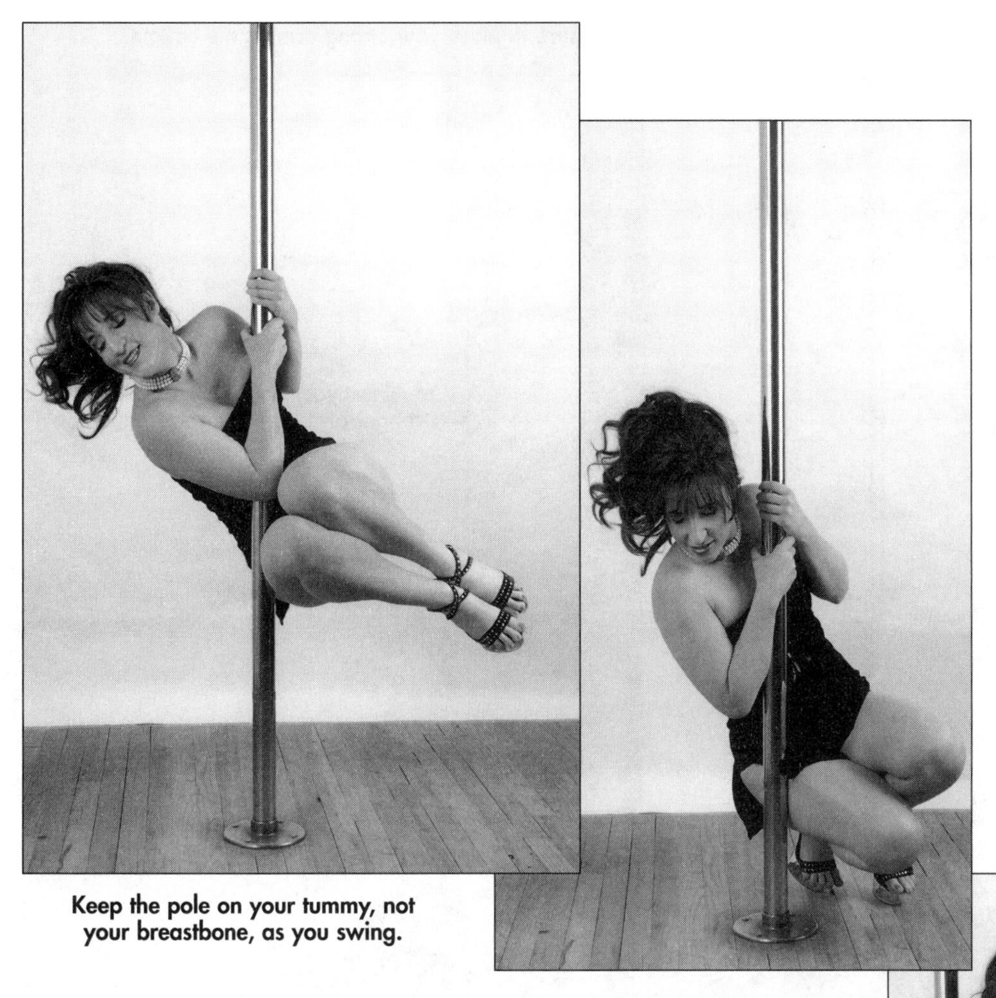

You can land on your feet or go all the way down to the floor.

Keep the pole on your tummy, not your breastbone, as you swing.

If you land on your feet, pivot them both around and stand up butt first.

Be sure to place your strong arm on the bottom.

You'll get your body up higher as your stronger arm supports you from below.

Keep your legs together and your body in a tight fetal position as you swing around.

Savannah Swing

This very skillful-looking swing is actually incredibly easy. Put your strong arm up on the pole about 6 inches above your head, lock your arm in straight, and lean to the side. Step with your inside foot away from the pole and swing your outside leg around, giving a little jump on to the pole.

Wrap your outside leg around the pole, and grab on to the pole with your other hand.

In your first rotation around the pole, bring your other leg up *over* your knee that's wrapped around the pole so you're crossing your legs.

Then as you come down, the foot that's wrapped around the pole will touch the ground. When that toe touches the ground, swing your straight leg around clockwise and drag your toe in a large circle as you come back up into a standing position.

If you do this just right, your dragging toe will spin you around until you come to a complete stop. Just remember not to go down too far, or it will be harder to get up. Use your toe touching the ground as your cue for your outside toe to arc around.

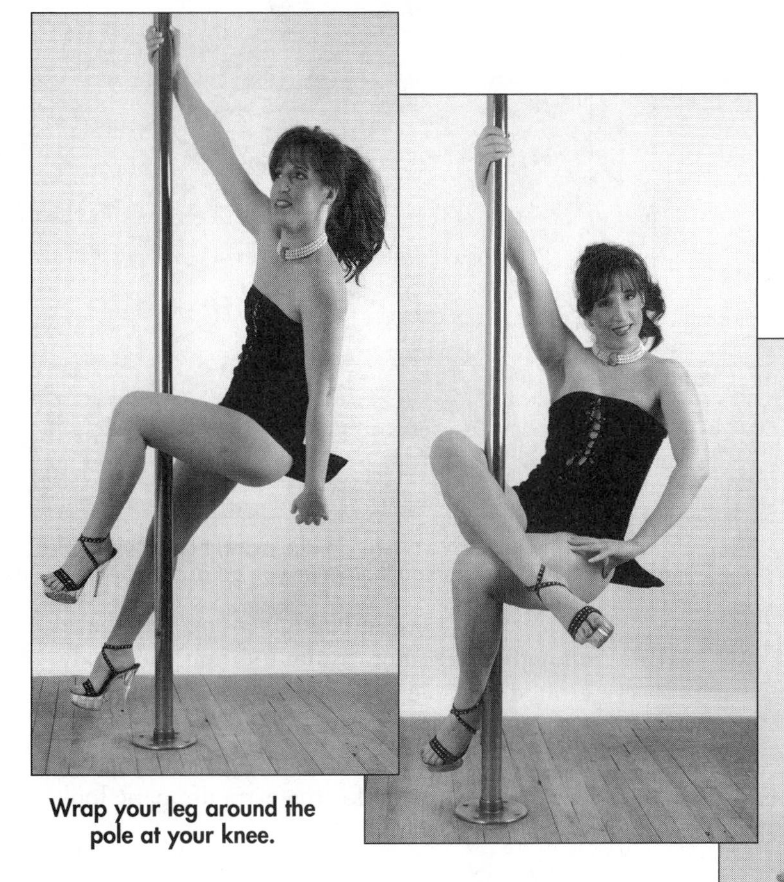

Cross your other leg up and over as if you're sitting cross-legged.

Wrap your leg around the pole at your knee.

When your right toe hits the floor, uncross your leg and let it slide around until you're standing up.

Aurora Swing

This is one of the prettiest and most dramatic swings I do. Some women who can't do the ankle swing get this one right away.

The point of this swing is to reach behind your body with one arm straight up and one arm straight down. The only way you can grab the pole with your arm straight down is to get those pesky legs out of the way. And the only way to do that is to kick them up!

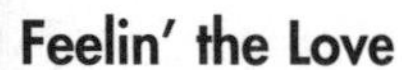

Feelin' the Love

After a glass or two of wine at my house, every dinner party ends with a pole dancing demonstration. I can't help it. Everyone funnels up to the bedroom, and we each take turns swinging around the pole—even the men. It's more fun than it is sexy—everyone loves [his or her] first time around the pole.

—Jennifer Solow, author, *The Booster*

First grab your pole with your stronger hand and fall forward, swinging your legs up to about hip-length and out in front of you. There's no real jump with this one, it's almost as if you're swinging around the pole holding on with one hand.

When your legs are away from the pole, reach around and grab the pole with your other hand so your fingers are facing down. Be sure to keep your body facing forward—you're not turning like all the other spins.

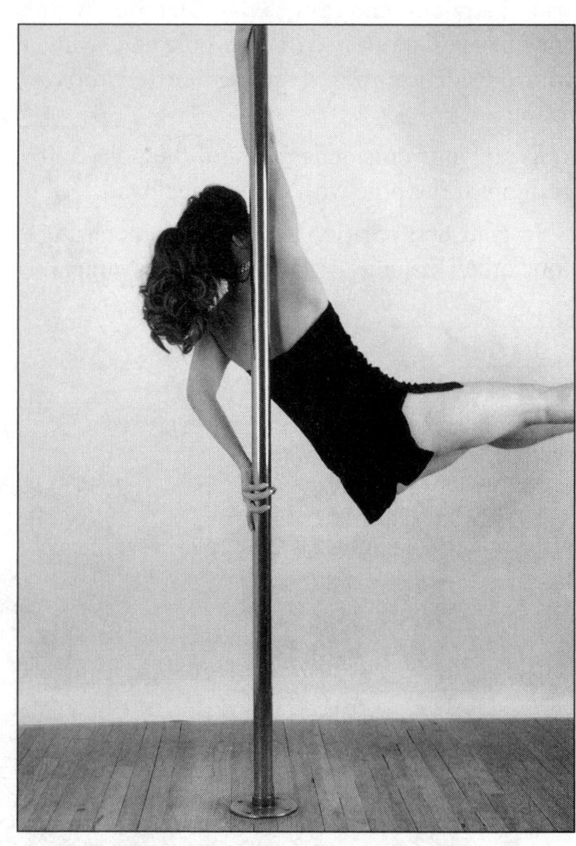

The higher your legs go, the more momentum and spins you'll have as you go around.

Your legs need to be high enough and have enough gentle momentum to bring your body around the pole; otherwise, you'll just slump to the floor. When your body does come around, bend your knees as you gently glide to the floor. Keep your neck up for the extra dramatic look.

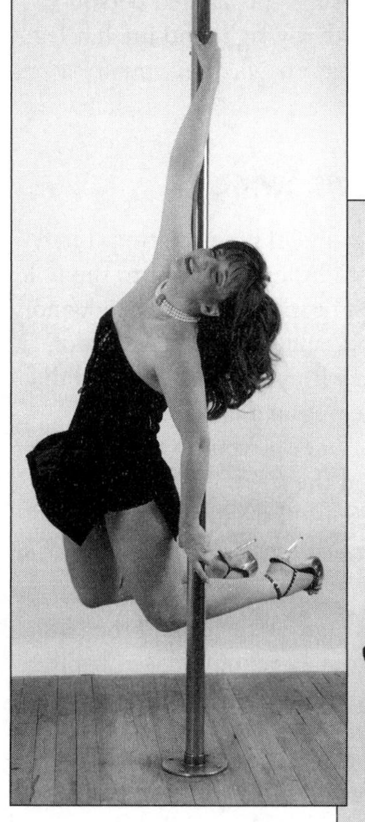

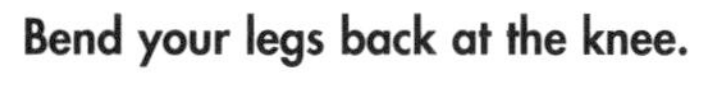

Bend your legs back at the knee.

Keep both arms straight as you come around.

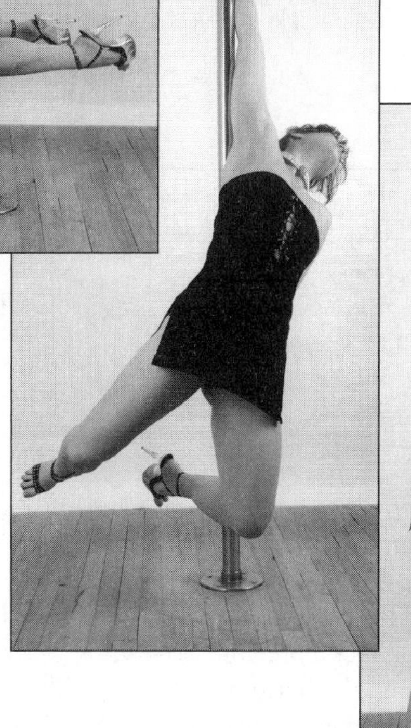

Keep your head back for added drama.

You can land gently on your knees or even on your feet and pull yourself back up—butt first, of course.

This one may take a lot of practice, but the main point is to kick those legs up gently and about 4 feet off the ground *before* you try to grab the pole with your other arm straight. If you try to grab before your legs are out of the way, you'll be bending your elbow when you grab it. Not only will that not work, it will hurt, too!

Upside Down and Inside Out

Okay, so you don't really turn yourself inside out with these moves, but you do go upside down! It's really not that hard, although it does take a lot of arm strength because you heave yourself up with your arms as you kick your leg up. There are many, many pole tricks, but we'll stick with the easiest and most practical ways of getting yourself upside down. When you perfect the basics here, I highly recommend Fawnia's DVDs on pole work, as she really gets into the detail and has more than 60 pole tricks for you to master!

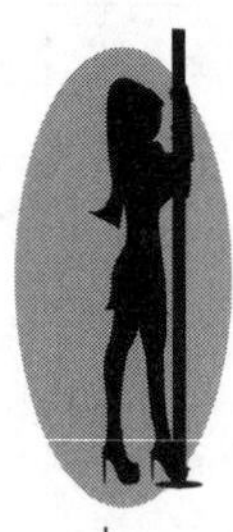

Slick Tricks

You might want to have a friend spotting you during upside-down moves to help you kick your ankle around the pole. He or she may have to just hold your body and place your ankle around the pole so you can feel what it's like.

You won't go smashing to the ground because you'll be holding on with your hands. The worst you'll do is slide down, and even then, girls I train always slide down slowly. However, if it will make you feel more comfortable, put some pillows around the bottom of the pole—and be sure the homeowner has insurance!

I find that even as a right-handed person I can kick up with both my right and my left leg, so I don't think it matters whether you are a righty or a lefty.

JoJo Upside-Down Swing

This swing reminds me of pole vaulting. First, kick up with your right leg. Hold on to the pole about shoulder height with your left hand, and as you step into the swing with your left foot, grab onto the pole with your right hand, and swing your right leg up in a large sweeping motion. Bend your knee as you do this so your ankle comes around the *front* of the pole. Even today when I dance and I do this move, all I'm thinking is *Ankle around the pole, ankle around the pole.*

Don't try to get your ankle around the pole without bending your knee; otherwise, you'll end up smashing your right hip against the pole.

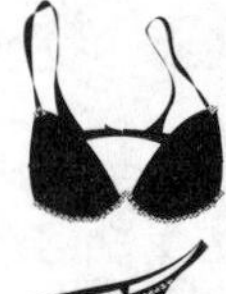

Behind the G-String

I made this mistake when I began going upside down, which led to the most beautiful, picturesque, kaleidoscope-colored bruise I had ever seen. I mean it was Christmas card worthy. (Were I not so lazy and actually sent Christmas cards out, this would have been the cover.)

This will take you several tries, but when you get that ankle around and you feel what it's like, it's pretty fun. Your other leg can also wrap around the pole as you slide down slowly, although I find it looks just as nice to stick the other leg out straight and point your toes as you come down.

When you perfect this move, you can do it in a spin and come down spinning, which also looks very professional.

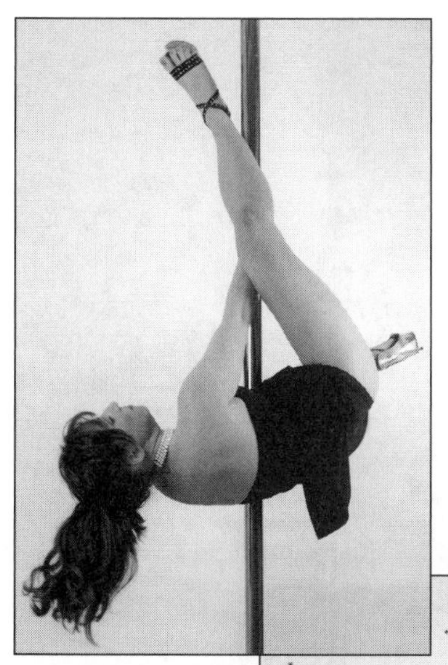

Use your arms to heave you up, but concentrate on bringing your ankle in front of the pole when your leg kicks up.

You can stick your free leg out straight, arch your back, and gracefully bend that leg at the knee, wrap it around the pole, or whatever you want. It's just ornament.

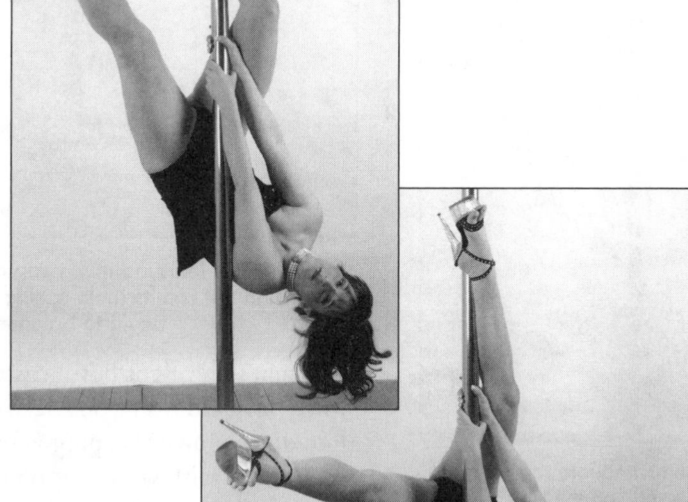

Let yourself slide gently down the pole.

When you reach the floor, slide yourself up into a sitting position so you're ready to go into your next move.

St. Kate

This pole move looks best if you can do it in one fell swoop, but while you're learning, it's best to start by swinging your leg up like in the JoJo upside-down swing.

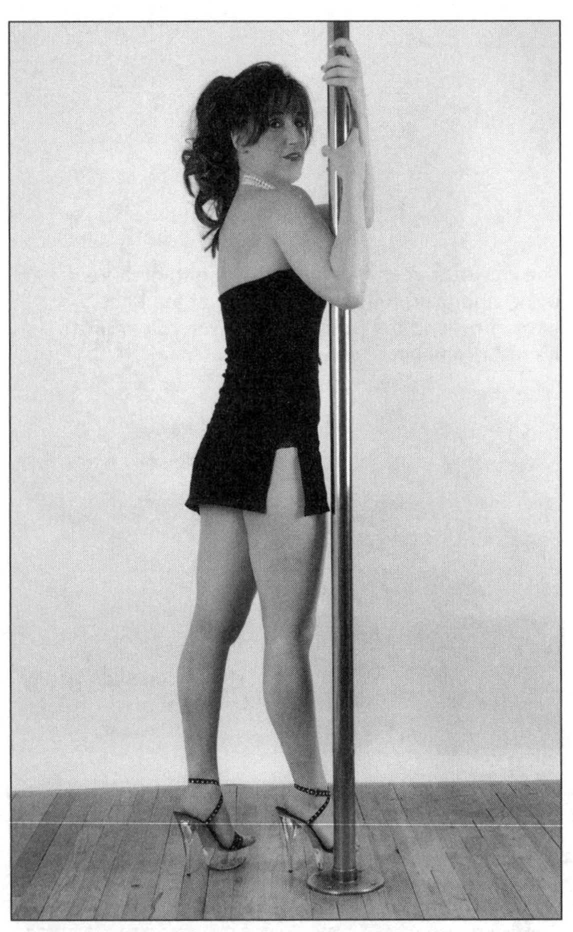

Start this move with the pole tucked into the crook of your right arm, both hands on the pole.

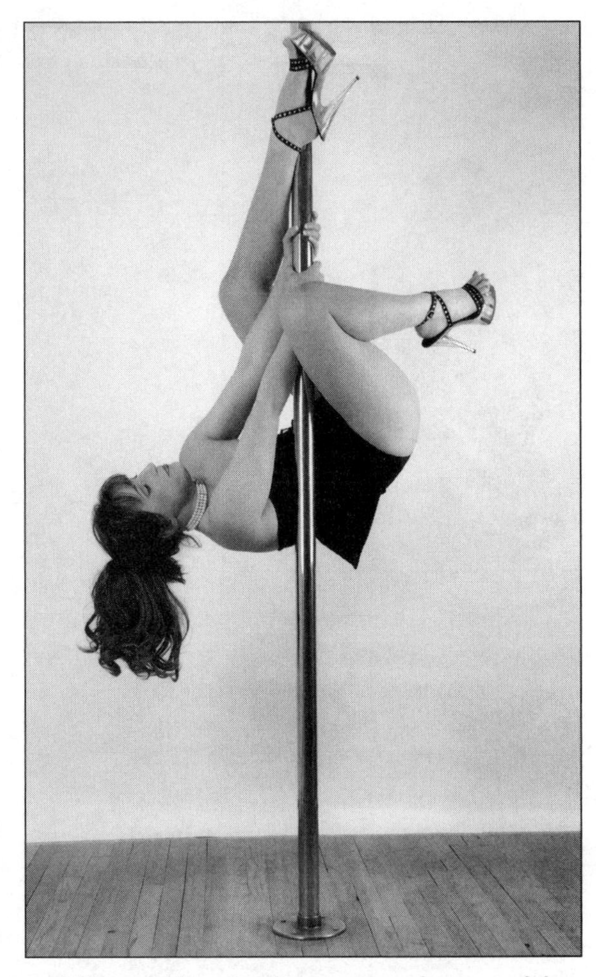

While you're learning this, wrap one leg around the pole and get comfortable upside down before you begin to balance.

When you've got both legs up, release them slowly forward over your head. Let yourself slide down slowly, keeping your legs out straight to the sides with your toes pointed to the walls.

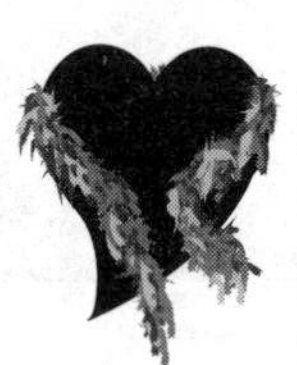

Feelin' the Love

When you get injured by the pole—there are very few people you can tell ….

—Nancy, student

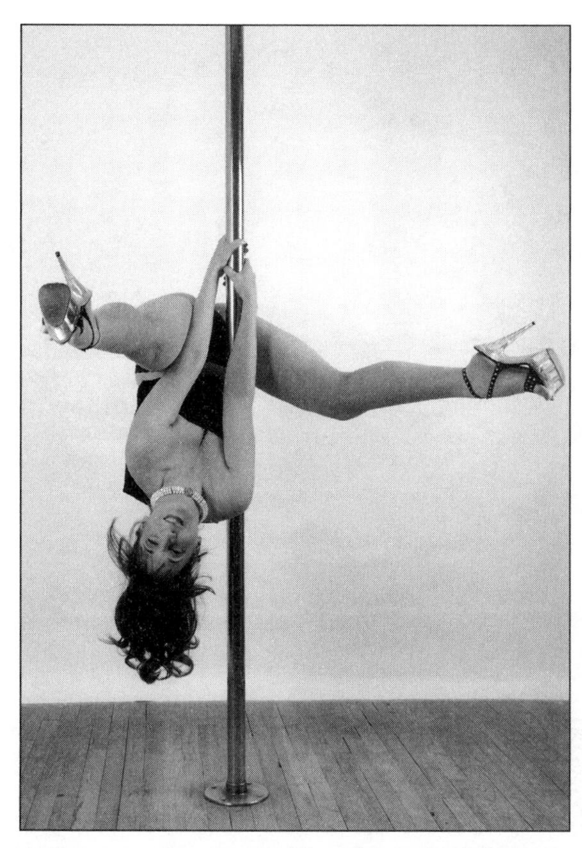

Balance your legs out straight, and gently slide down the pole.

When you feel your head touching the floor, ease your upper back forward until about a quarter of your back is on the floor. Using serious muscle control, gently bring your legs together and roll over onto your side, ready for your next move!

The St. Kate is quite a balancing act, so until you truly feel comfortable doing it in one move, it's best to do it in steps. Eventually you'll be able to go up and over in one swing. Then, when you're really good, add some spin by swinging your legs up and into the move, as opposed to just jumping straight up. Now that's impressive!

The Least You Need to Know

- Always lean out to the side when you begin to jump.
- Use your outside leg for momentum. The swing's the thing.
- Your arms hold you up, not your legs. Your legs are there more for getting the momentum going and decoration.
- Use a spotter when first trying to go upside down. It might help, too, to place pillows around the base of the pole—just in case!

In This Part

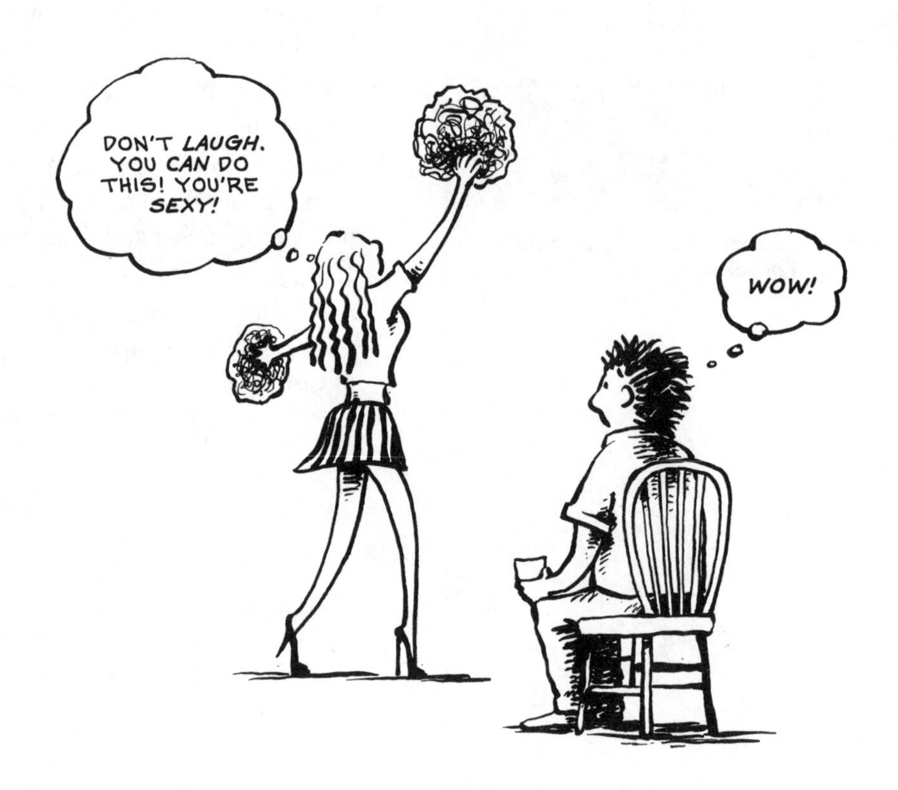

Part 3

It's All About You, but Include Him, Too!

Now's your chance to show off everything you've learned, and by saying that, I don't mean you're going to do a dance for him … you're going to do a dance for *yourself*—and let him watch! This is where you take complete control over how much he sees, when he sees it, and where he sees it. Now that we've unleashed your inner diva, release your creativity and think "outside the bedroom"!

Everything you've done so far has been about you, but now you're including him by giving him the gift of a lap dance. In this part, you learn how to really get him aroused by teasing with your clothing, your moves, and your body language.

You can do this without cracking up laughing if you just follow it through. Just remember that he's on your side and he'll be so amazed with the effort you're putting into this for him. And if you mess up, so what? Chances are he won't notice, and if you do fall on your face, laugh at it. This isn't life or death, so have fun with it!

In This Chapter

- Lap dancing—it's more than just the lap
- Crawling up and crawling down
- Backward, forward, and upside-down tricks
- Your attitude—what really makes a sexy lap dance

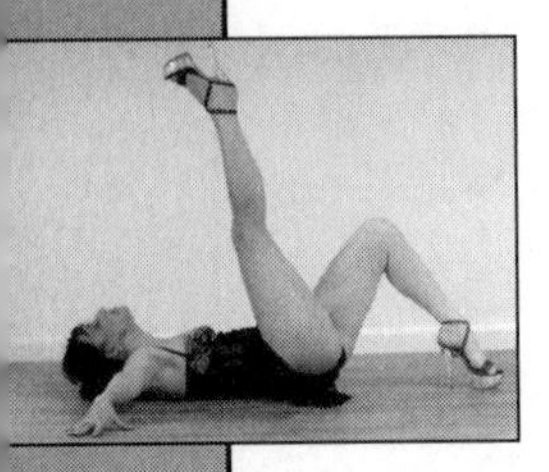 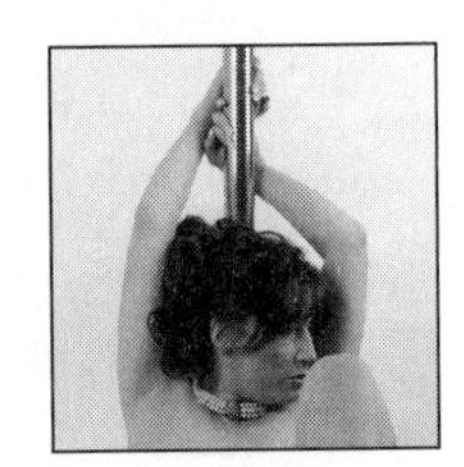 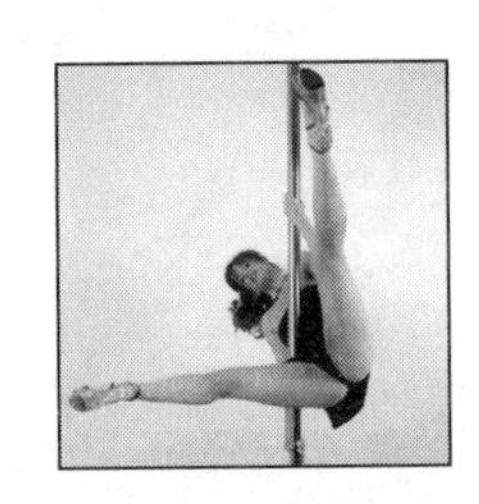 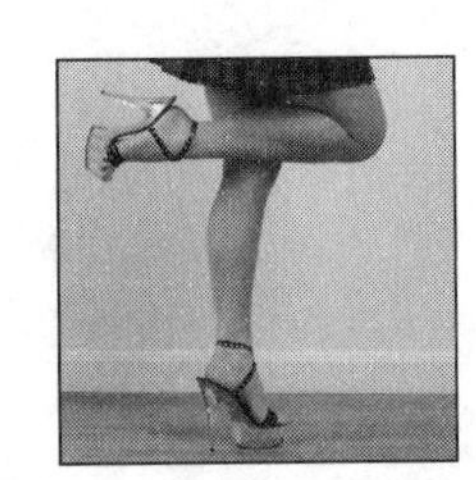 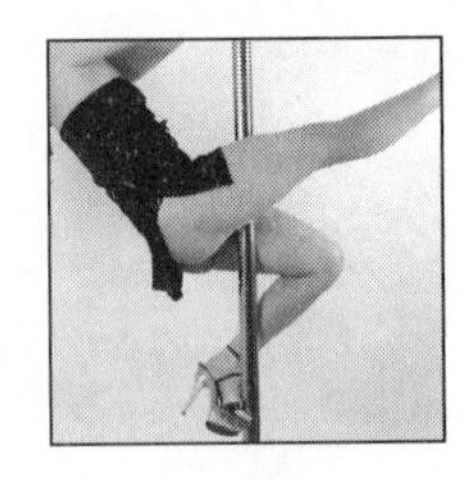 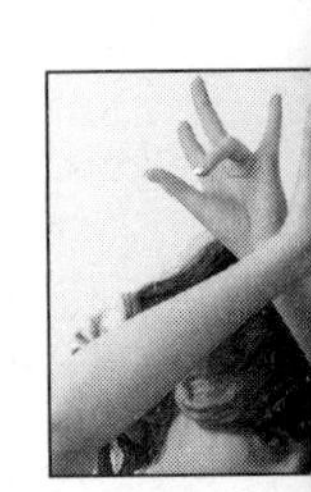

Chapter 10

Sit On It!

Lap dancing is one of the sexiest dances you can do for a man, and it's actually a lot easier than you'd think. It all comes back to my favorite phrase: sexy is a state of mind. But by now you already know that, so let's get on with the fun physical aspect of lap dancing!

It's Not Just the Lap

Lap dancing includes the show *in front of* your man as well as the actual dance *on* him. And just because you're going to be physically touching him doesn't change the main belief behind your dance, which is that you are still dancing for *you*, and he is just lucky to be there. Nothing will turn him on more than to see you performing for yourself.

So ignore him during parts of your lap dance. Take a few measures of the song to do your own thing as if he doesn't even exist, because men, as we all know, want what they can't have, including your attention. So if you ignore him several times during your dance, he'll just want you even more and pay closer attention.

Incorporating Floor Work

When you begin your dance, don't just walk up to him and plop yourself on his lap and start gyrating around. There's no warm-up there, no challenge. Just like sex, you need some foreplay to really get into the act before the actual act itself.

So you'll saunter in, admiring yourself (remember, don't prance right up in front of him and start dancing as soon as the music starts because you'll look too anxious to please him), as you step, step, pause … step, step, pause … then shoot him a sexy look. Look him up and down, grin (remember to not have a stone face), and continue to glide your fingers admiringly on yourself.

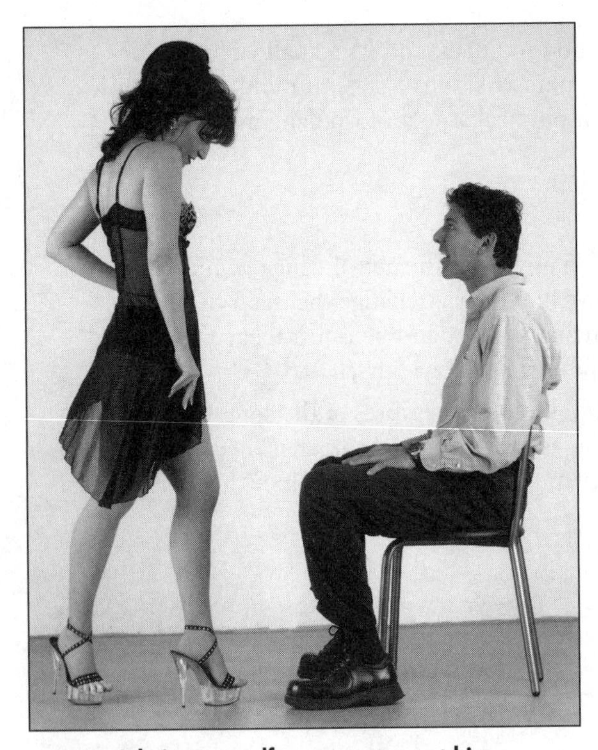

Admire yourself as you enter, not him.

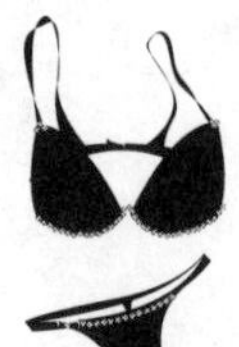

Behind the G-String

I once taught a class of five women how to lap dance on their boyfriends. To start, I did a lap dance on one of the men. When I was done, I asked him what he thought was the sexiest part of the dance, and he said, "The eye contact and the confidence." We women were all pretty floored to hear a guy say that, but he insisted that what turned him on the most was my looking at him in the eye and how confident I was as I danced.

When the song lyrics start (remember to whisper lip-sync the lyrics when appropriate), come down to the floor and do a measure or two of floor work. (Men love a butt in their face!)

Emotion in Motion

When you feel ready, crawl up to him so you're on your knees, with your arms straight up and your fingernails clawing at his chest.

This is the *only* time you should look at him as if he is your master, like you are there to please him. Stare longingly into his eyes, but not for too long—that gets creepy. Break it up by rolling your neck, looking down at yourself or at your hands as they move around him or you.

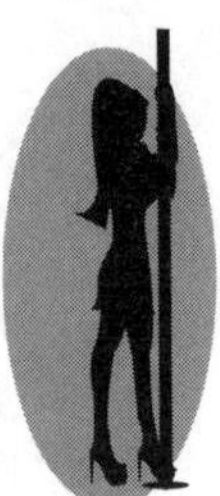

Slick Tricks

Don't actually touch his "manhood." Instead, go around it delicately with your fingers—it'll drive him wild!

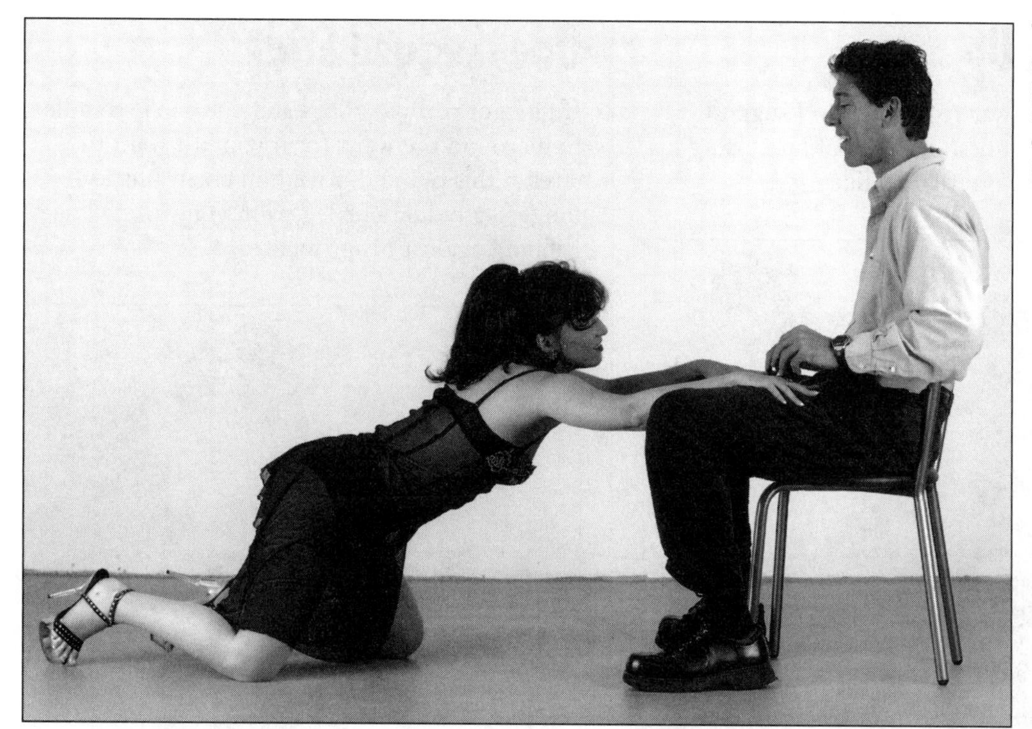

This is the only time you should look at him as if you are there to please him.

You can claw at his chest or tease him with delicate caresses of your fingertips.

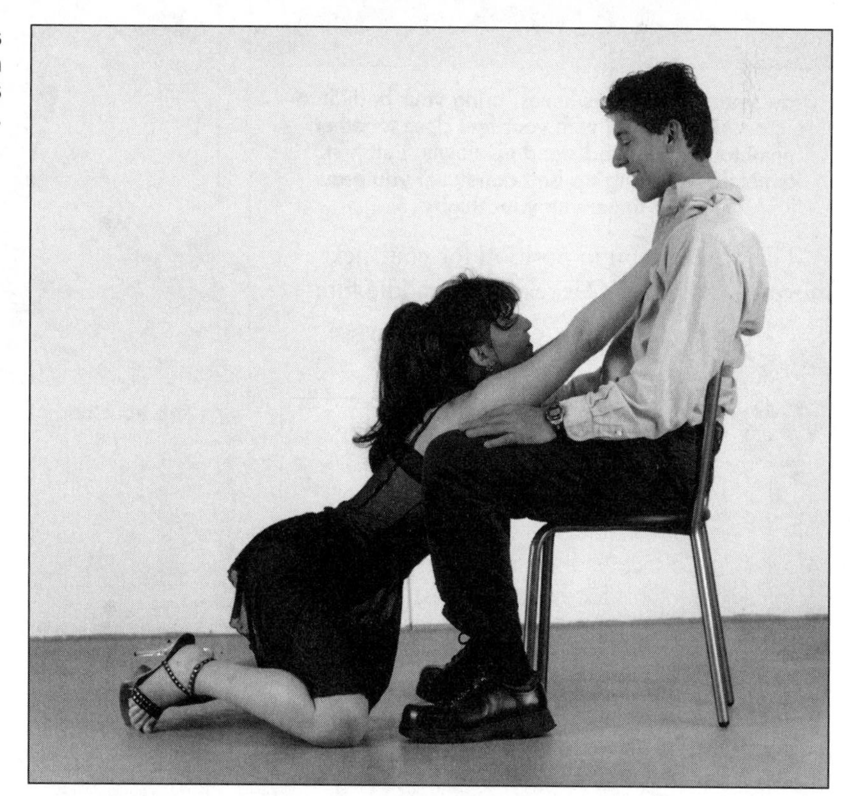

Standing Up

There's no easy way to do this, so I suggest standing up, butt first, in front of him, using his knees to balance on if you'd like.

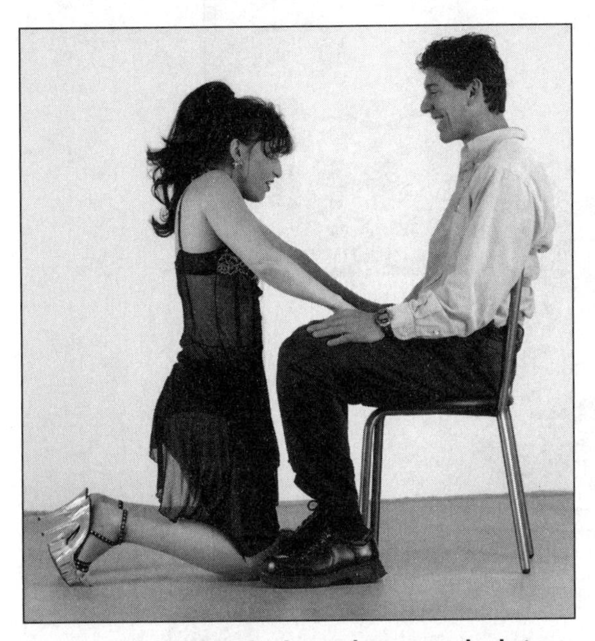

Draw your hands to his knees, bring your body into a crouching position with your feet close together, pivot to the side, and stand up slowly, butt first. Remember standing up isn't done until you draw your fingers up your thighs.

This will get you in position for your next moves—on his lap! Get ready to straddle him!

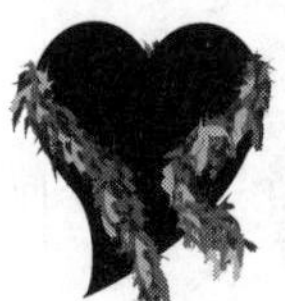

Feelin' the Love

Tonight went great … the man's in bed now, snoozing like a baby! He was utterly stunned and speechless. He wondered if I've been lying all this time about what my real night job is! The look on his face was priceless!

—Peaches, student

One-Legged Slide

If he's got really big legs and you can't straddle him around the waist (or if you just want to stretch this out and drive him crazy a little longer), straddle one leg, with your inside knee rubbing against his groin area.

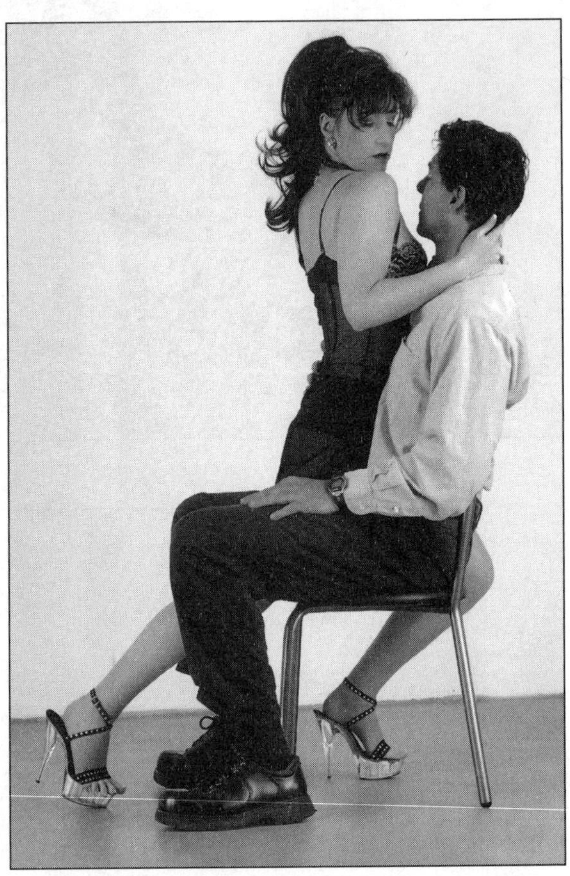

Rub your body up along his chest as you grind on his thigh.

Straddle

Then lift one leg over him and straddle him, sitting right on it. If you're on a sofa, it might be difficult to actually sit on it, but act like you are anyway. If he's in a chair (obviously without arms) you'll be able to maneuver a little more … creatively.

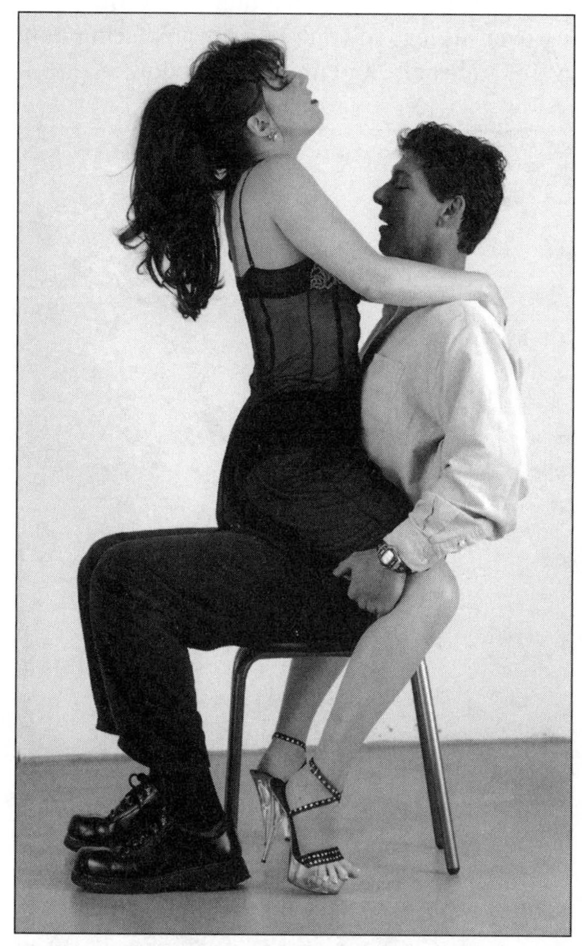

Don't be afraid to sit right on those things—you can't hurt them. And if you do, then what's a little pain for a whole lot of pleasure?

Rotate

While you're straddling him, rotate your butt around with the music or pump it up and down. Your hands, meanwhile, are gently tugging at the back of his hair, and you are breathing in his ear, giving it soft kisses, etc.

Draw Up and Down

Now draw your body up against him and either stand up if you can or extend up on your thighs so that you're coming up lengthwise from your head to your tummy. (I always thought it would be funny to wear a long dress with a ton of huge buttons, so when I drew my body up, the buttons would catch on his nose—*ping ping ping ping ping*—kind of like in a cartoon)

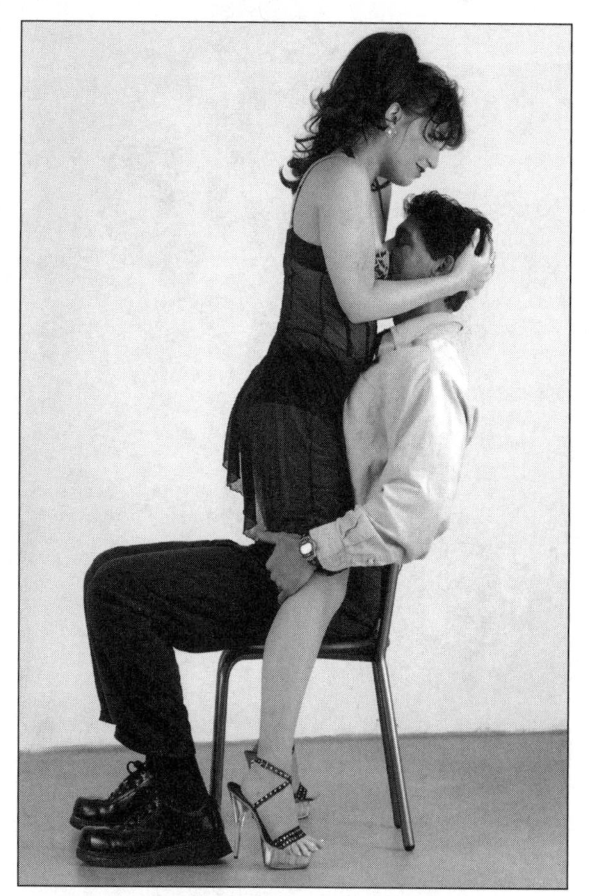

Rub your whole body along his as you slide all the way up and then all the way back down.

Now come down, again drawing your body right against his, and rotate a little more.

Getting Off (Him)

There are a few ways to get off him, and the simplest, most direct way, is to simply stand up, lift one leg off and over his lap so you end up on his side. You can also lift one leg off, step back, step back with the other leg, and slink back a few steps to your floor dancing area.

If he's sitting in a kitchen-type chair, lift one leg off and pivot around (similar to the chair move) so you are in back of him, your hand massaging his shoulders, your head bending down breathing in his ear ….

You can also claw your hand down his chest toward his groin, but again, go around it and then claw your hands back up.

Walk another step or two around him, with your arm trailing on his shoulder, and then *wham!* Surprise him by slamming your other leg over his legs so you're on his lap, facing him again, and rotate and draw up and down.

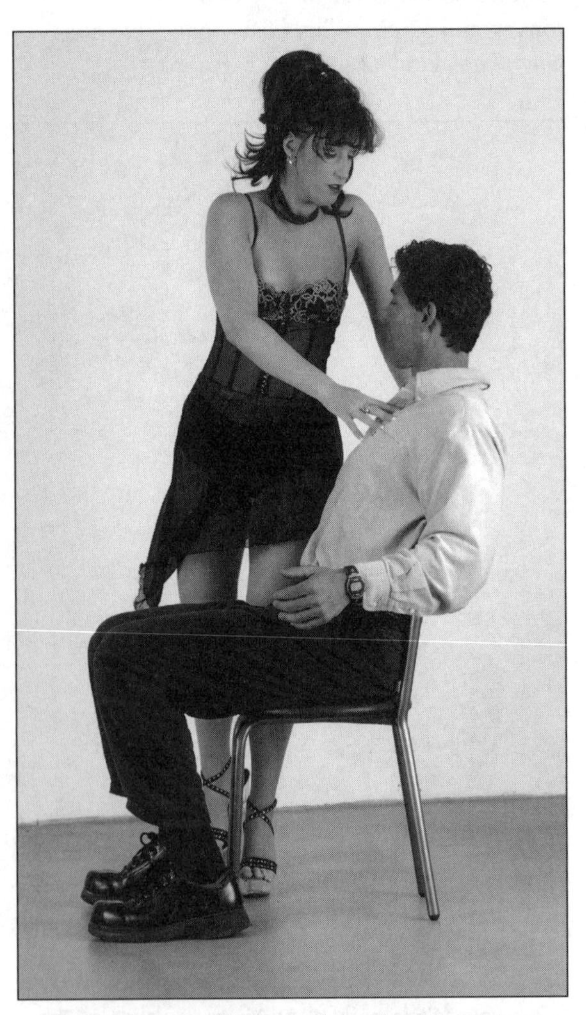

Lift your leg over his lap and step back, pivoting on your left foot to bring you around behind him.

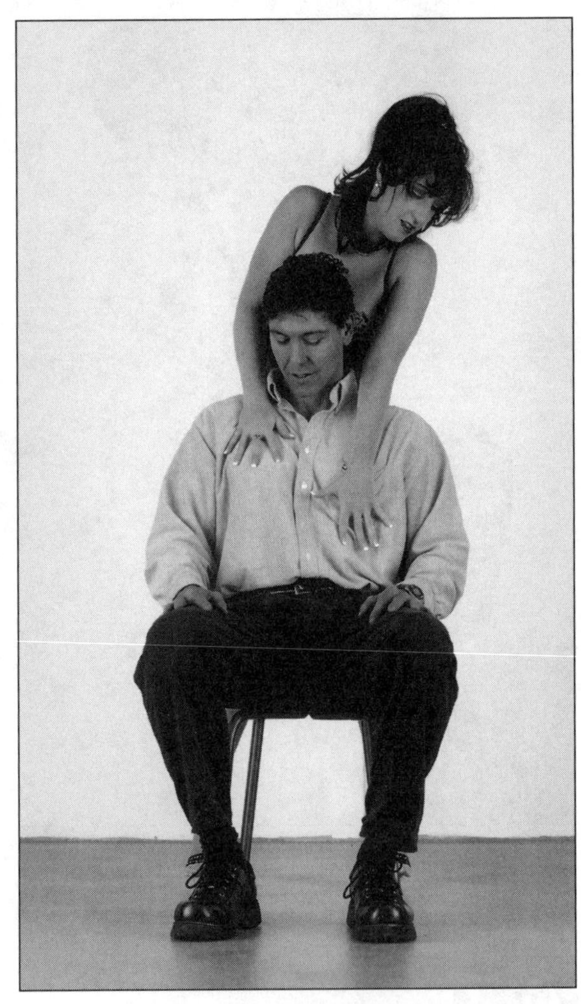

Claw your hands down his chest …

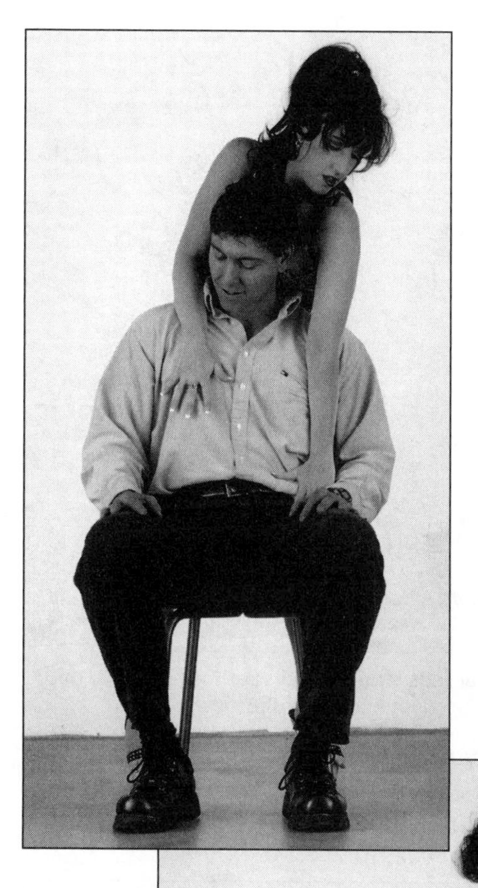

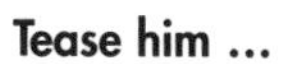

Tease him ...

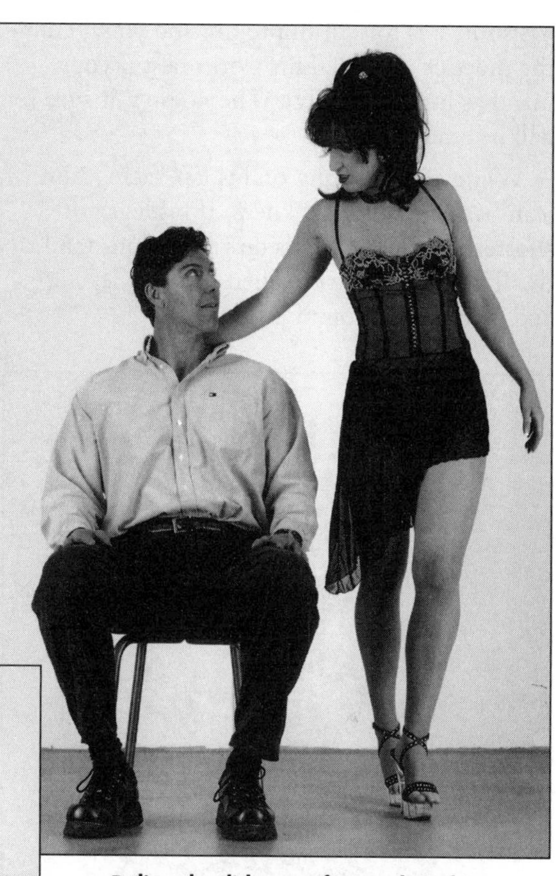

Delicately glide your finger along his shoulder as you walk around him ...

And then ... surprise him with a slam!

Leaning *Way* Back

This move is tons of fun to do, and you'll enjoy the practice as well! This works best if your man has longer legs, but if he doesn't, it sure will be amusing.

While you're sitting on his lap, facing him, lean back and grab his knees. If his legs are shorter, slide your hands down his shins (and to the floor, if necessary). Then lift your legs up and wrap them around his neck.

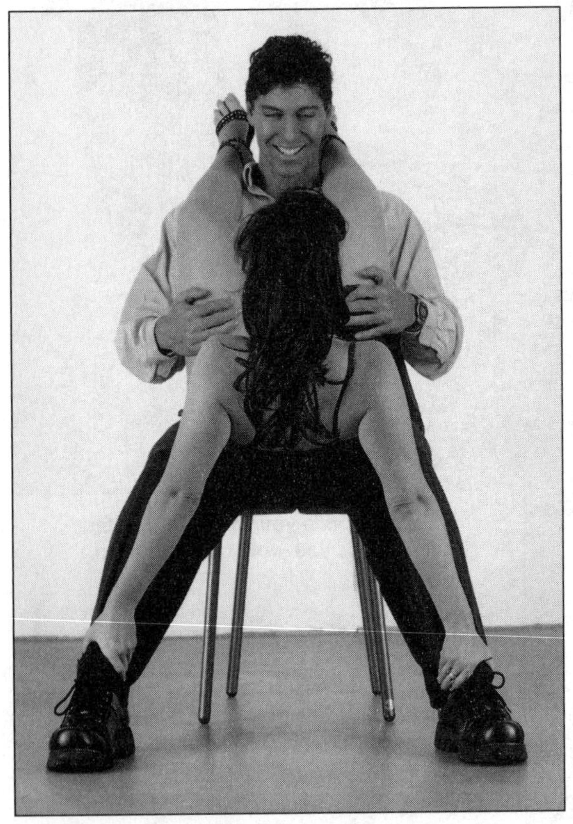

Grip either his knees or his ankles and then lift and swirl those hips!

While he's recovering from that bombshell, spread your legs in V legs. Talk about shock!

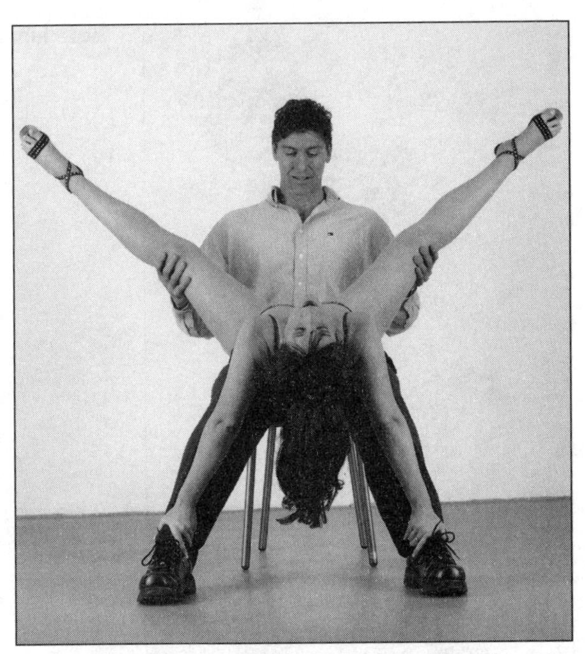

Keep your legs straight and your toes pointed, and let him enjoy the view.

Bring your legs back together after 3 seconds and then slowly ease your body down between his legs until you're lying on your back.

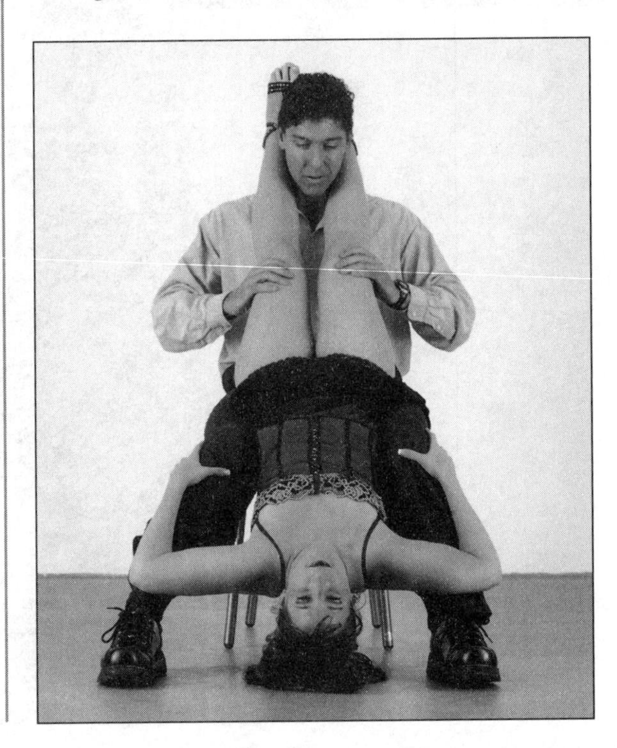

Hold onto his legs to help ease you down to the floor. Why not throw in one more V legs here for good measure! Then sensually roll into your next move.

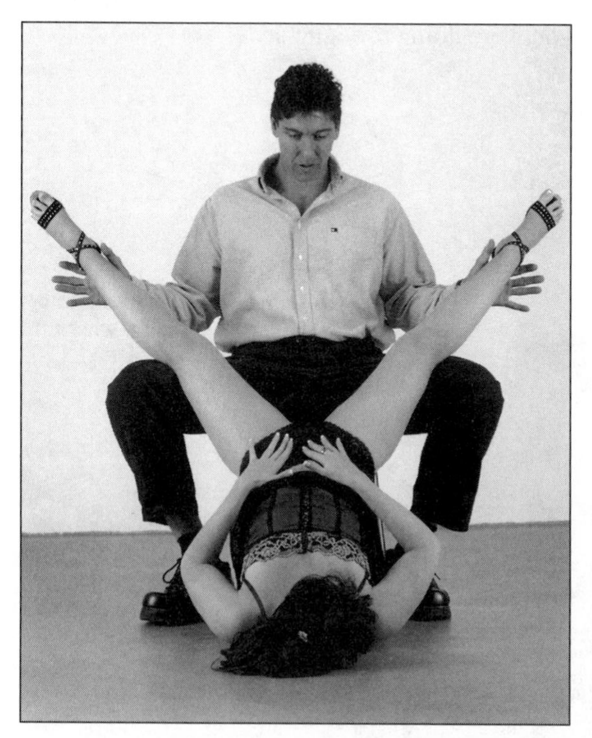

You can never spread your legs enough for a man!

Doing It Backward

When you step away from him, you can turn around with your back to him and continue to do your floor or chair work, whatever you'd like. When you're ready, stand up with your back to him, slowly back up, and then gently sit on his lap, rotating your butt around.

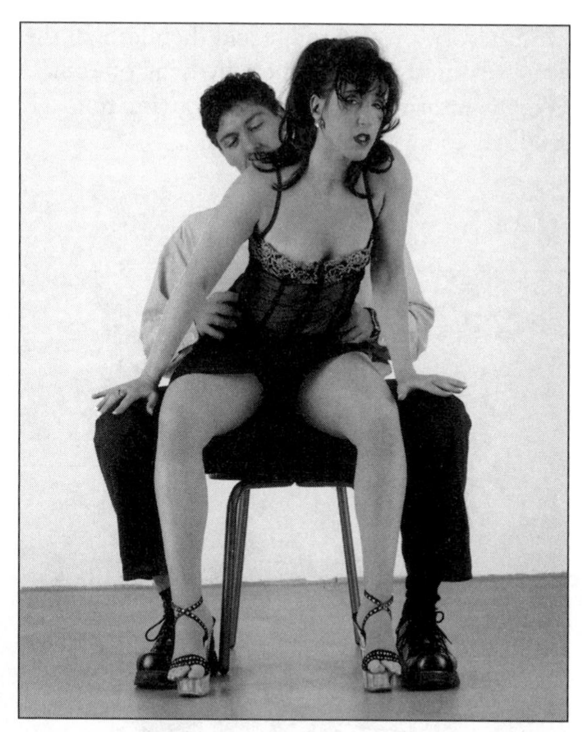

Use his knees to balance your hands as you grind into him.

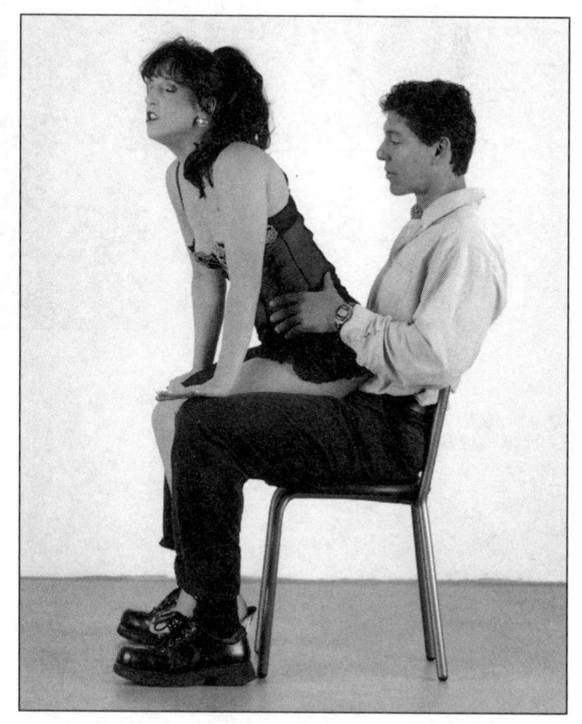

Lean forward and rotate around or rub your hips up and down on it.

Lean forward and rotate and then lean all the way back until you're essentially lying on him. Wrap your arm around his neck, giving him small kisses or whatever you'd like.

Then if you want, you can lean forward again and diva dive down so you're on the floor on your hands and knees, with your butt rotating in his face. (Men *love* this!) Now instead of rotating your butt, move it back and forth as if you were doing it doggy-style.

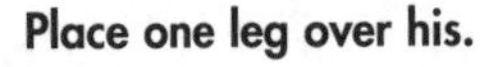

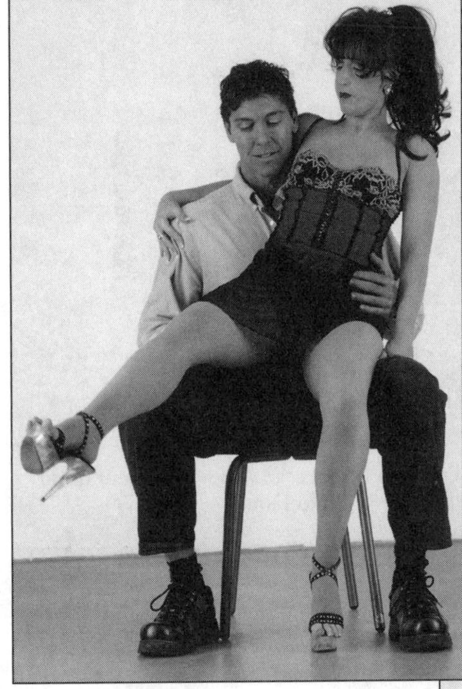

Place one leg over his.

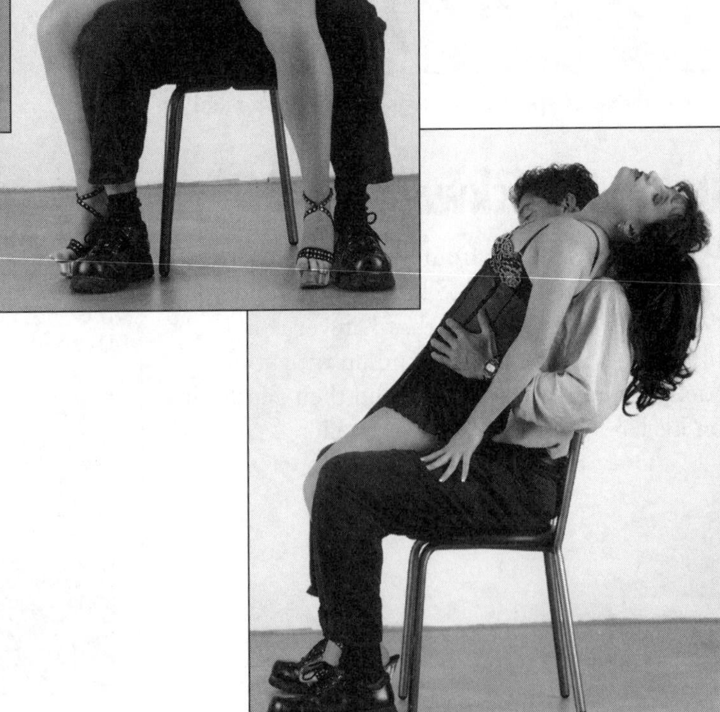

Lean back, take his hand in yours, and glide it where you want it to go!

Don't forget the drama!

Lap Crawl

Lap crawling doesn't actually take you anywhere like regular crawling takes you from point A to point B, but I don't think your man will complain ....

First sit on his lap with your back to him and rotate around. Now slide your hands down his legs while lifting your own legs up, bent at the knee so you're still on him yet in a crawling position facing forward.

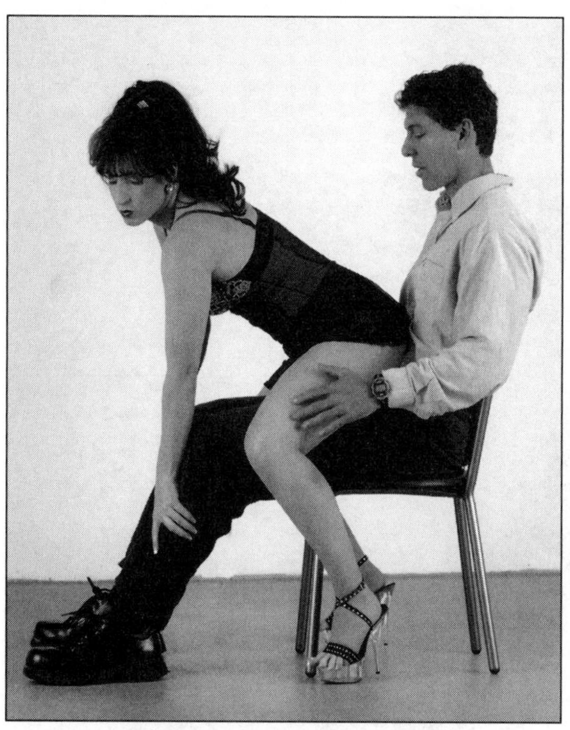

Close his legs and lean forward.

You'll have to maneuver his legs around, so take charge and do it! If he resists because he's not sure what's going on, say to him, "Let me move your legs." Rotate around in this position, leaning forward as you continue to pulsate your hips with the undercurrent of the song.

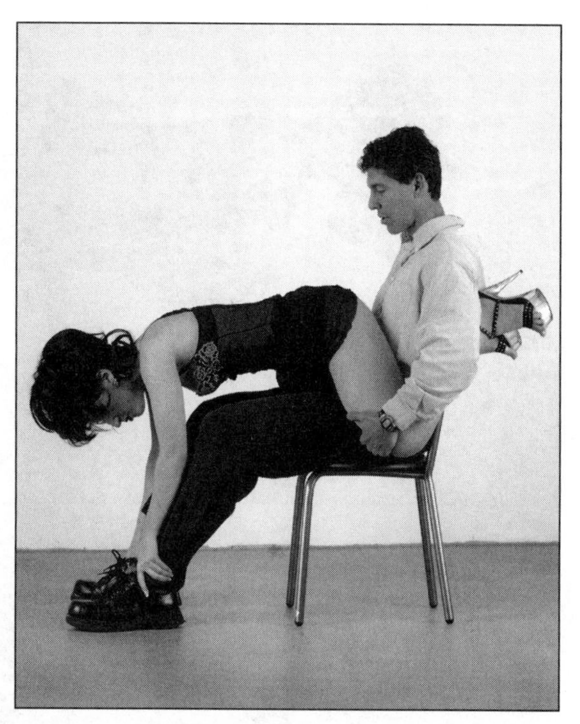

Slide your hands down his shins for balance as your butt moves farther up his chest.

You might have to tell him to hold your legs. Giving direction during your lapdance is essential because he will be so nervous and want to do everything correctly that he'll keep his legs stiff.

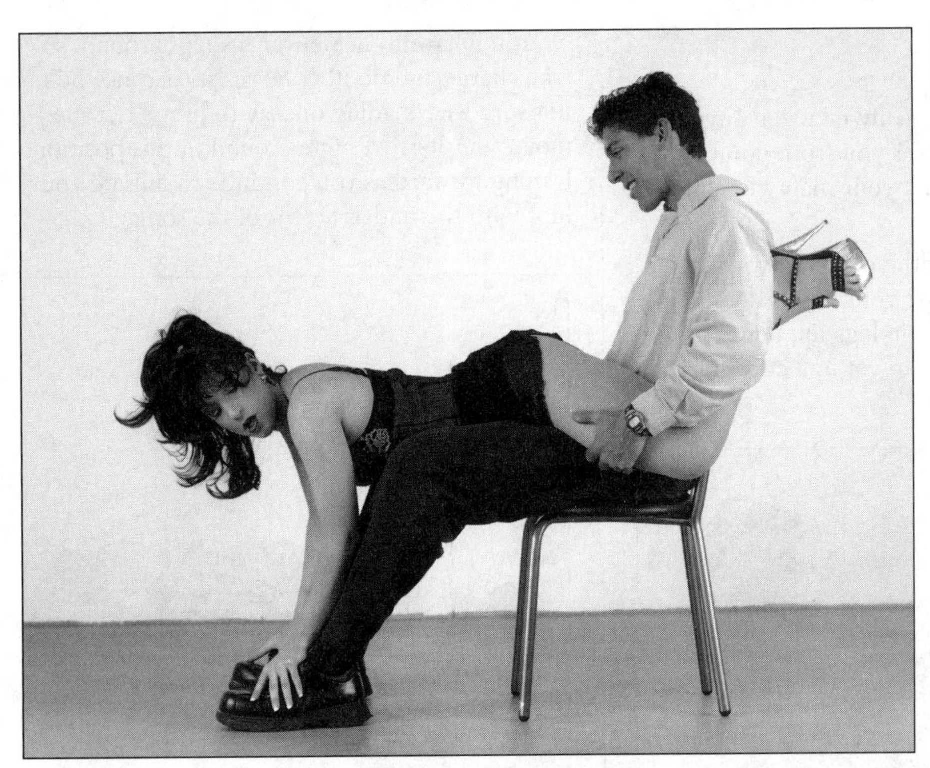

Lean all the way forward so your hips meet his.

Slide yourself up in one graceful move.

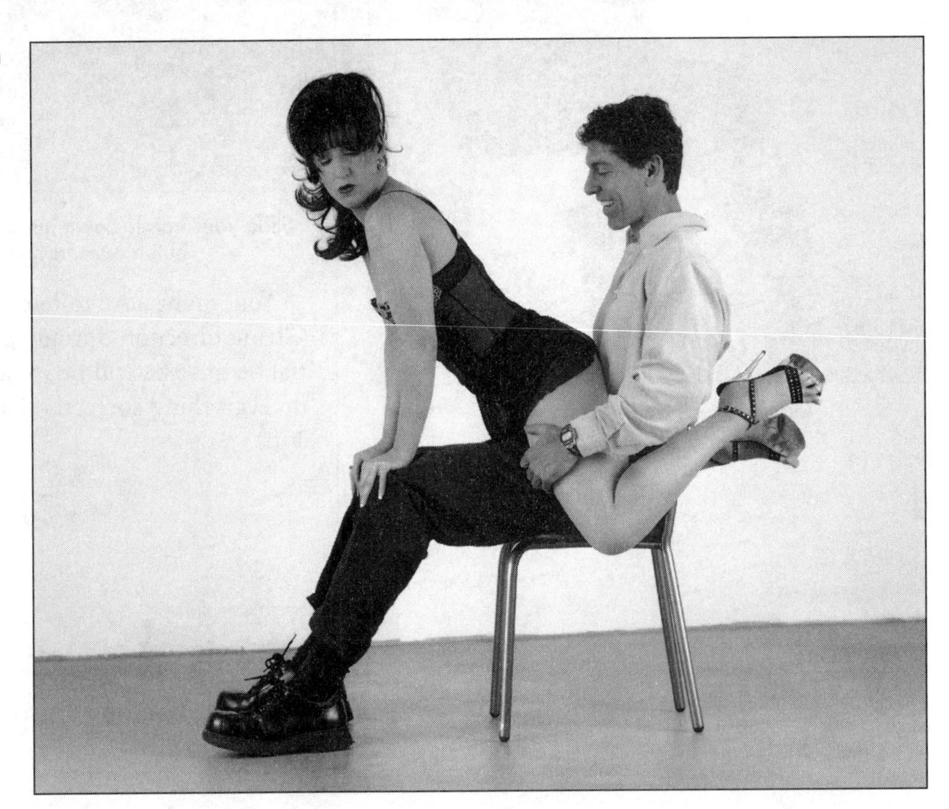

It's most comfortable to bend your knees so your legs provide a counterbalance, but just remember that your main focus is your arms. That's where all the pressure should go; your legs are just lightly holding on. Besides, if you dig your heels into his shoulder blades, it might ruin the mood …

Then, when you feel he's had enough, sit back up the way you started or crawl forward down to the floor. If you choose to sit up, this will take some muscle control because you want to do it in one fluid movement, not inch by inch. This will also instantly sit you back down on his lap, where you can grind some more before you slide off into your next move. That is, if he lets you go!

The Least You Need to Know

- As with other dancing, act like you're lap dancing for your pleasure, not his.
- When you're moving around him, keep your fingers lightly massaging the back of his neck, his chest, his legs, etc.—whatever's handy.
- Go *around* his "manhood" rather than touch it directly. He'll get more turned on.
- Don't be afraid to direct him during the lap dance.

In This Chapter

- Shirt, jacket, skirt, and dress teases
- Timing your striptease
- Humor: why you must use it

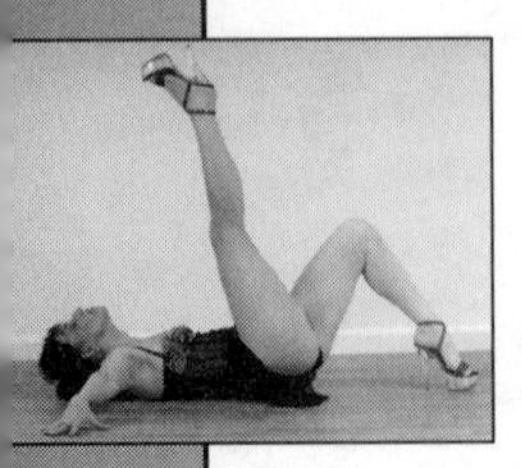
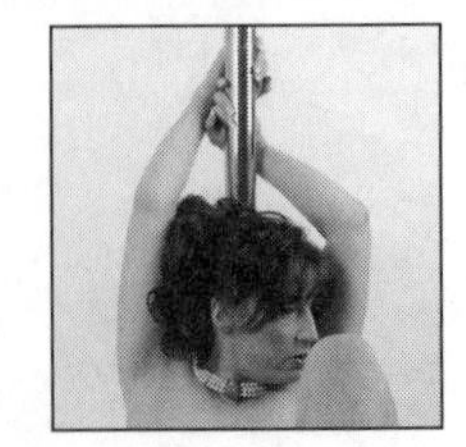
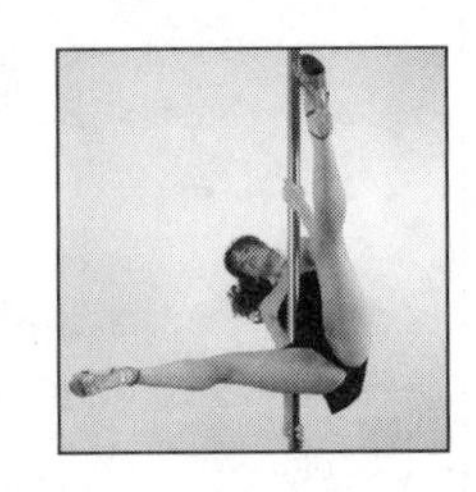
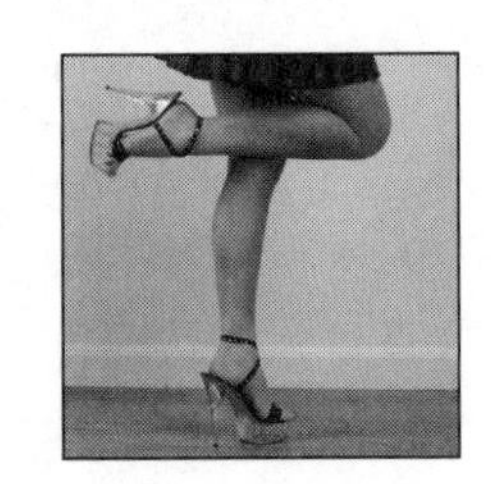
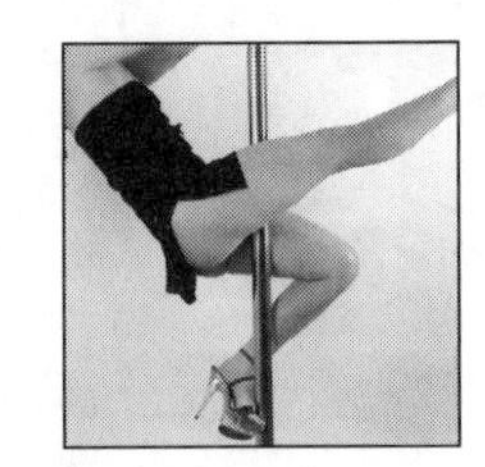
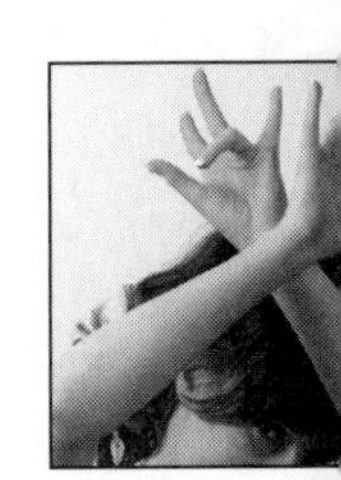

Chapter 11

Taking It Off with a Tease

Now the most important part of the whole dance (or at least the part your audience has been anxiously waiting for) … the tease! And the key word there is *tease*. People want what they can't have. They want to see what's secret. And guess who has the power to decide when … and if … they get to see anything at all? You do! Use that power to drive them crazy!

Seeing Double

This has got to be one of the sexiest tricks ever, and no skin is even seen! Just put on a pair of underwear or a thong over your real underwear. After your entrance and he sees how good you look, turn around so your back is to him. Reach up underneath your skirt and pull the decoy underwear down so it's above your knees.

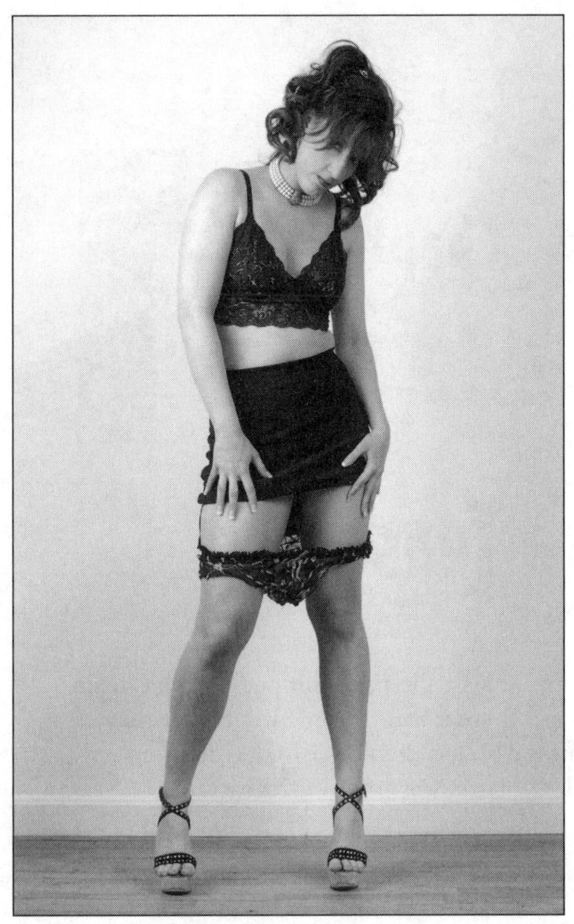

Bring your underwear down to just above your knees to be sure he sees it.

Now turn around and walk a few steps back and forth so he can admire the fact that your underwear is down!

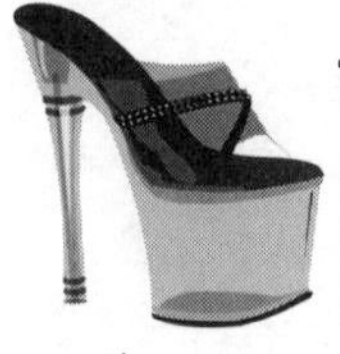

Trippin' Up

Be sure your decoy underwear isn't too loose; otherwise, it'll just fall right down, and you'll lose the effect.

When you're ready to take it off, turn your back to him again, stop moving, and put your feet together. Pull the underwear down so it's around your ankles and then step out with one foot so the underwear is still draped over the other toe. Kick the underwear into the air, catch it with your hand, and turn around to face him. You can either just toss the underwear away or at him, whatever you want to do.

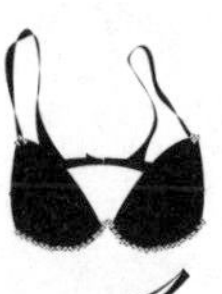

Behind the G-String

When I was a club dancer, I would pretend to shoot my underwear at the customers, and they'd all put their hands up like they wanted to catch it and looked disappointed when I faked them out. Then I would pretend to sniff them and declare, "Oh no, you wouldn't want these, they're stinky!" The guys would erupt with laughter!

Eyelet Tease

We all love our butt, don't get me wrong, but sometimes it's sexier if we don't see it all at once. Just show him a little now—and let him know you'll show the rest when you're good and ready!

Tan lines are incredibly sexy, so tease him with those, too. To him, he's seeing something forbidden.

Pull your skirt down in the back until just an eyelet shape of your butt cheeks is showing. If you've got hips, the skirt can rest on your butt while you dance around, so there's no need to take it off right away.

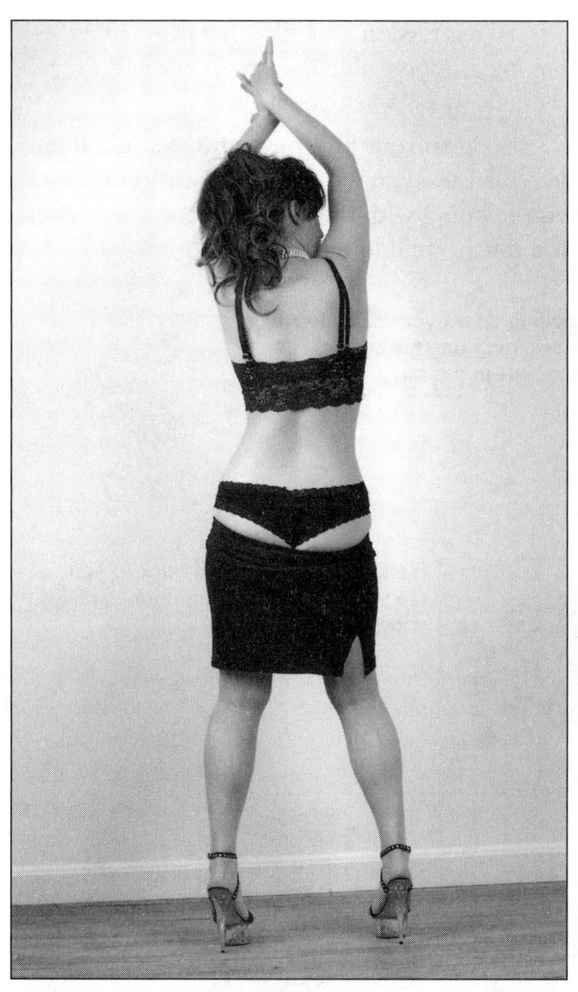

Reveal only a little of your butt, and make him wait for the rest!

Dance around a bit more and then continue peeling. When you're finally ready to take it off, put your legs together, either facing him or not, and lean over, alternately bending one knee while the other is straight.

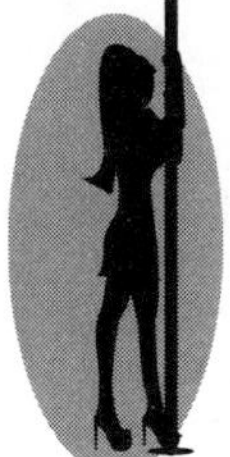

Slick Tricks

I prefer to do this not facing, and thus not acknowledging, my man because then it's like he's secretly watching me take off my clothes.

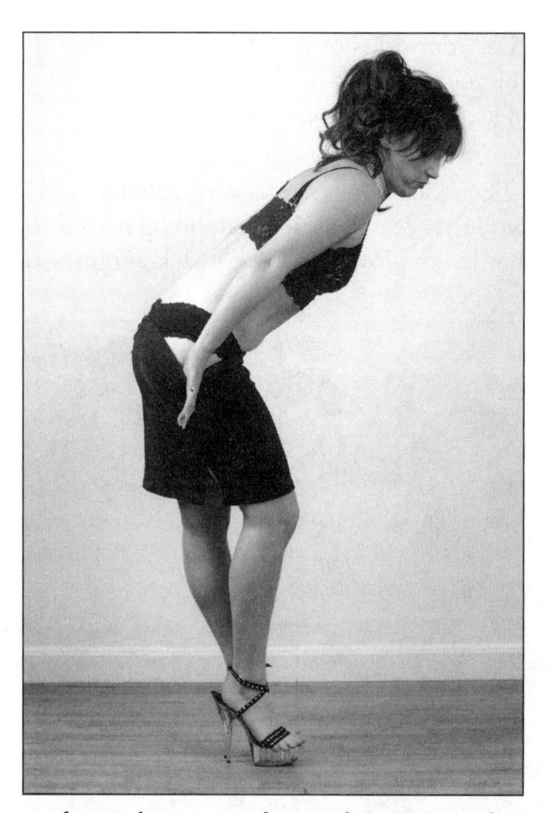

Lean forward as you work your skirt over your butt.

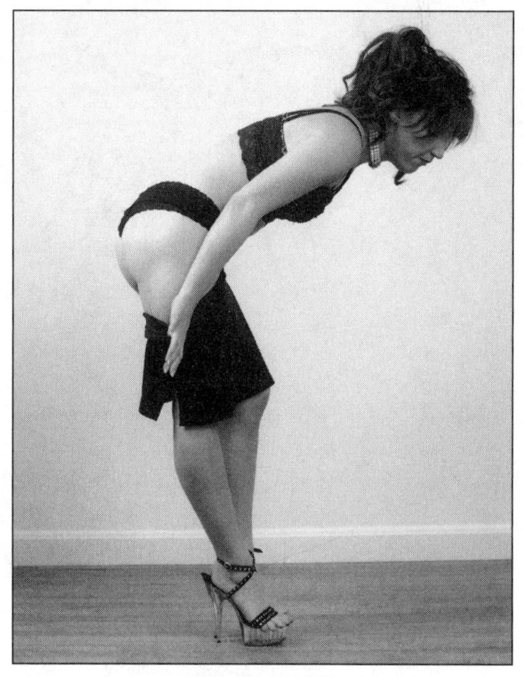

Keep your feet together and stop dancing as you lower your skirt.

Let your dress or skirt fall to your ankles (you might have to help it down if it's tight), and step out with one foot, leaving material over the other toe.

Then kick up the dress/skirt, catch it, and whip it between your legs, grabbing it with the other hand. Now slowly look back at him with a facial expression that says, *You wish you were this dress*, as you slide the dress back and forth seductively between your legs.

Also keep your butt pulsating to a minimum here because you want him to focus on what you're doing with the dress. If your butt moves too much, we'll lose the effect.

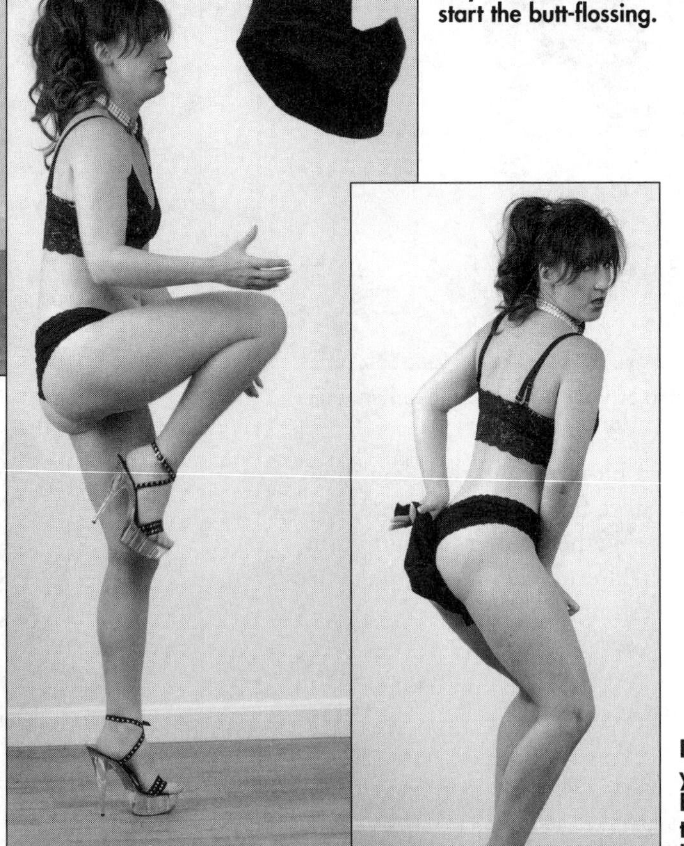

When pulling down your skirt, leave some fabric over one toe so you can kick your skirt in the air.

Kick your skirt up and back to you so you can catch it, and immediately start the butt-flossing.

Don't saw yourself in half! Be sure not to sway your butt too much because you want him to focus on what you're doing.

Jacket Tease

The sexiest outfit you can ever wear is a business suit. Period. It's strong, it's sexy, and it leaves a lot to the imagination, particularly when you're teasing with your jacket.

You can also do this trick with a man's shirt or any other kind of button or zip-up-style piece of clothing. When you want to begin taking off your jacket, unbutton one button and show him some cleavage. Dance around a little more until you're ready to undo the second, and the third. (Never button more than three buttons with a jacket.)

You also don't want to open up just one side completely, because then it looks like you're selling stolen watches on the street. In fact, wrap your jacket around you tighter. He knows it's undone so he's expecting to see something exciting, so drive him crazy and act shy.

When you're ready to reveal, slide one side of the jacket to the side, exposing one breast and the side of your body. Take care not to expose your whole tummy, and keep the other side of the jacket covering up everything except the exposed breast and your side. Now you can do the same with the opposite side, again making sure you cover your tummy and reveal just a boob and a slice of skin.

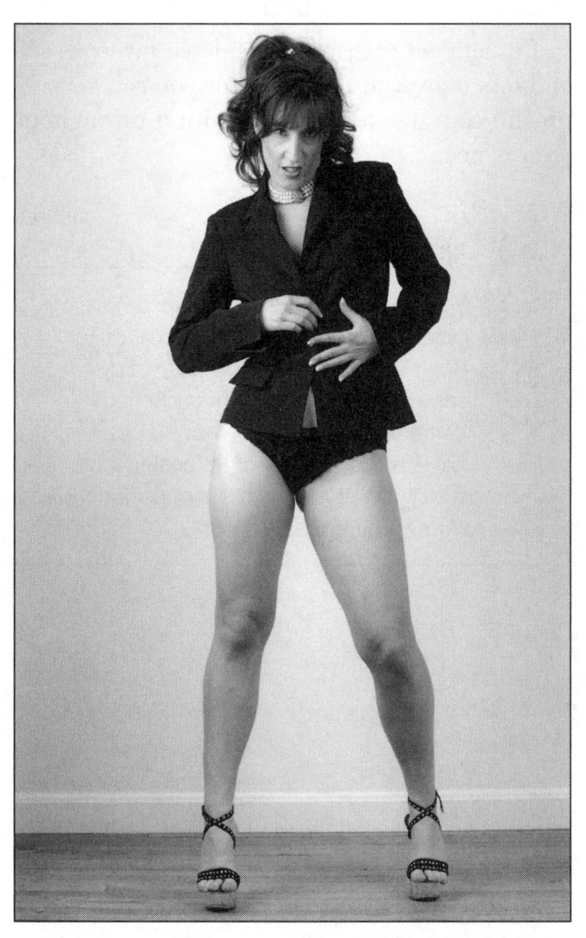

When your buttons are undone, don't just open up the jacket and let him see everything!

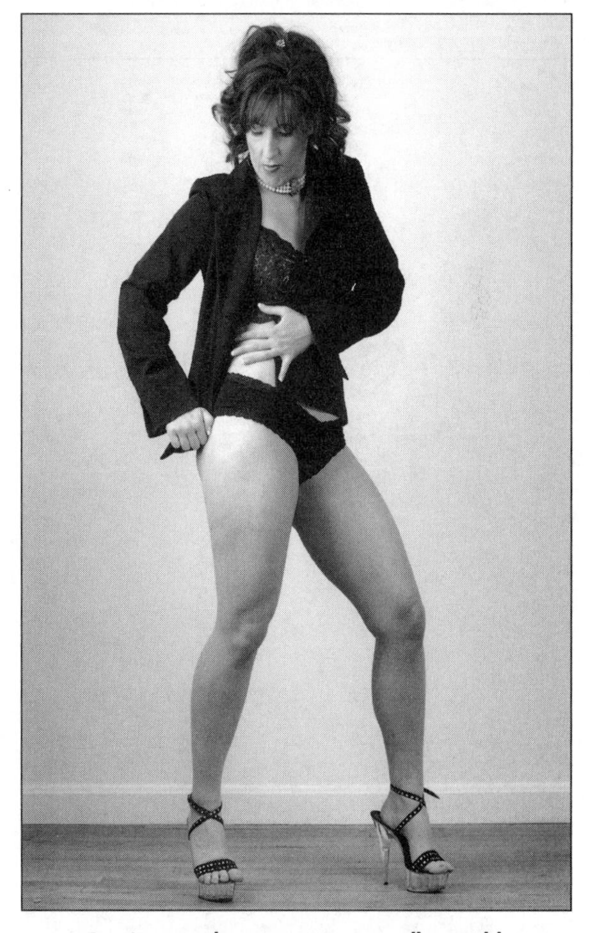

Continue to dance as you normally would, which means you can let go of the jacket and let the sides go wherever.

Now here's a tease that will completely drive him wild! You'll need to be sure you're wearing the V-shaped booty shorts; otherwise, for this trick to work you'll have to make a wedge with your underwear.

Turn so your back is facing him, and using the opposite hands for the opposite arms, reach over and pull your jacket down to your elbows. Let your bra straps fall with it. This works best if your bra straps are the same color as the jacket, so in the dark lighting he can't tell where the bra ends and the jacket begins.

If you've got long hair, try to swish it so it rests on your chest, because we really want to expose as much of the back as we can here. Be sure that jacket is down to your elbows.

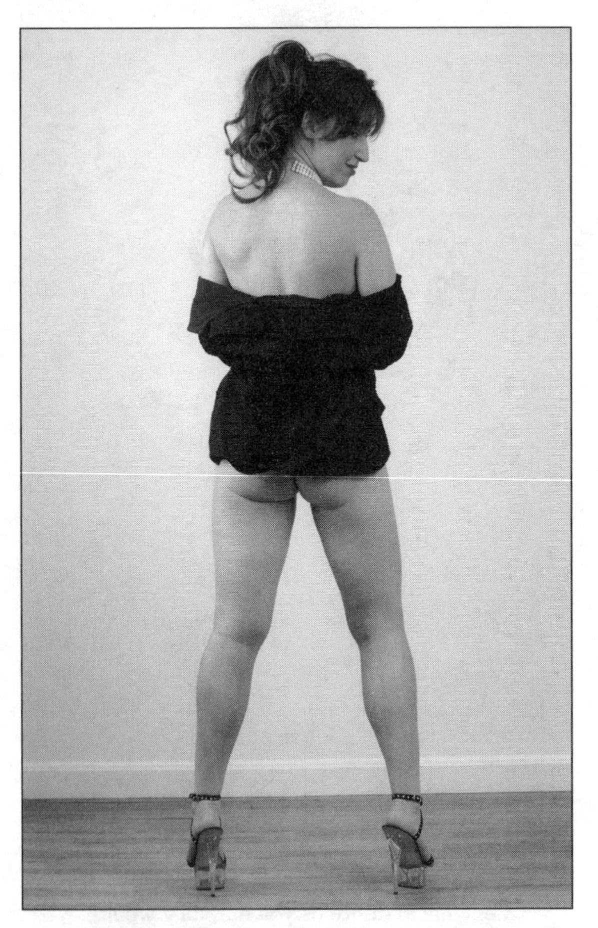

Depending on how long the jacket is depends on if you have to subtly pull it up or pull it down.

Regardless of the jacket length, you want just a hint of your butt showing so that from behind, you look naked. Practice this in the mirror until you can bring your jacket down smoothly, with your bra straps, to your elbows, as well as so you know how high or low you have to adjust your jacket to get that perfect hint of butt.

Roll your shoulders now, one at a time, and look over your shoulder at him with a super sultry expression.

Now shoulder roll turn around, your hands still clutching the sides of the jacket. Saunter up to him so he can see your cleavage, and maybe draw one of your fingers along said cleavage (while still holding on to the jacket).

I usually let the jacket ride down my arms and toss it away at this point, or you can keep it on and continue to tease him with it throughout your dance.

Slick Tricks

When you unbutton or unzip or unsnap anything, particularly a shirt or jacket, don't just open it up for the world to see. Keep hiding what's underneath. Remember, he wants what he can't have, so tease him by exposing one breast and covering the other and then vice versa. Keep him guessing!

Make 'Em Big!

You can make cleavage! It's really easy. (This is the only way I can do it.) Bring your bra or dress straps down over your shoulders and then insert your fingers, bending them so your knuckles are down by your nipples.

Now push your boobs up and together and roll only your hands, *not your shoulders*, as you lean forward.

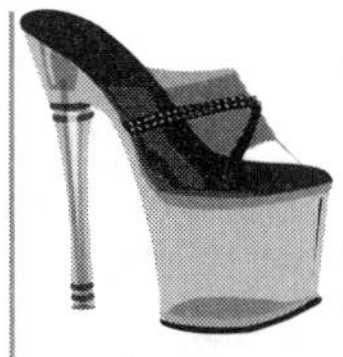

Trippin' Up

Be sure that when you're making the cleavage, you aren't covering up your boobs with your hands.

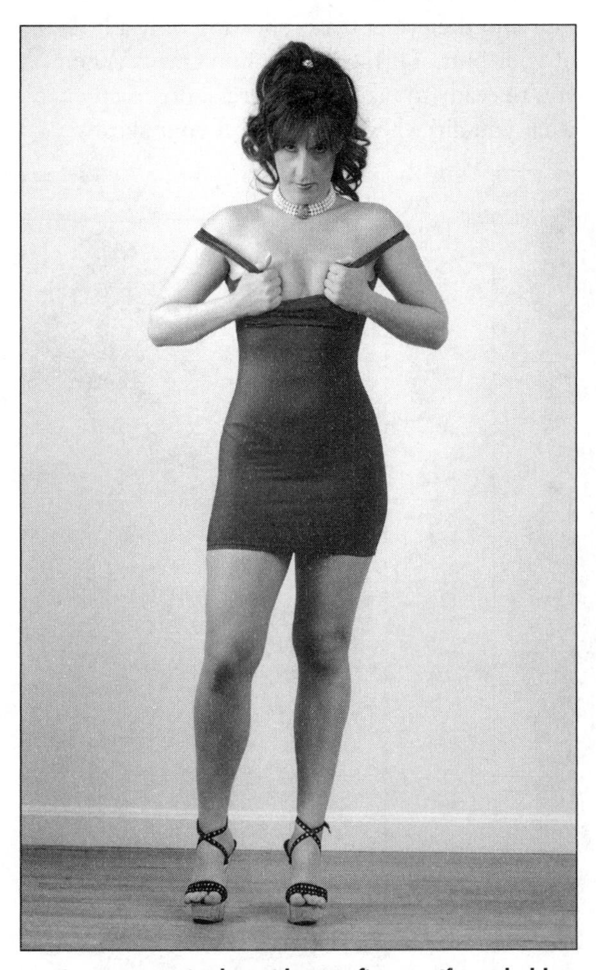

Cover your nipples with your fingers. If you hold them any higher, you'll hide the cleavage.

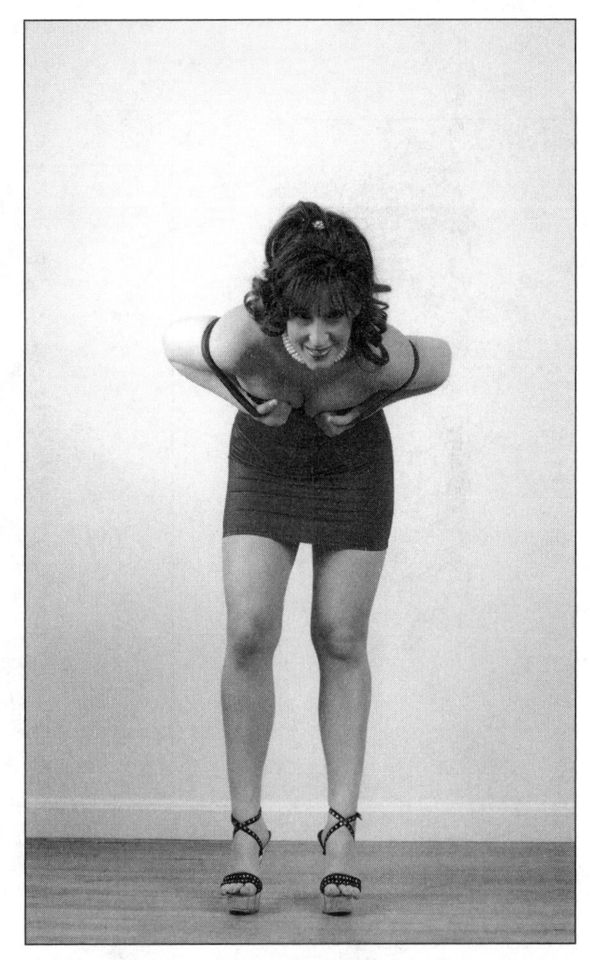

Push your boobs up and in, rolling only your hands, not your shoulders.

Slow Peel

When you're wearing a dress, you always want to peel it down. Very rarely do you want to take anything off over your head (because in doing so you're just inviting havoc, especially if you're wearing a fake ponytail or large earrings).

When you're ready to peel off your dress, use one arm to take the other out of its sleeve as seductively as you can.

Then just leave it. Yes, I said leave it.

Then do the same with the other arm, and peel your dress down slowly so that you've got a skirt and bra effect. Now as intelligent women, we would think, *Oh, a bra and skirt.* Men, however, think *Peeled-down dress!* … and that which is forbidden turns them on. Dance around for a while with the peeled-down dress because that keeps them intrigued … yet they still have seen nothing, and it is up to you when—and if—they will be so lucky to see anything at all.

Now you can peel your dress down just a little more do the eyelet tease, showing only a little bit of your butt. This will drive him crazy! When you're ready to take off the dress, do exactly what you did when stripping off your skirt.

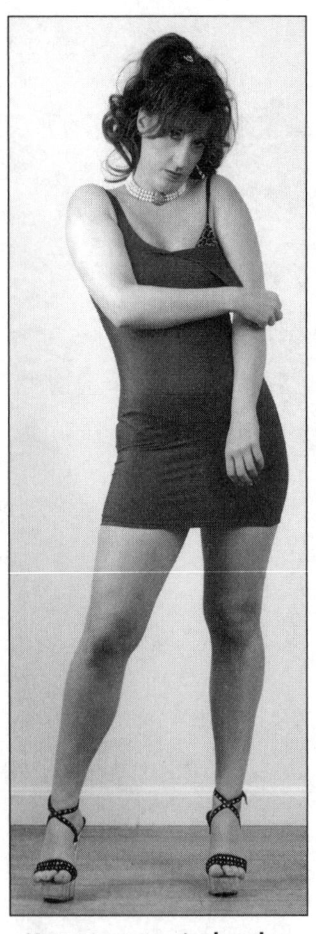

Use your opposite hand to pull your sleeve down.

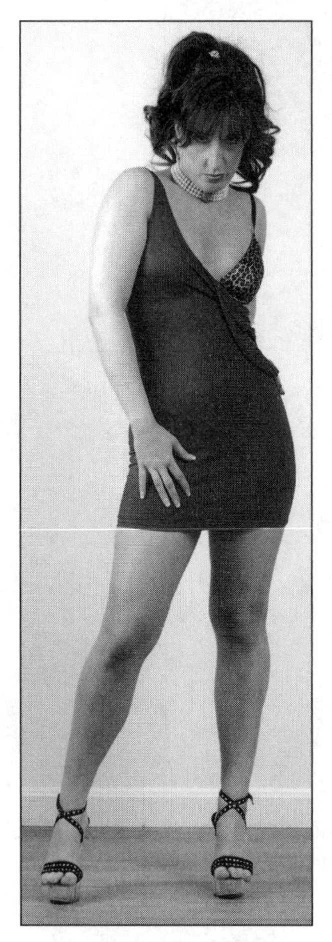

Leave one sleeve off, and continue your dance.

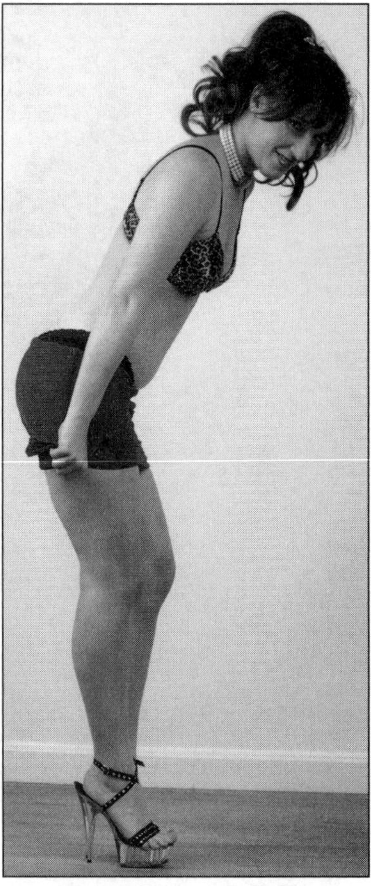

Treat your dress as if it was a skirt, and continue with your eyelet tease.

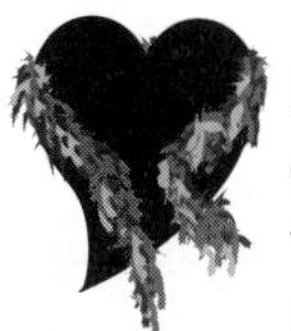

Feelin' the Love

When I auditioned at the O'Farrell Theater in San Francisco, I wore a beautiful tight white velvet Betsy Johnson dress that just happened to have a slight turtleneck. When it came time for me to remove the dress, I got my head trapped under the tiny dress neck and had to run backstage to take it off!

—Rose Mittleman, pole instructor, Slinky Productions, San Francisco

Skirts, Shirts, and Shorts

I'm sure you know this already, but one of the sexiest outfits, in a perverted sort of way, that 99 percent of guys love is the schoolgirl uniform. So here's the obligatory schoolgirl striptease, which is a great example of how to do a tease out of any kind of combination skirt/shirt costume.

There are so many teases with this costume, one of the sexiest being the shoulder tease. Use your opposite hand to slide down both the shirt and your bra strap, and rotate your shoulder around. Be sure to remember your bra strap; the shirt itself doesn't have the same effect unless you expose your whole shoulder.

The schoolgirl uniform can have any number of skirt variations, from zippers to buttons to elastic to Velcro. The uniform I'm wearing comes with a Velcro skirt, which adds a lot of unique striptease moves to this dance.

As with any skirt strip, you want your audience to see that you're considering taking off your skirt, so you want to stand so your clasp mechanism faces the audience. Slowly peel back the Velcro, and you'll have him eating out of your hand!

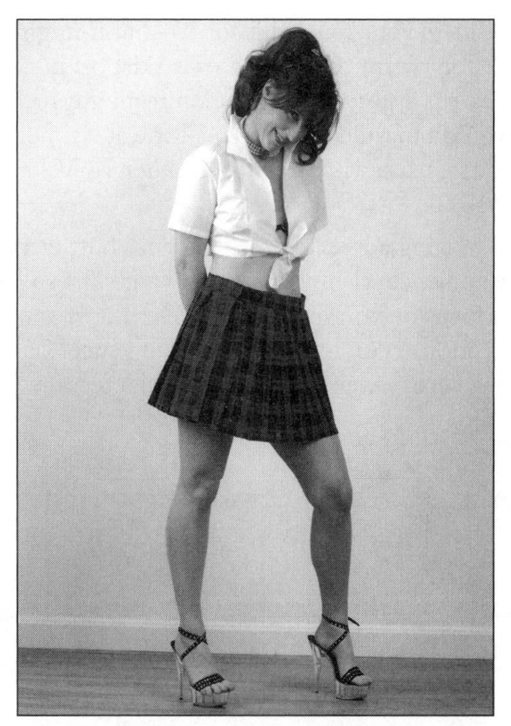

Men just love the innocent schoolgirl uniform!

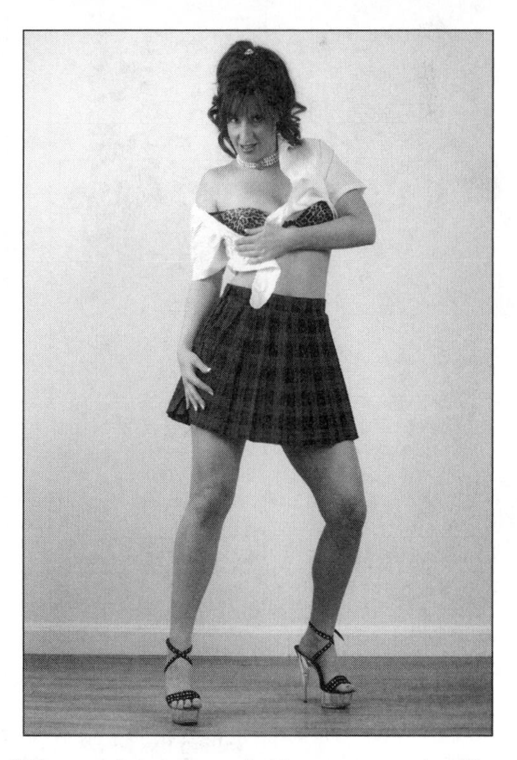

Slide your bra strap and shirt over your shoulder.

Unless your song calls for it—and it might—you don't want to just tear your skirt off in one quick rip. I got a great reaction from guys when I would unfasten the Velcro a little at a time, or undo it, tease with my hip, and then re-Velcro the skirt.

I'm a big advocate of having your butt facing the audience when you take off your skirt so he can focus on your butt, and a Velcro skirt is no exception. With my back to the audience, I undo the Velcro, lowering it into an eyelet tease.

Let him admire that little bit of skin for a few moments and then continue to play with your skirt. Let one side fall completely, and use the skirt as a scarf to slide all over your shoulders or even between your legs.

You can coyly wrap your skirt around you as if you're suddenly Little Miss Modest, or you can tease your man with it, wrap it around his neck, or even go down onto the floor and dramatically slide it over your legs, thighs, or anywhere else that turns you (and him) on!

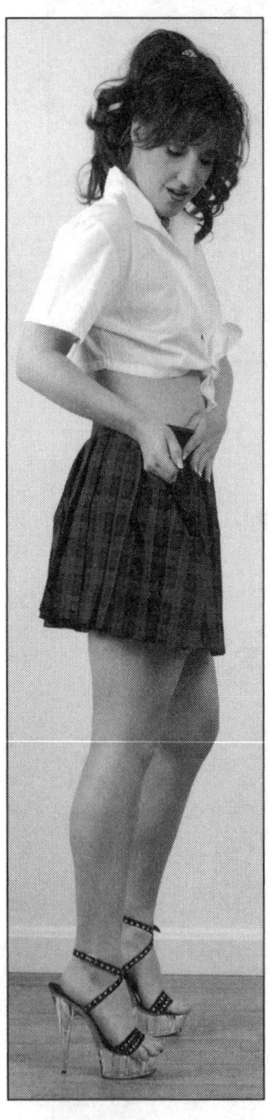

Be sure he sees that you're contemplating removing your skirt.

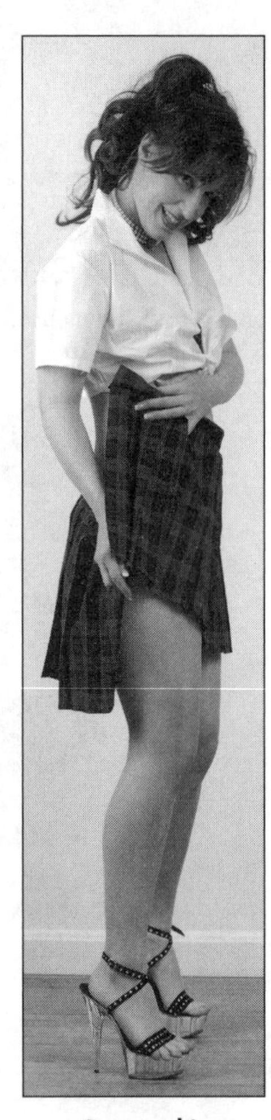

Capture his attention by not taking the whole skirt completely off at once.

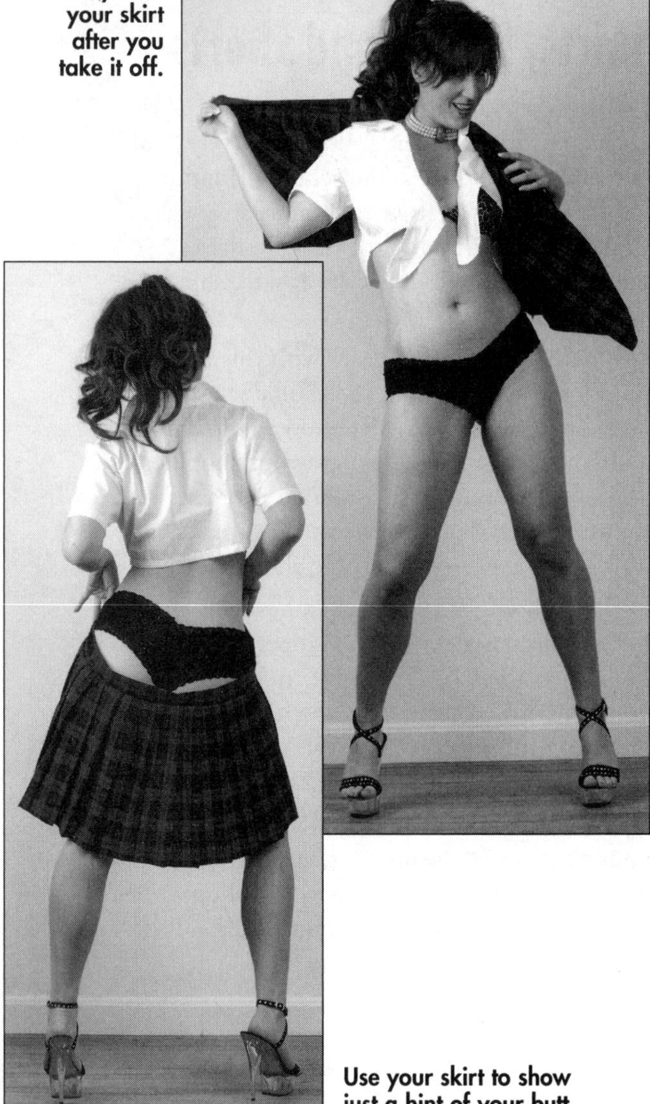

Play with your skirt after you take it off.

Use your skirt to show just a hint of your butt.

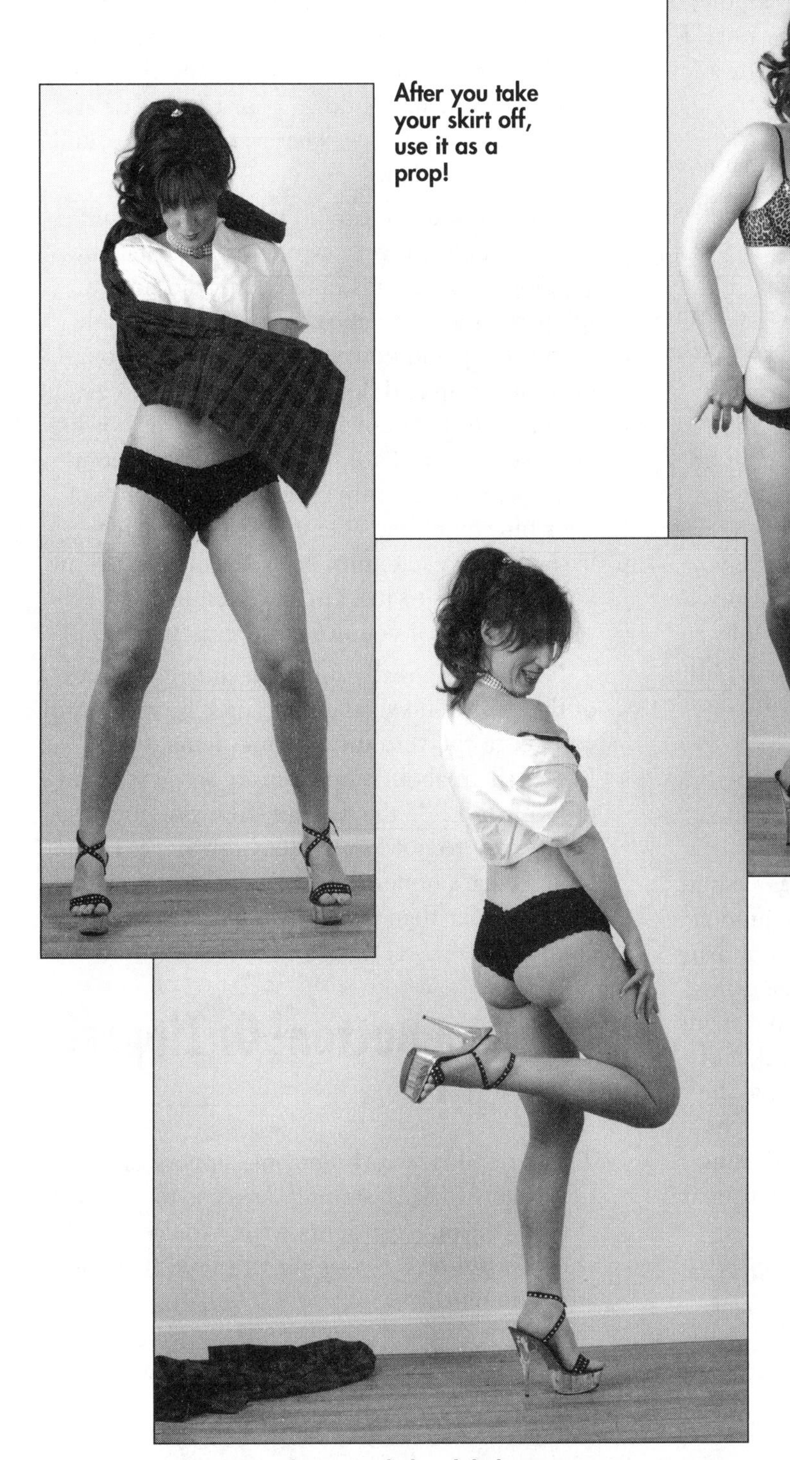

After you take your skirt off, use it as a prop!

Leave your shirt on a little while longer so you can tease all the way to the end!

Be sure to lift your panty sides alternately, about 4 or 5 inches above or below where they would normally rest.

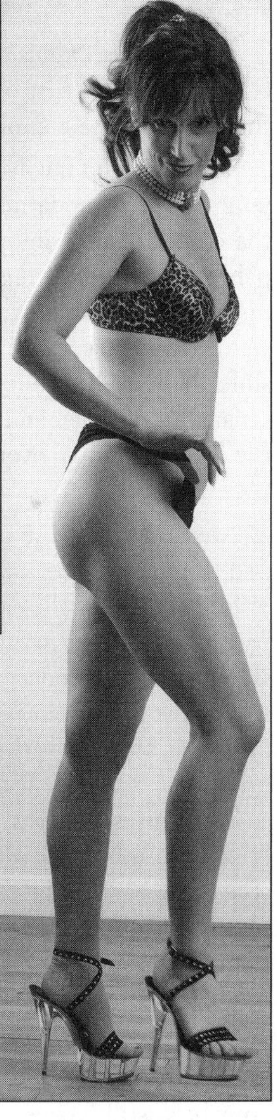

Lift your panties about an inch away from your hips, with just your thumb entwined, to ensure for smoother sliding.

Now that your skirt is off, you still have your shirt to play with. When I wear this costume, or any costume with a button-down or tie shirt, I tend to leave it on for the whole dance for a few reasons:

- The audience never forgets your character.
- It gives you something to do as you dance.
- It's sexier to continuously tease.

There are all kinds of fun ways to tease with bras and panties that will drive your man crazier than if you were completely naked.

The first one involves just your bra. Slide your hands up underneath the cups, lifting up the cups and covering your nipples with your palms. Be sure to bring your pinkies all the way up to the bottom of your nipples, because you want to show as much "bottom boob" as possible. Now rotate your hands so your boobs rub sensually together, and when you're ready, bring the bra back down over your boobs so he hasn't seen a thing!

Another sexy tease that also involves the bra and the panties starts with your back to him. While you're swirling your hips, lower your panties so you've got about 1 inch of your butt showing. Next, undo your bra from behind and toss it away. Continue swirling, raise your arms in the air and caress them as they come down, or whatever you want to do for a few moments as he admires the view of your bare back and butt. Again, he's not seeing anything vital, but a strap-free back and just a hint of the your butt, plus knowing that you're now topless (but he can't see your boobs) will have him bursting at the seams.

Now back up toward him, moving with the undercurrent of the music, and sit on his lap, your back still facing him. Take his hands and place them on your breasts as you rotate your butt right on his groin area.

Now stand up, cross your arms over your chest to cover your boobs, walk a few paces forward, and then turn around. Keep those boobs hidden for another few moments and then you can slide your hands down your tummy, or arc your arms into the air, whatever you'd like, and continue your dance.

A sexy tease you can do with just the panties is very simple yet very, very effective. Start by slipping your thumbs underneath the sides of the panties as you dance, and alternately slide each side up and down. Be sure you go about 4 or 5 inches up and down on either side to get the effect of this move, which is you're showing glimpses of your bare hips. Even though your booty shorts may only cover about 2 inches of your hips on either side, to see a completely bare hip will excite him because you don't show your bare hips to just anyone (well let's hope you don't, and if you do, be sure they tip you!).

Now for the really fun part: slide both sides of the panties down together, inch by inch, until you get to the very top of your "female stuff." Lower them about 1/2 inch more so he sees just the tip, and slide the panties from side to side, taking care to not lower them any more. He knows what's under there, so giving him just a peek is sexier than if you just pulled them down completely.

Cute as a Button! Or Zipper! Or Snap!

The general rule with buttons, zippers, snaps, ties, or any other fastening device is to *not* look at them as you're undoing them. You're a pro, after all. But do let your audience see that you are undoing them.

For example, if you have an article of clothing with the zipper on the side, turn that side to the audience and show him you're unzipping, up and down, nice and slow, and leave the zipper open for a while as you dance around.

Buttons can be tricky because there's always one button that refuses to come undone. Regardless, buttoning three buttons on a shirt normally is sufficient or if you've got a dress with all buttons down the front, leave a few open at the top and the bottom—otherwise, you'd be unbuttoning all day!

If you do have a rogue button, exaggerate the fact that it's giving you trouble and you know it, so when you finally get it undone you can make a point of victory because you triumphed over said button. That way you're not embarrassed, and your audience isn't embarrassed for you. Then get right back in character and continue.

Behind the G-String

I was dancing at the Flags in Slough, England, wearing a business suit with a skirt that I knew would be a struggle to get out of gracefully. I knew that if I tried to take if off and ignored the blatant fact that my butt was too big for it that I'd look like a fool … so I used humor (just a sophisticated way of saying that I have no shame). I pretended to really struggle getting it off, grunting and essentially wrestling the skirt off. When I finally got it to my ankles, I kicked it up, caught it, held it up victoriously for all to see, and yelled "Yeah!"—much to the delight of the crowd who cheered me on in my victory over the villainous skirt.

Unless your pants (or slacks, as my mother would say) button or Velcro up the side for easy escape, I'd avoid stripping out of them because pant legs are just too tricky to take off without some kind of mishap.

But if you're determined to wear jeans and don't want to cut and Velcro the sides, then my advice is to take them down to just under the crown of your butt. Get yourself down on the floor on your back, bring up both legs, and use your hands to take off the jeans around your feet.

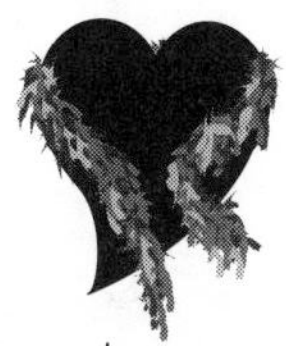

Feelin' the Love

Never wear anything with a tight neck and never wear pants that are tight at the ankles if you plan to gracefully remove these items!

—Catherine Rose Mittleman, pole instructor, Slinky Productions, San Francisco

The Least You Need to Know

- Don't take it all off right away. Stretch out the fun.
- Play with your clothing when it comes off. Toss it around—or at him!—or find other creative uses for it.
- Undo it, but keep it hidden. That's why this is called a *tease!*
- Only button about 3 buttons on a jacket or shirt. You don't want to spend all your time unbuttoning.

In This Part

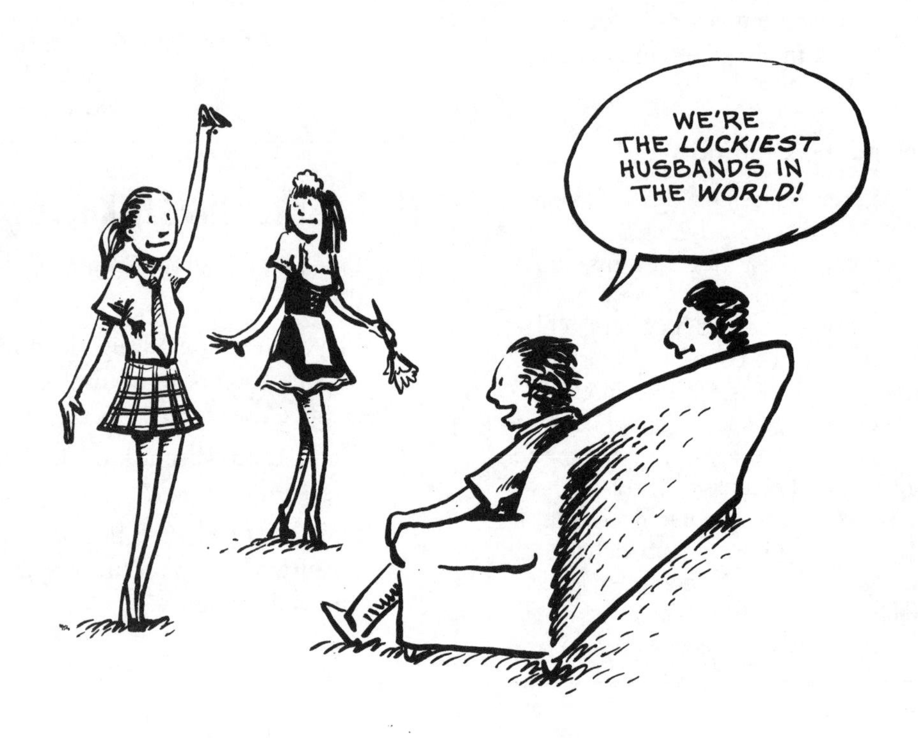

Part 4

Putting It All Together

Now it's time to put all you've learned so far into practice. In Part 4, to really start those creative wheels turning, I've suggested songs, both slow and fast, that make me feel sexy when I dance. (Beware, a lot of them are from the 1980s!) What songs make you feel sexy? Think back to songs you loved in high school or songs you love now.

Once you've got your song, it's time to decide what to wear, so I also give you ideas for fun costumes you could experiment with, either matching them to your song or matching them to your man's career. From there I've suggested several creative ways to start your dance for him, whether it be in the kitchen, bathroom, office, living room, or ….

But say you want to do more than just one dance for your husband because now you've become addicted to exotic dancing, but you don't quite want to go work in a real strip club. Gather your friends and read the final chapter, where you'll learn how to plan and put on a fun, noncompetitive show that will show off what sexy, powerful women you are!

In This Chapter

- Striptease theme ideas
- Matching costumes with music
- Location, location, location

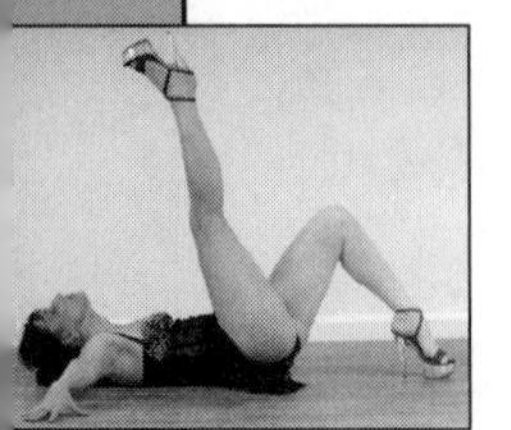
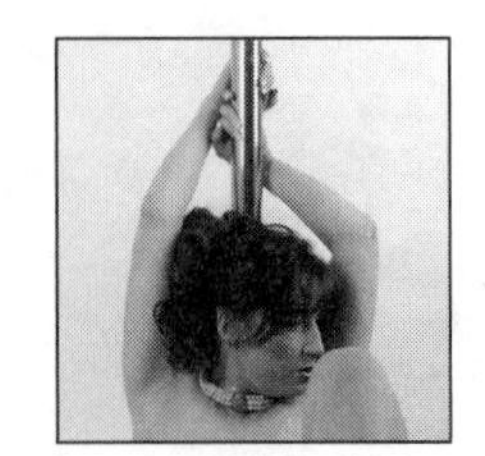
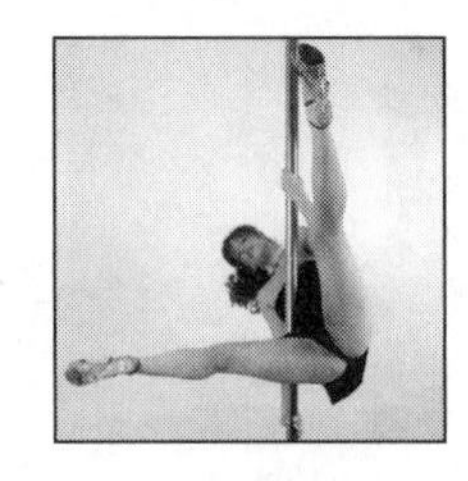
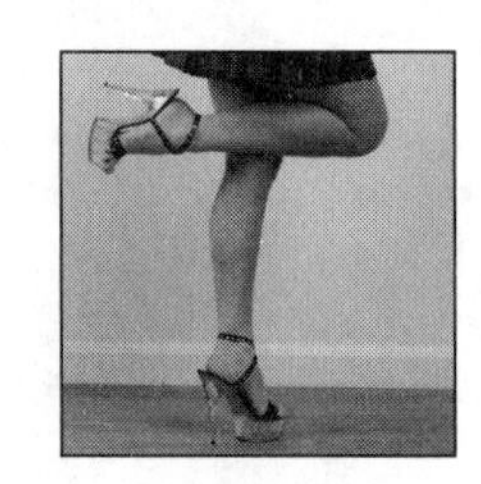
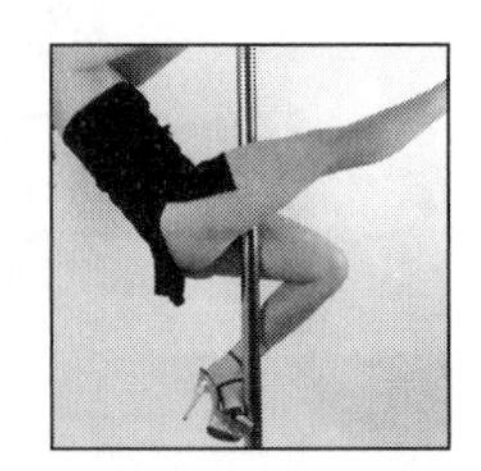
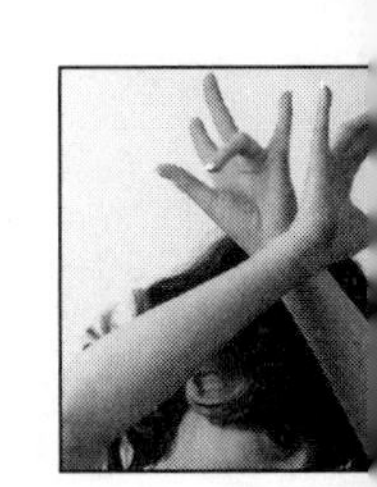

Chapter 12

It's Showtime!

Now that you know what to do and how to do it, let's get creative! Although you know your man will love a sexy lingerie striptease in the bedroom or living room, there's no need to restrict ourselves to the "typical" striptease.

Forget NASCAR Dads—Hello NASCAR Moms!

So many men love NASCAR, and if your man is one of them, why not treat him to something a little … racier? You can easily find variations of a sexy racing suit. Find one you like and feel most comfortable in. Be sure it's easy to strip off, too!

For example, you could wear a racing jumpsuit, skirt/jacket combination, dress, or short set in a racing theme. What would be really cute would be to get a large, one-piece gray mechanic-type uniform and wear your sexy racer outfit underneath for a little surprise! If you get a set of uniform pants, you might want to cut the legs up the sides and Velcro them in spots for easy fast or slow removal.

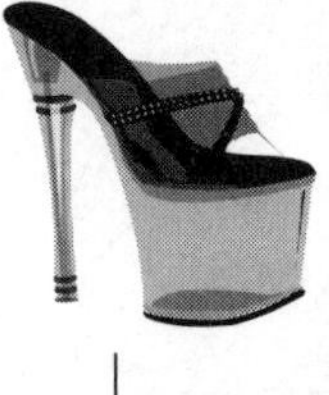

Trippin' Up

Stripping off pants can be very difficult. Don't attempt to take something off over your feet unless the bottoms are very flared and will fit over your feet (or shoes) easily.

As for music, you could choose something car or racer related:

- "I Can't Drive 55" by Sammy Hagar
- "Little Red Corvette" by Prince
- "Pink Cadillac" by Bruce Springsteen
- "Get Out of My Dreams, Get Into My Car" by Billy Ocean
- "Freeway of Love" by Aretha Franklin

If he works on his car in the garage or in the yard (depending on the neighbor situation, of course), you can surprise him in these locales. And trust me, he'll love the break! Use the hood of the car to do floor work, be creative with some of his tools (the ones he uses on the cars!), and slide down the side of the car as if it were your wall. Check out his workspace when he's not there, and let your creative juices flow!

Sex-retary

Most white-collar men love the whole secretary fantasy. The twist here, however, is that when he asks you if you are his secretary, you say, "No, I'm the CEO!"

My sexiest outfit ever—at least the one I got the most compliments on—was my business suit, a nice, form-fitting jacket and miniskirt. There's so much teasing to be done with a business suit that you'll have him hanging on your every move!

The obvious place to accost him with this theme is in his office. Be sure to begin your dance by taking charge. Sit him in his chair, and if he's already in a chair, strut in, put your CD in the player, and tell him to sit … tight. Press play, and you're on! If he's in the home office, saunter in with your pad of paper and a pencil, and sit seductively on the edge of his desk. He'll ask you what you're doing, and you can tell him you're here to take … dictation. Then, because you of course have your remote control handy and already put the correct music in the stereo, you start the song and start your dance.

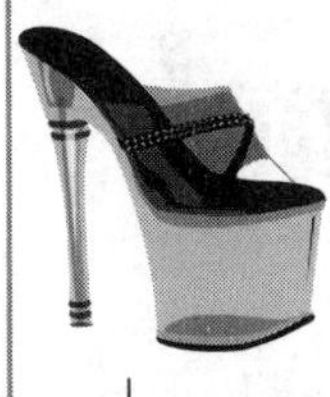

Trippin' Up

Take care not to ruin the moment by sitting on the keyboard, deleting his files, or crumpling that important contract on his desk!

You can use his office chair, start with a lap dance, be creative with his mouse (insert your own cat-related joke here), or if you know he really, really loves you, you can just swish everything off his desk and get on it yourself!

As far as song suggestions go, you can pretty much go with whatever song moves you because although this is an office theme, it's open enough to do either a slow or fast song (see the later "Music to Dance To" section).

Ma'am, Yes Ma'am!

If he's a military man, camouflage is always a sure and sexy bet, and with any military jacket, you can do the ever-sexy jacket tease. I'm all for using real clothing in your costumes, so check out your nearest military surplus store for uniforms and fun props. Camouflage fabric is very popular, but you don't have to stick with just the ordinary green or beige. Go for hot pink, blues, or even fiery reds! If he's an officer, go for the crisp, clean officer look, which is sexy and strong. Or don a sailor uniforms if that's what he is. Just be sure that no matter what kind of military costume you get, you can easily peel it off.

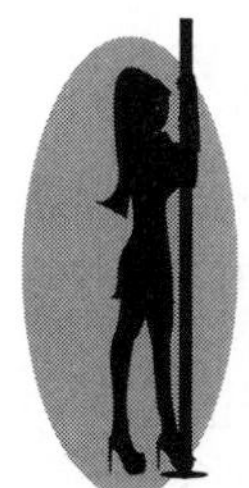

Slick Tricks

As soon as that costume is on, you are on, too. He'll love if you take charge. Tell him, "At ease, soldier!" as you order him where to sit, and make him address you "Ma'am, yes ma'am!"

I'd use "Born in the USA" by Bruce Springsteen for a military-related dance. It might not sound like a sexy song now, but sit down, listen to it, and think of creative things you can do, and suddenly this song becomes very, very sexy! Even Neil Diamond's "America" can make your military man very, very proud to serve his country … and you!

When I wear my sailor outfits, I try to use a water-themed song like "Take Me to the River" by either Annie Lenox or the Talking Heads. Even if you don't use a military-themed song, a sailor costume is very versatile and can be worn with any sort of song—be it fast, slow, or in between.

Time for Dessert!

If he loves cooking, go for a chef theme and get him while he's preparing the meal (but before he starts actually cooking, as that could lead to some … unpleasantness). If there's an island in the kitchen, use that to do your floor work. For props, put the food and some of his utensils to work—his kitchen utensils! You'll look so yummy that he'll forget about eating the real food!

Try a uniform store for a chef's jacket and hat. You can even go so far as to have your little sexy pet name (Honey, Sugar, Cooki, etc.) embroidered on the breast pocket. Underneath you can wear standard lingerie—or no lingerie at all! Or you can also get really creative and make your own costume for your kitchen striptease—completely out of food! Thread some fruit together, like strawberries or cherries, and make a fruit bra and thong. Or while your kids make their dried macaroni projects … well, you know where this idea is going!

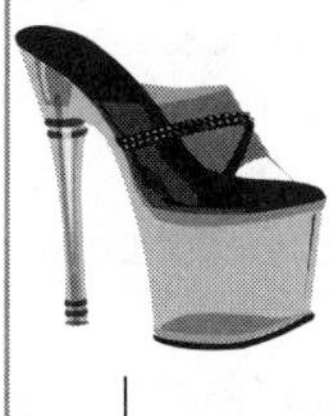

Trippin' Up

The kitchen is a natural place to get out the can of whipped cream and have a little fun, but be sure not to get that or anything else sugary in "female places."

"Pour Some Sugar on Me" by Def Leppard and "Cherry Pie" by Warrant are two sure hits with this kitchen theme.

You can begin by dimming the lights, stepping out of the shadows, and declaring … "Welcome to Hell's Kitchen!" Start the music, sweep off the counter, and start cookin'!

Workout Wonder Woman

The home gym can be very erotic. I don't think I even have to tell you how much fun some of those weight benches could be! Do be careful timing your dance, though. You don't want to appear just as he's lifting 500-pound dumbbells!

As for a costume, you have your pick of sexy boxing and workout costumes. The music is up to you on this one; almost anything would fit, particularly "Let's Get Physical" by Olivia Newton-John. That might be an old song, but it's still incredibly sexy and will make you want to really work it!

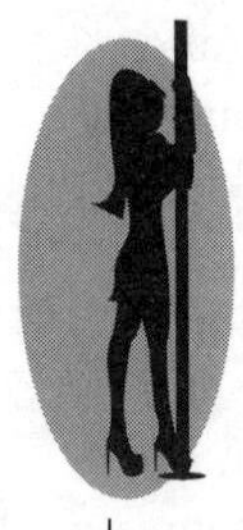

Slick Tricks

For some added fun, secretly switch the lightbulbs in the room to red ones. When he turns on the lights, he won't know what's going to happen … until he hears the music and sees you, that is! Then he'll be the one turned on!

Worshipping His Goddess

Picture it: he's just getting out of the shower. The bathroom is full of steam. He can't see much in front of him. But then the steam clears … and there you stand in your Greek goddess costume, looking as if you stepped right from the clouds of Mount Olympus!

You can dry him off, and seat him on the rim of the tub or the toilet (be sure the seat is down!) or even the sink or countertop! And before you strip off your white costume, you can even step into the shower yourself and turn on the water. He's sure to appreciate that!

Magical-sounding music might work best with this theme. Something from Enya might be appropriate. You could even choose instrumental music with no lyrics to get in the way.

Health-Care Harlot

This goes without saying: if he's a doctor or an EMT, he'd surely love the sexy nurse theme or even the in-charge hot doctor theme. You could start by wearing loose scrubs with something hot underneath or even jump right in with the sexy nurse uniforms you can find everywhere. Try your nearest uniform store for a real doctor's lab coat and then get your stethescope, rubber gloves, and pen, because girl, you are about to write a prescription for love!

As far as music, any kind, fast or slow, will work. The "hair" bands of the 1980s did a few doctor-related songs and then there's the standard "Doctor Doctor" by the Thompson Twins, which is incredibly sexy.

To Protect and Serv(ice)

For your city's finest, the sexy cop outfit is always a hit—or you could take it the other way and be his sexy prisoner. You can find lots of different styles of police and prisoner uniforms online, from rompers to two-pieces to dresses. Choose what best becomes your body.

In London, I used to use my London bobbie outfit with the song "Hotstepper" by Ini Kamooze, although the police officer costume is general enough that it can pretty much fit with any song you choose.

Begin your dance by heralding, "Assume the position!" and go from there. Use as much of his uniform and gun belt accessories as you can, although you can provide your own fuzzy handcuffs.

If he's a fireman, you can find plenty of fire-themed outfits. Many different varieties of sexy firewoman costumes are available, usually with a longer fire jacket, which makes teasing in your dance so much fun. If you have access to his actual fire jacket, don that with your black platform boots.

"Burning Down the House" by the Talking Heads or "Hot in the City" by Billy Idol were two of my favorites when I was a firewoman, or even "Hot in Herre" by Nelly. You really can't get a much more appropriate "hot" song than that!

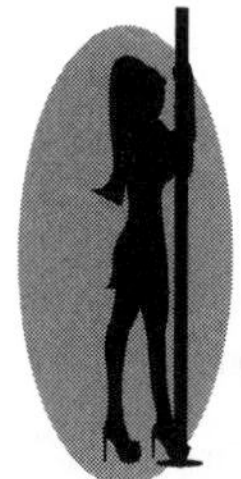

Slick Tricks

If you're doing a firewoman dance, have a squirtgun handy. Use it to keep him cool during your dance—while you just keep getting hotter and hotter. And if you want to turn it on yourself, it will likely turn him on more, too!

Ignorance Is Bliss!

If he's an educator, you've got all kinds of themes to go with: sexy cheerleader, innocent schoolgirl, or even bossy teacher. And what guy doesn't have a sexy librarian fantasy? All that primness and properness, her hair pulled back in a bun, her no-nonsense glasses, reading her scholarly reference book, *The Deaths of the Popes: Comprehensive Accounts Including Funerals, Burial Places, and Epitaphs* (okay, okay, that's my other book!). But then … off come the glasses, the hair falls loose around her face, and prim and proper go right out the window!

Even if you don't wear glasses, get a pair with plain lenses. He'll know something is up when you walk in and peer over the top of them at him.

Fun songs with this theme would be Van Halen's "Hot for Teacher," "Don't Stand So Close to Me" by the Police, or "Buttons" by the Pussycat Dolls.

Biker Babe

Whether he rides or not, I don't know any guy who wouldn't appreciate a biker babe theme. Sexy Harley-Davidson costumes go without saying; you could even just wear his leather jacket (with your sexy platform boots!). Put on his favorite song, and you're set for a dance on and around his bike!

Any kind of "tough" song works great here, particularly "I Love Rock and Roll" by Joan Jett, "Bad to the Bone" by George Thoroghgood, or even "Girls Girls Girls" by Mötley Crüe. Quiet Riot, AC/DC, and Ozzy Osbourne songs will also get you ready to ride!

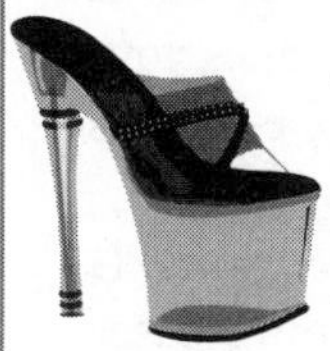

Trippin' Up

Be very careful not to knock his bike over if you're using it in your dance. That might upset him a little, and you don't want to ruin the moment (or have to run for your life in your platforms!).

Fiancée Fantasy

So you're gonna get married … lovely! Give him a prewedding show with a crazy wedding dress you'd never wear at the real ceremony. Or you could don some sexy white bride lingerie—or just a veil and nothing else!—to get him thinking about the honeymoon.

You can have real fun with this one dancing to Madonna's "Like a Virgin" or "Chapel of Love." "White Wedding" by Billy Idol is also fun. Of course this would be great for a sensual dance as well, and any love song will really put both of you in the mood. But be careful: after you do this dance for him you may not be able to wear pure white on your wedding day!

Dirty Minds

Cleaning day? Perfect! The French maid with her feather duster is always a popular costume, and it will certainly clean out his dirty mind … or just make it dirtier! You'll find so many variations of a French maid costume that it may take you a while to decide which one works best for you.

It would be fun to start dusting, in your costume, while he's watching TV. Don't say anything at all; just keep dusting until you get to the TV and then turn it off. Purr something intriguing, like, "Let's dust that thing off," or "Ready for some cleaning action?"

"I'm a Slave 4 U" by Britney Spears is a great song here, or go with anything that makes you feel sexy. The French maid outfit is one of those general outfits that get the same sexy effect even if you don't have a cleaning-based song. (I don't even know if there are any cleaning-based songs!)

Music to Dance To

If none of the song suggestions I've given you earlier in this chapter really inspire you, here are a few more suggestions:

Sensual and sexy:

- Anything by Barry White
- "Feelin' Love" by Paula Cole
- "Erotica" or "Justify My Love" by Madonna
- "You Can Leave Your Hat On" by Tom Jones
- "Fever" by Madonna or Bette Midler
- "Red Light Special" by TLC
- "Slow" by Kylie Minogue
- "Wicked Game" by Chris Isaac
- "Diamonds and Pearls" by Prince (Really, anything by Prince will work!)
- "Private Dancer" by Tina Turner
- "In Your Eyes" by Peter Gabriel

Classic hot stripper:

- "Don't Cha" by the Pussycat Dolls
- "Free Your Mind" by En Vogue
- "I Want Your Sex" by George Michael
- "Lady Marmalade" by Christina Aguilera, Pink, Mya, and L'il Kim
- "Goodies" by Chiara
- "Nasty Girl" by Vanity 6
- "Get Off" by Prince
- "Head Like a Hole" or "Closer" by Nine Inch Nails
- "Sadness" by Enigma

Devilishly cutesy:

- "Rag Doll" by Aerosmith
- "Oops I Did It Again" by Britney Spears
- "Cream" or "Raspberry Beret" by Prince
- "That Girl" by Shaggy
- "True Blue" by Madonna

Inspirational/Powerful:

- "Bittersweet Symphony" by the Verve
- "Vogue," "Express Yourself," or "Ray of Light" by Madonna
- "Always" by Erasure
- "Safety Dance" by Men Without Hats
- "What I Am" by Edie Brickell
- "Human Behavior" by Björk
- "Sisters Are Doin' It for Themselves" by Annie Lenox and Aretha Franklin

Choose a song that really makes you feel sexy; go online and find an outfit; and practice, practice, practice!

No matter what the occasion, your sexy dance for him is something he will always remember. So give him the ultimate gift—your very sexy self!

The Least You Need to Know

- You can find almost any costume theme online. From biker babe to sexy CEO, you can find the perfect costume to surprise him when he least expects it!
- You want to do this right, so match your music with your costume and location for an extra special treat!
- Start by choosing a song that motivates you and then build on that song and feeling with the costume and location.

In This Chapter

- Introducing … you!
- Learning a step-by-step choreographed dance
- Taking what you've learned so far and mixing it up!

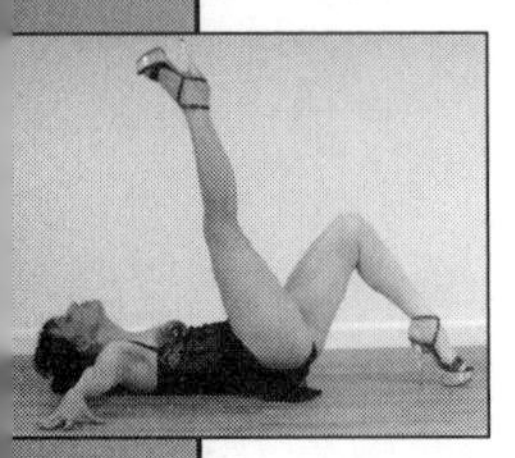
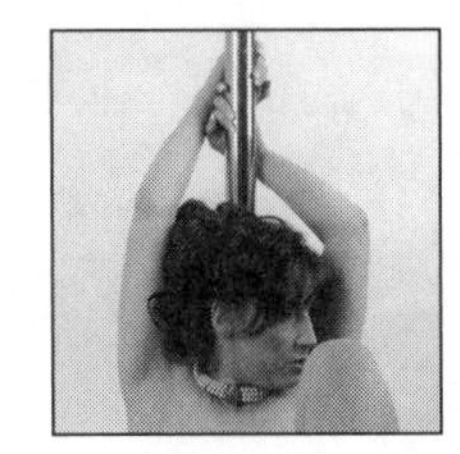
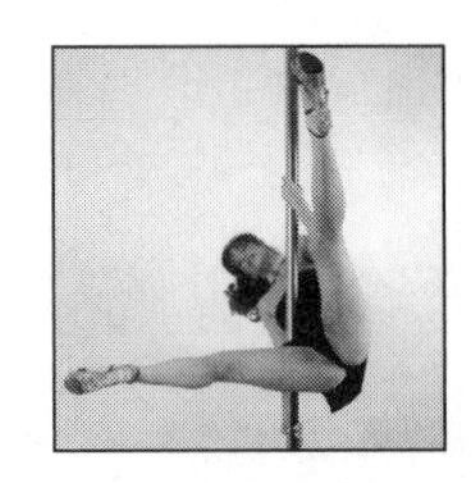
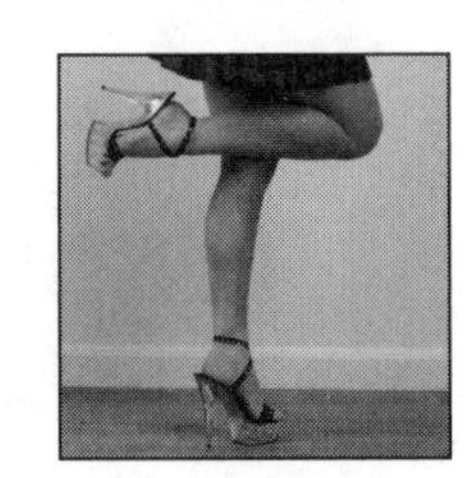
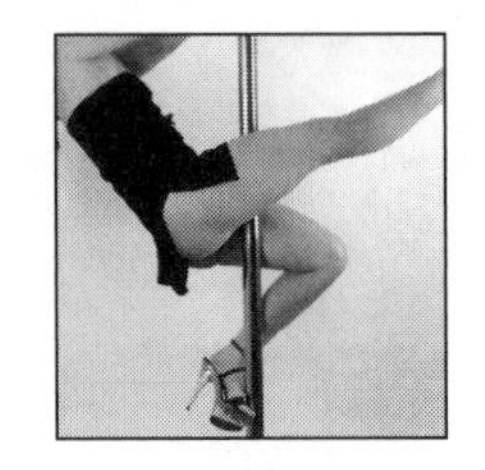
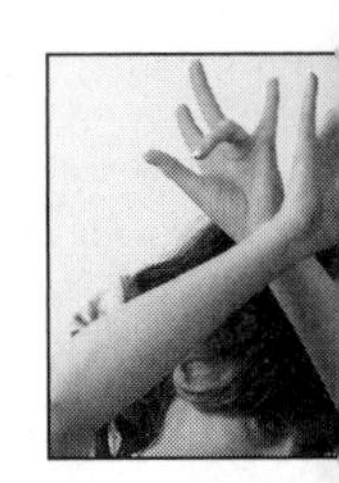

Chapter 13

A Little Choreography Help

You've practiced all the moves, the pole is your friend, and the chair is your lover. Now it's time to show *him* how sexy you know you are.

But where do you start? How do you put together everything you've learned so far so you look like you know what you're doing—and follow through without breaking up laughing? And what about attitude? Is yours ready to rock? Remember, the dance moves alone won't turn him on. Your *attitude* is what will turn him on and what he'll remember overall about your dance.

Some women dance better and feel more secure with a choreographed routine to follow, so for those of you who that applies to, this chapter is for you. Use the routines in this chapter as a guide to help you keep moving as you practice. Practice three or four moves at a time, transitioning into them until you feel comfortable. Then you'll have a handful of mini-routines under your belt and feel more confident when you dance. Add in your music—music that makes you feel strong and sexy—and your body will move on its own.

Follow my suggestions or adapt them as you like. This is just a guide of what you can do, and if your music tells you to do something else, do it! Do what feels natural. If it doesn't feel natural to you, it won't look natural to him. Soon you'll be so confident with your dancing you won't need my help!

A Step-by-Step Routine

To help you remember what you're doing and what you do next, I've arranged this first dance in six "stations":

1. Introduction
2. The approach
3. The chair
4. The pole
5. The routine
6. The lap dance

In each station, I've grouped several mini-routines so you can get comfortable with your knew, sexy self one routine at a time.

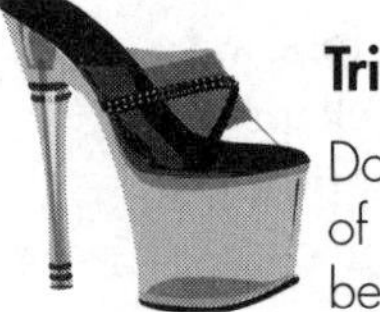

Trippin' Up

Don't choreograph every little detail of your dance, because then you'll be thinking about your routine while you dance, not about how sexy you are. Also if your routine is too tightly choreographed and you make a mistake, it'll throw off your whole dance.

Every woman will interpret a song differently, and songs are various lengths and tempos—some have long introductions, some have almost no introduction; most use lyrics, but you might choose to use a song with no lyrics. So to choreograph a song, even in mini-routines, and have it fit right with the length, tempo, and lyrics of your song is impossible. Adapt these mini-routines to fit your song, and move some routines around to make them work for you. Remember, *it's all about you!*

Introduction

Are you ready? I hope so, because the second your song starts, you're on!

When you've got him seated where you want him, either push play on your CD player or use a remote to press play and then toss the remote aside. (Remember to set the correct volume beforehand so you don't have to fidget with it when your music is on!) Take a deep breath, close your eyes as your regular self and then open them as your sexy self.

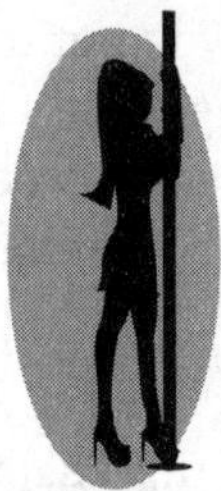

Slick Tricks

You really need to have a distinct cutoff between "regular you" and "sexy you." Eventually these two people will blend into one, but for right now, concentrate on a distinctly sexy you.

Now feel the undercurrent of the song for a few beats. Let the beat go from your brain down to your toes and back up. Raise your head and take that first step. Remember to take your sweet time with the introduction because he'll wait—and he'll like it!

Take a step toward him. Take another step. Then pause. Caress yourself slowly yet deliberately as you do your walking orgasm (turn to Chapter 6 for a refresher if you need it). Step, step, pause. Step, step, pause.

Look him up and down with a sly grin, as if you're taking mental notes on him, and then go back to admiring yourself. You can even turn around so your back is facing him, which is definitely going to show him that this dance is about you, not him.

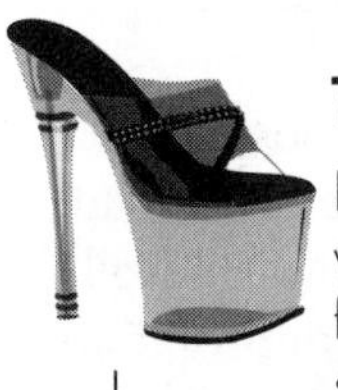

Trippin' Up

Don't glare at him continuously when you walk in. That's very freaky. Break it up and look at yourself, because this is about you, not him!

Keep pulsating with the undercurrent of the music, but don't go immediately into the dance moves. Keep it simple until the lyrics start and then begin your dance.

That's the introduction part of your dance. Practice this part until you're comfortable and can do it without fear. Don't look like you're looking for his approval! This is *your* performance!

The Approach

When you begin dancing, don't forget to lightly lip-sync with the song, too. That'll ensure you don't have a stone face and will help you look like you're doing this song specifically for him.

To begin your dance, roll your shoulders and then shoulder roll turn (Chapter 6) down onto your knees. Move into a thigh pumper, keeping your neck rolling and going with the undercurrent of the song as you pump. Lean back on one side and love your leg (Chapter 7). Keep your leg straight, point your toe, and draw your fingertip down your leg slowly. It will feel too slow, but it will look right.

Move on to *buttus smackus* (Chapter 7). Cup your hand, and smack it like you mean it!

Roll over on your tummy next, and pump that floor (Chapter 7). Arc your arms out and around to push up your butt. Do a butt circle (Chapter 7), keeping your head down and your butt in the air swirling it at his face.

Crawl to your chair, keeping your elbows bent and your front end down. Next up: the chair portion of your dance!

You've definitely got his attention now! Practice these approach moves over and over until you can do it automatically and feel comfortable before going on to the next block of moves.

The Chair

I placed the chair portion of this routine just after the approach because it's an object to play with and might help you feel more secure, particularly at the beginning of your dance. (All these moves, unless otherwise noted, can be found in Chapter 8.)

Facing the chair, place your hands on the seat. Straighten your legs and slide them behind you, keeping them apart, and pump your butt.

Now slide your legs up and to the sides so your knees bend and so you're in a sitting position with your back to him. Push the chair underneath you so you're sitting, still with your back to him.

Roll your shoulders deeply and look back at him over one shoulder. With your opposite hand, pull your bra strap/dress sleeve down over that shoulder. Glide one finger around your sexy shoulder, and slide the sleeve/strap back up (Chapter 11). Butt circle until you're standing up.

Practice this sequence so you can do it smoothly, making sure you can easily slide the chair on the floor or carpet and judging how much space you want between you and him.

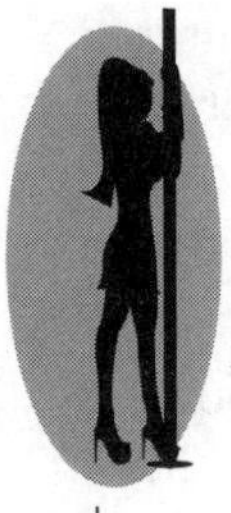

Slick Tricks

When you're done with your chair, either kick it out of your way or gruffly place it where you want it. Don't just move it, because that's a technical move that will break the spell of your dance.

Snap your right foot out and up onto the chair so your back is still to him, your butt still swirling with the undercurrent of the song. Let go of the chair with your hands.

Kick your right leg over the chair to the left and follow through so you're facing him, swaying to the undercurrent. If you lose your balance, don't worry. Just make it look like another move, like you *meant* to do it. He won't notice.

Facing him, snap up your left foot onto the chair, so the inside of your thigh is facing him. Step into a chair swirl, sitting as you fling your hair in a full circle. Remember to sit with your legs open and your hands placed strongly on your knees.

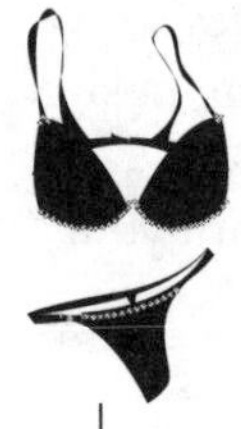

Behind the G-String

You'll definitely want to practice this series a lot, particularly the kick over the chair so you can get comfortable balancing with gravity.

Now, scoot your butt as far forward on the chair as you can and lean back. Shock him with the V legs pose, and hold it for 3 seconds.

Bring your legs down and together. Kneel down on the floor, lean your back against the edge of the chair seat, look up at the ceiling with your best orgasm expression, rotate those hips, and keep those fingers gliding all over you.

We'll pause for a break here so I can remind you to review that set of chair moves again, so you know what to expect when you lean back on the chair. You don't want to be in the middle of your dance, get to the chair portion, and have your chair slide away from you! Now, when you're ready …

Diva dive (Chapter 7) down with your butt rotating, and remember to keep your head tucked in so you're looking through your legs. Slide up dramatically into a princess pose (Chapter 7), remembering to keep your neck up. Come down slowly and try not to "plunk." Roll over onto your back so your body is in profile to him—think mud flap pose (Chapter 7).

Impress him with your swirl and slide (Chapter 8), but remember not to scoot your butt over if the chair isn't positioned exactly how you want it. Position your right foot so your arch rests on the side of the chair pad, your heel beneath the pad, and your toes above. The other foot should be resting entirely on top of the chair pad. If you need to maneuver the chair, use your feet to do so.

Slide onto your hands and knees, and stand up slowly, butt first. Take your time, and remember to draw your hands up on the inside of your thighs (Chapter 6). Turn to him, massaging yourself deliberately, rolling your neck, and admiring your own body (Chapter 6).

Slowly back up until your back is against the pole and your arms up (Chapter 9).

The Pole

He was wowed by your chair moves. He'll be floored by your pole routine—wishing he was that pole by the time you're through! (You can find the following moves, unless otherwise noted, in Chapter 9.)

Turn around so you're facing the pole, and slide your hands down so your butt is sticking out and your legs are spread. Swirl your butt. Pole strut around the pole, making sure to bend your elbow.

Hop into the Xandra swing, and go all the way to the floor. Get up gracefully, bringing your butt up first—slowly.

Step to the front of the pole so you're facing him, and pole slide. Keep your neck up and in the drama and point your toes as you slide down.

Practice this simple first set to get used to using your friend the pole in an actual dance. For your next mini-routine ...

Bring your legs together and roll over so you're on your hands and knees. (Be sure to stay close to the pole when you roll.) Draw your arms up and flip your hair. Holding the pole with your inside hand, go into a squatting position with your feet together. Pivot on your toes so you're facing the opposite direction and then stand up slowly, butt first.

Step around the pole while you massage it and tempt him with your eyes. Pole strut around the pole, bending your elbow as you walk. Step into the Veronica (cross-legged) swing. Don't look at the floor as you prepare to swing, and keep your head back for the drama. When you land, come up butt first, massaging the pole.

Continue to go over this part of the routine until you're confident in your moves. Now, for your next pole tricks:

Take a few steps into the Marilyn (backward swing). You must keep your momentum, so lean forward into this swing and keep your head dramatically up as you go around.

Lean on only one elbow so you're on your side, not your back, and windmill your legs over the pole (Chapter 7).

Roll over on your hands and knees, staying close to the pole. Get up gracefully, butt first, and take your time coming up into a pole massage with your fingertips. Pivot your feet, peek at him with your sexy "come-hither" look, and point to him.

Strut around the pole quickly to gather momentum, and fly into the Harley swing and then get up gracefully.

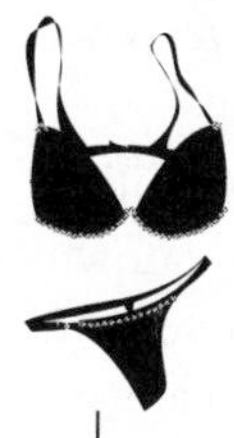

Behind the G-String

You don't have to get up as I say word for word. As long as you make an effort to get up in a sexy, slinky kind of way, it will work. Just never stand straight up!

This part of the routine puts two swings together back to back so you can get the feel of doing them smoothly, as opposed to one swing, then another swing, then another swing. Remember to always sway your butt with the undercurrent of the song.

Next, take a few steps and launch into the Vixen swing, landing on your toe and making a nice, wide arc around with the other toe. Then, turn to wall, and assume the position!

Practice these three swings together in order, without stopping, without looking at the floor as you walk around, and without thinking about them. To avoid thinking about your swings (I can't even do them if I think about them), remember just the first step of each swing and as you go into it your body will remember what to do, I promise! So for example, with the Marilyn swing, you only have to remember, *Step on the inside toe*, and because you know the swing, your body will do the rest automatically.

The Routine

Now it's all you. No chair, no pole. Just you and your dance. He'll be glued to your every move. Have fun with it! (All these moves can be found in Chapter 7.)

Play with the wall for a few beats, squatting down, pivoting on your toes, and coming up slowly butt-first. You can even turn so your side is against the wall and arc your arm straight out and all the way back as you arch back, sweep your arm back up, or whatever you'd like.

Take some time to really play with the wall. When you're ready, turn around and slide down the wall (Chapter 6). Remember to remove your arm from the wall as you turn and then lean your upper back against the wall as you follow through with the passion of the song on your face and sway down, your hands seductively caressing your body.

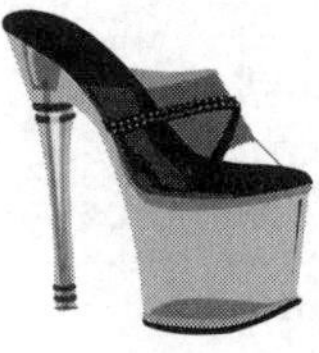

Trippin' Up

No pointed elbows or palms out!

Diva dive forward. (Use a small dive with your hands, not a diving-board dive.) Butt circle, keeping your butt in the air and your head down—you want him to focus on your butt here.

Crawl toward him, remembering to keep those elbows bent at all times. Do not let your arms come up completely straight. Take your time and have fun with it—swirl your hair, do a desperation pump, roll your shoulders, etc.

Really practice your crawl in this routine. Crawling does not feel sexy—I know, I know. It feels clunky and stupid but trust me, it looks great!

Rise up on your thighs, drawing your fingers along the inside of your thighs as you swirl your head dramatically. Move into thigh pumper. Roll your neck, close your eyes, and breathe in through your mouth, all while your fingers are slowly caressing your body.

Strike a princess pose. Swing your right leg all the way over so your foot touches the back of your left thigh. Sit *back*, not straight down, with enough muscle control so you don't plunk on the floor. Then ease onto your back, your hand caressing and your butt undulating to the music at all times.

Bring your legs up straight together, hands on your thighs. Open your legs slowly and give him the V leg shocker. Keep your legs straight and open for 3 seconds.

Continue going over these sequence until you can do it smoothly and without thinking. Make it all blend into one.

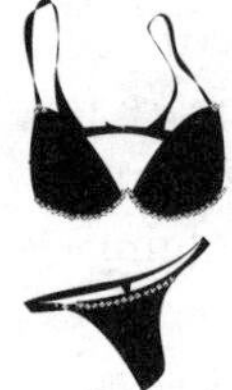

Behind the G-String

You don't have to do each and every move in one single dance. Don't try to cram something in. Save it for another dance, and just let it flow.

Next, close your legs and cross your feet. Place your arms out to the sides and strike the mud flap pose—only this time with your feet crossed. As your legs come down, shift your feet to the side.

Windmill next. Lean completely on one side, propped up by your elbow, and land on your other elbow. Arc your legs up and over one at a time, not together. The second leg has to have just as much momentum as the first.

Roll smoothly over onto your hands and knees. Butt circle, sliding your arms out straight in front of you and tucking your head under. Keep your thighs spread. Your butt is facing him now, so after a swirl or two, move your butt back and forth in a pumping action. He'll really love that!

Do that sequence till it's smooth, ladies! Then move on for more!

Slide your legs out straight in back of you, with your arms straight out front, and pump the floor. Roll over onto one side, and prop yourself up on your elbow. Love your leg. Do this slowly and stare at your finger as it glides down your leg. When your finger gets to your butt, your leg should be down as well.

Show him how much you are in awe of your own body. Don't look at him as you do this. Concentrate on yourself.

Next, *buttus smackus!* Swirl one finger delicately on your butt and then slap it like you mean it! And cup your hand when you smack to really get is attention. No wimpy slaps!

Roll over onto your back so you're sideways to him, and go into a mud flap pose, starting with your head back and your back arched, one leg straight and one leg bent. Draw your arms up your tummy, to your chest, and out to the side. Now relax your back, lift your straight leg up, and use it to bring your body up slowly with your head back. (Remember to glide your arms up from behind; they do not ever lift off the floor.) Keep your pose for 3 seconds.

Roll over toward him so you're on your hands and knees and then crawl right up to him.

Make that series of moves nice and smooth, and be very wary of your expression. Lightly lip-synch, wink at him, point to him, blow him kisses, whatever feels right. And now for the part he's been really waiting for …

The Lap Dance

Practicing lap dancing can be tough without a model, so if someone is willing to be your guinea pig, that's great. If no human is available, you could even put a stuffed animal in the chair, just so you have a point of focus. If you have neither, just use the empty chair because you still need to get a feel (so to speak) for the lap dance.

Here's how you do it (all these moves can all be found in Chapter 10):

Crawl up to him, and when you get right to him, crawl up his legs, caressing his legs with your hands. Place your hands on his knees to balance and then get into your crouching position. Pivot your feet to one side and stand up butt first so he really gets the effect of your butt.

Using one leg at a time, straddle him and sit on *it.* Rotate around, and pump up and down. Run your fingers through his hair and roll your neck, all while keeping in your dramatic character.

Draw your body up tight against his until you're standing over him. Push his face into your chest, and wiggle it around in there. Then, slide tightly down him again, continuously pumping or rotating on his lap.

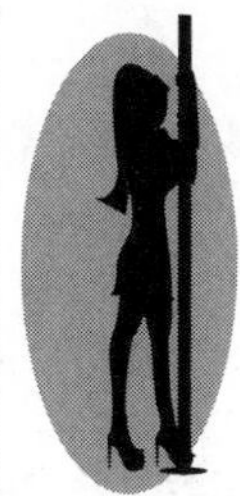

Slick Tricks

Don't be afraid to act. Just follow it through, and he'll really, truly, believe you are completely enveloped in ecstasy.

Practice this sequence as much as you can, and concentrate on your confident attitude, particularly because you'll be so close to him. Now, for more …

Lean back, placing your arms on his knees for support. Roll your head back in ecstasy as you continue to swirl your hips. Bring yourself back up, and place your hands on his shoulders.

Lift one leg over him to get off, and step around the chair so you're behind him. Slide your arms down his chest to his inner thighs.

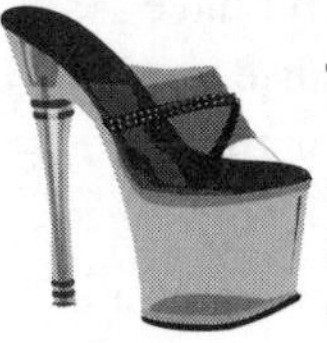

Trippin' Up

At this point in your chair dance, don't actually touch *it*. Instead, go around it—it'll drive him wild!

Breathe softly in his ear, and draw your arms up, back to his shoulders. Let your hands caress the top of his back and his shoulder as you step around him.

Then, catch him off-guard by slamming your leg over his lap so you're straddling him again. Rotate around on it, and slide up and down.

Go over those moves again until you've got a good beat going with your song because remember, you still want to move with your song, not just do moves to do them.

Now, using one leg at a time, step off him, turn around, and walk away with your back to him. Raise your arms, sway your butt, caress yourself, all with your back to him. This is showing him that it's still all about you, and you know he'll want what he can't have.

Slowly back up to him and sit on his groin area, rotating your butt and leaning forward. Maneuver his knees so you can hold onto them, lean forward, and bring your legs up in back. Now swirl that butt right in his face!

From here, you can tell him to straighten his legs and you can slide down and roll over into your next move. Or you can use your body to swing back up (which will bring your feet back to the floor). Lean back onto his chest, wrap your arm around his neck, and continue to pulsate against him.

Stand up and twirl around so you're facing him. (This should bring you near to the end of your song, and I always thought it's great to end a song on a lap dance, facing him.) Straddle him again, rubbing your body and swirling your butt, kissing him, or whatever else you'd like to do. The rest is up to you!

There you have a very basic dance comprised of several smaller chunks of routines to practice. The more comfortable you get with these smaller routines, the easier the whole thing will be when your song is playing and he's sitting there drooling over what's to come. Have fun!

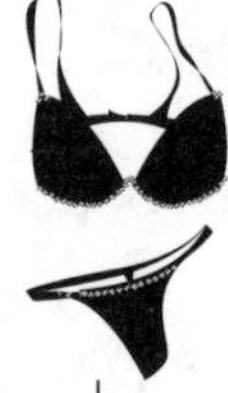

Behind the G-String

If your song ends on a definite beat, you should end on a definite beat, too. This wraps up your dance nicely and looks incredibly strong. If your song fades out, keep your end position until the music fades completely out.

Mixin' It Up

If you want more of a mixed choreography, I've got that covered, too. The following instructions are particularly helpful with transitioning from one move to the next. This dance, as I did it, was to a faster-tempo song than the previous dance.

This dance is more mixed up, too—it has more transitions from move to move to move. One of the most important things to remember in any dance is that when you transition, just roll into the next position. There is no right or wrong. Just do it. Trust me, he's not going to say, "Hmmm … that transition should have been smoother. Now I'm completely turned off." It's not really how you get there that counts; it's your attitude while you're getting there that he'll remember.

Introduction

As with the preceding routine, your introduction should be well paced. Never look too anxious to begin; don't rush up in front of your man and just start dancing. Take your sweet time, because he'll wait … and he'll like it! Take a beat or so to get into your song. Close your eyes, take a deep breath, open them, and you're on!

Step, step, pause. Massage yourself deliberately. Step, step, pause. Look him up and down. Continue pulsating to the undercurrent of the music and admire yourself, while ignoring him.

The Approach

As in the slower dance, you need an approach to him. In this faster-paced song, your approach will be stronger and more in his face!

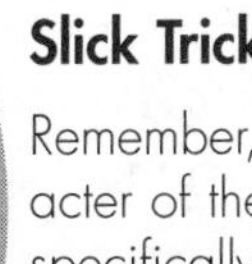

Slick Tricks

Remember, you're taking on the character of the singer, so you're talking specifically to him. Lip-sync at least the key words to add some animation in your face and make the song more personal for him. Just be careful not to overarticulate on your lip-sync because that can be distracting.

Strut right up to him. Point to him, and beckon him with your finger. Act like you're about to sit on him and then abruptly turn around. Take a few steps, stop, and look at him over your shoulder. Then do a twirl or strut to your chair (Chapter 6).

Show Him You're the Queen!

Here's where the real dance starts! Snap your leg onto the chair. Get your butt into it with big butt circles first, followed by little butt circles (Chapter 6).

Snap your leg off the chair, take a small step and then a large step behind the chair, and slide your left foot to meet your right. Stay close to the chair as you do this, and be sure to bend over at the hips so your butt is prominent as your right foot slides over.

Slide over behind the chair and delicately stroke the sides of the chair as you tempt him with your sexy eyes. Crouch down, look through the bars of the chair (or peek over the top if your chair doesn't have bars), reach through (or over), and beckon him.

Turn to the side and come up butt first. Step to the side of the chair, and kick it out of the way. If the chair is on a rug and falls over when you kick it away, let it go and stay in character. Don't apologize for it!

Strut to the pole and jump on with an enthusiastic Xandra swing with one leg out in back (Chapter 9). Go all the way to the floor. Get up sexily—as long as it's butt first you'll look great. Approach him with a walking orgasm (Chapter 6). Turn to the side for a body roll (Chapter 7).

Face him for the sunset move to the floor (Chapter 6). Be sure your palms sweep against your shins as you lean over so you get the full circle effect.

Slide your arms up and flip your hair. Bring your bra/dress straps down, fingers inside your bra/dress, and push up your boobs (Chapter 11). Roll your *hands*, not your shoulders. Lift your straps back up.

Slide your body to the side on the floor so you're facing him, extend one arm out, and roll toward him so you're facing him (Chapter 7).

Next, love that leg (Chapter 7)! Stare at your leg, not him, and bring your finger down slower than it seems like you should, even with a faster song. Roll onto your back so you're in profile to him, and assume the mud flap pose (Chapter 7). Keep your neck back, and glide your arm up from behind. Come up slowly.

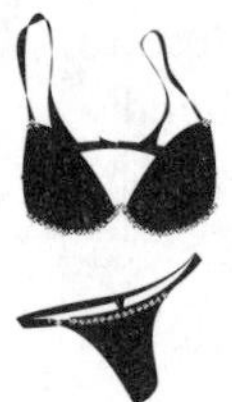

Behind the G-String

The higher the arch in your back, the prettier mud flap pose looks.

Roll over on your hands and knees, and crawl to him (Chapter 7). Keep your elbows bent and your front end down. Place your hands on his knees and draw them up his thighs (Chapter 10). Don't touch *it;* just go around it.

Stand up, butt first, using his knees to balance if you have to (Chapter 10). Abruptly turn around and strut toward the pole. Stop midway to the pole, and look back at him over your shoulder. Swirl your butt and smack it! Smack it like you mean it—no weak spanks here.

Strut to the pole and do the Savannah swing, reaching around and grabbing the pole from behind with your knees up (Chapter 9). Landing on your knees, step in to a crouch, pivot your feet, and stand up butt first (Chapter 7). Hide behind the pole, look at him from one side of the pole to the other as you massage the pole with your fingertips and pivot your feet (Chapter 9).

Step in front of the pole and slide down (Chapter 9). Roll forward onto your hands and knees and then stand up butt first (Chapter 7).

Strut to him, straddle him, and sit right on it. Rotate around and up and down with the music. Draw up and down, running your fingers through his hair. Lean back and place your hands on his knees for balance (Chapter 10). Rotate your hips, and roll your neck back.

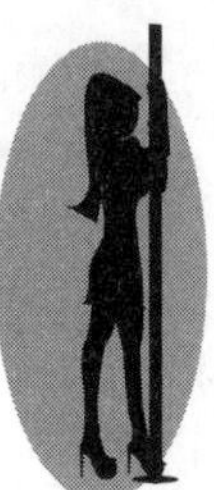

Slick Tricks

Don't be afraid to tell him how to position his legs. This is your song, he'll do what you tell him, and he'll like it!

Slide your arms down his shins and spread your legs. Let your body slide down until your back is on the floor. Place your legs together and roll to the side, tucking your head under as it swirls around (Chapter 7).

Roll over onto your hands and knees so you're sideways to him (Chapter 7). Suck in your tummy and do the desperation pump (Chapter 7). Keep your hands at uneven lengths, and don't rest completely on your forearms.

Next, draw up your arms and flip your hair. Stand up butt first (Chapter 7). Back up or saunter over to your chair without making a straight beeline to it (Chapter 6). Position your chair so the back of it is facing him.

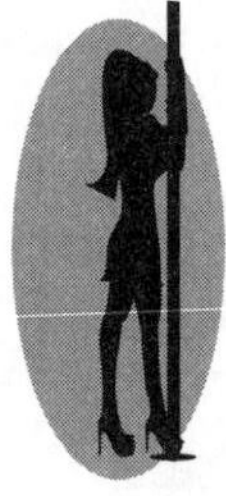

Slick Tricks

Don't just move the chair; stay in character and use force to position it where you want it. Even slam it down on the floor for extra effect.

Sit on the chair backward, facing him. Roll your shoulders and lean back. Come as far forward as you can. Holding the middle of the chair back, bring your legs up into V legs. Keep them open for 3 seconds, point your toes, and glide your fingertips up and down your thighs. Keep your head back, too.

Bring your legs together and pivot your body sideways into the prettiest pose ever. Do not bicycle, and keep your head back! Slowly, if even at all, rub your legs together.

Roll your legs 1-2-3, and let the force of that bring your body up. Kick the chair out of the way if you have to, and strut to your pole.

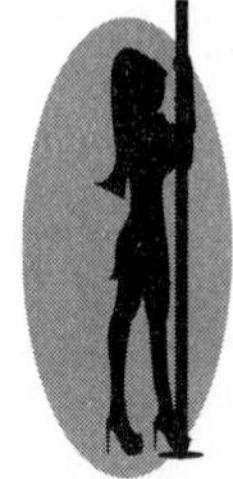

Slick Tricks

If there's a lot of distance between here you are now and the pole, strut, stop, and look over your shoulder at him. Roll your shoulders and strut to the pole.

With one hand facing down and the other up, go into a sideways swing and come up butt first (Chapter 9). Step around the pole, walking orgasm toward him (Chapter 6). Roll your shoulders and come down on your knees (Chapter 6). Slide over onto one side and windmill (Chapter 7).

Smack your butt and windmill back. Roll over on your hands and knees, with your butt to him. Butt circle, draw your arms in, and roll your neck up (Chapter 7). Lean back so you see him, upside down, while rotating your hips.

Slide your legs underneath you and out to the side so you're in a crawling position. Crawl to him. Take your time, swirl your hair, rear up on your thighs, dive down, etc.

When you get to him, use his knees to balance as you stand up butt first. Sit on him with your back to him (Chapter 10). Lean forward and grind it. Using his knees to balance your hands, bend your knees and swirl your hips in his face. Bring yourself up, still grinding. Place his hands on your chest, and lean back and wrap your arm around his neck. Come forward and butt circle up.

Walk away from him like you could care less what he does (Chapter 6). Look back at him over your shoulder and wink. Strut to the pole and do a final spin, landing gracefully on the floor as your music ends (Chapter 9).

Remember the overall purpose of your dance, which is to show him how sexy you know you are, not to impress him with physical dance moves. You're here to show him that you're in control, so you do what *you* want to do, when you want to do it.

Believe in yourself as you do this dance. Stay in your song, stay in character, and be proud of what you're doing. Follow it through until the end. Of course you might giggle, but don't just stop midway through and say "Oh I feel so stupid." Your man is on your side; he wants you to do this; he wants you to follow through until the end. He is not criticizing you, he is admiring and adoring you. And if he ever—God help him—does criticize you, you'll never dance for him again, and you'll make no apologies.

That's the main theme here—no apologies! No apologies for cellulite, fat, stretch marks, or anything else you might think you have wrong with you. You are a woman, and all women have those things so tough, he can deal with it. And if he doesn't like it, then "Buh-bye! Leave my stage. Don't need ya!"

So go easy on yourself. This dance is all about you and primarily for your enjoyment so you can feel sexy. And always remember the cardinal rule: he's lucky to be there!

The Least You Need to Know

- The purpose of your dance is to show him that *you know* you're sexy.
- If you must choreograph, do it very loosely so you'll remember where to go, but not so tightly that a slip will throw you completely off.
- Keep going if you make a mistake—trust me, he won't notice.

In This Chapter

- Planning a show with your friends
- Making sure everybody stays friends
- Sharing responsibilities and setting some ground rules
- Dancing for an audience—and collecting tips!

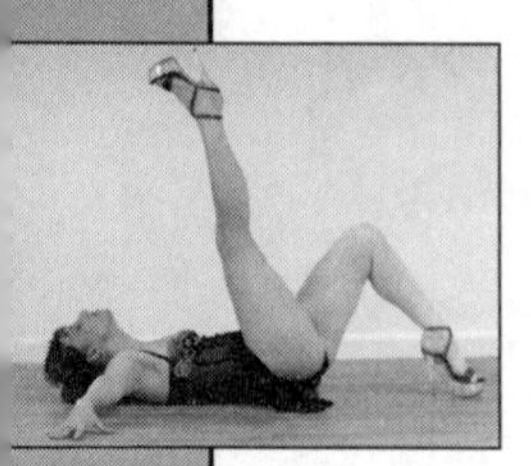
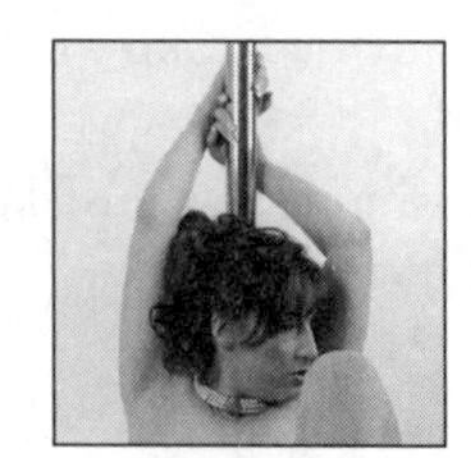
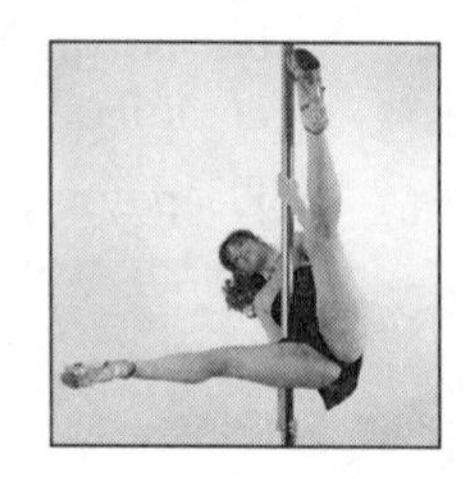
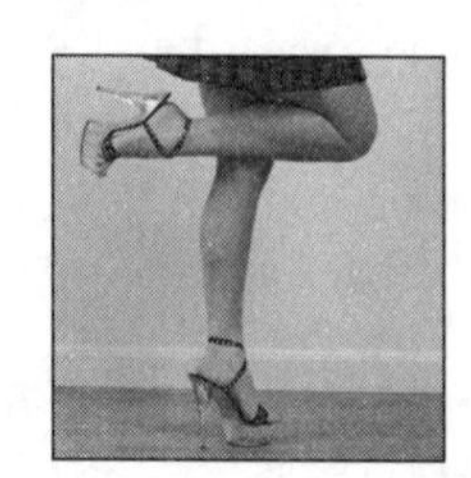
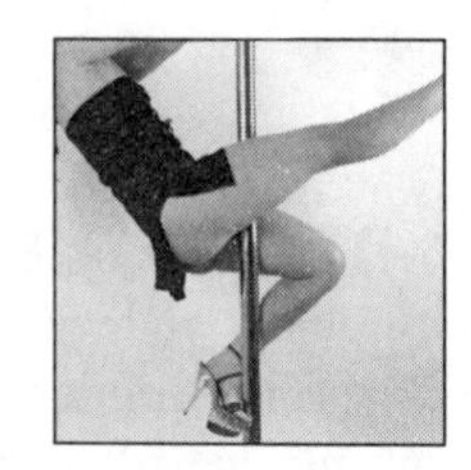
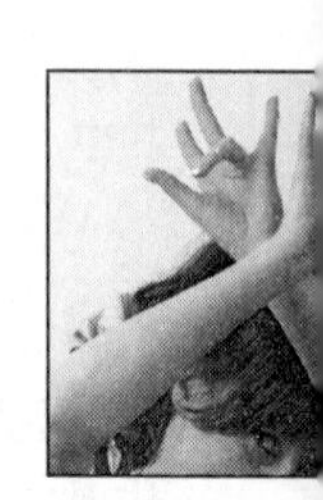

Chapter 14

Showcase Showdown!

You've done your dance for your man, and he's *floored*—and wanting to know when you'll do it again! Naturally, you tell all your girlfriends how much fun it was to dress up, strip, command the show, and wrap him around your little finger, and now they want to do it, too. But you think, *There's power—and money—in numbers. Let's all put on a sexy showcase for our guys and make them tip us!* As the proverbial wheels begin to spin, a sly grin spreads across your face ....

In this chapter, I walk you through how to plan a showcase in your own home, from the very beginning to the very end, covering every possible aspect associated with a grand performance. You learn how to handle all the egos involved, set up your showcase so every detail's covered, perform for a mixed audience, and most important, deal with dancing in front of your friends' spouses so you all remain strong friends after the show.

Girls' Night *In*

First, you've got to get everyone excited about doing a show, but you can't come right out and say, "Let's do a striptease show!" If you do, your girlfriends might run for the hills and never speak to you again. You must start gradually.

Kick the men out of the house, invite a bunch of your girlfriends over for some wine (if anyone doesn't know someone else, formally introduce them immediately so no one feels awkward), and casually say, "Hey, you guys have to check out this DVD I got. It's on pole dancing and chair dancing and striptease stuff, and the girl who teaches it is so pretty and funny. She's amazing at what she does!" Then pop in this book's DVD and watch, laugh, and try some of the stuff yourselves. Maybe you can even show them some of your favorite moves as you're watching the DVD, especially if you have a pole in your house. Seeing the fun you have as you swing around on the pole might be just the thing your shy friends need to get onboard with the idea.

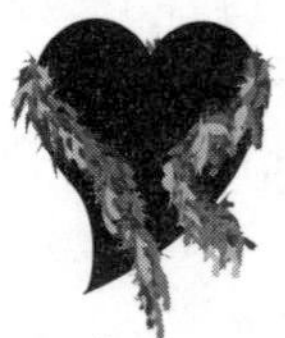

Feelin' the Love

I just wanted to say thanks so much for planning the recital … and asking me to be a part of it, I had *such* a blast. I can't believe I was ever nervous about it in the first place!

—Sasha, student

And then say, "And look at all these costumes!" as you pull out your stack of costume pages you've printed out, in color, from www.catdancerz.com. (I find they have the best variety for the lowest cost.) Or if you've bought a few already, run to your closet and grab them!

Now, assuming your friends' reactions so far are enthusiastic (how could they not be?), propose doing a show, just like in a strip club, but at home, with just you girls. The thought of performing usually scares girls, so assure them you won't "show anything," it'll be fun, and you can make the guys tip you!

Expect to hear, "Oh no, I could never do that!" Like a Girl Scout, be prepared. Answer with, "I'm not saying we'll do it tomorrow. We have to all practice first and pick a song and a costume. It will be so much fun!"

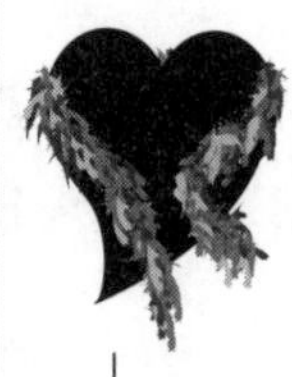

Feelin' the Love

Dancing in my first showcase was the biggest rush of my life!

—Meredith, Gypsy Rose instructor

Most likely you'll also hear "Oh, but my butt's too big," "I hate my stretch marks," "I hate my thighs," *blah blah blah*. This is your moment to take command and say "No apologies! The lights will be dark and you don't even have to take anything off. You can just dance. And who cares if you have stretch marks or cellulite? You're a woman—you're supposed to! Besides, some or all of the rest of us do, too. Who cares!"

To this, you're likely to get some sort of mumbled "I don't know," but then you can come in with the clincher: "We're doing this for *us*, not for them! And we'll make money from it, too!" Really stress the fact that this is all about you girls, not the men in the audience.

Remind them that exotic dancing is all about girl power and showing the guys who's who. Share with them what Vixen, a Gypsy Rose instructor, says about it: "A showcase is not only empowering and invigorating to those participating, it is also empowering and invigorating to those watching. (My mother spun around the pole during the intermission!)" If you've got some doubters still, loan them your copy of this book—or if you're afraid you'll never get it back, tell them where they can get their very own copy. Let them read a few chapters and watch the DVD, and I bet most if not all your friends will soon come around to your way of thinking!

Remind them what a fun, challenging project this can be:

- You can do programs. (Surely you've got some friends who scrapbook or otherwise get creative with design or card-making computer software.)
- You can pick fun stage names.
- You can dance to any song you want, be it a sexy slow number, "your song," or a sexy R&B number you know gets him in the mood.

Feelin' the Love

No one else in the audience knew that my song had a very special meaning to my boyfriend John and me, but the minute the music started, he knew it—and it made the experience phenomenal.

—Vixen, Gypsy Rose instructor

- Shopping for costumes! Enough said.
- You can get your hair and nails done for the show. Think of it as a predance spa day!
- With all the rehearsals you'll be doing, your body will likely shed a few pounds and tone up in some spots.

And so on and so on.

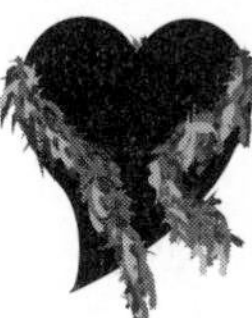

Feelin' the Love

I was so nervous before my dance, and I wanted everything to be absolutely perfect. Just as I was starting my first butt circle, I realized my music was skipping. Luckily, I had brought a second copy of my songs, but I had to run off the stage, through the crowd, to the bathroom and dig through my bag to find it. Even though I was horrified by the mishap at first, I was able to laugh about it, and it completely relaxed me. By the time we got the music straightened out and I got up on stage to start again, I realized my performance wouldn't be—and didn't have to be—perfect. I was there to dance, have fun, and show off what I had learned!

—Juliana, Gypsy Rose instructor (who has danced in nine recitals)

In fact, you don't even have to mention doing a show at first. Instead, tell your friends what a great workout dancing is, and invite some of them over and to dance with you as fun exercise. Tell them to wear something that makes them feel sexy, because sweatpants and sneakers are boring. After a few weeks of dancing together, and when you can sense their confidence in their dancing is up, casually mention the show thing. You might be surprised how many takers you get!

Filling Your Showcase

The showcase should be a positive experience for everyone, not a drama-queen floor show no one enjoys. This should be a fun, sister-power experience, not a negative, competitive disaster.

It might go without saying, but I have to say it anyway: you've got to be sure all the girls you invite to do this are *normal.* Seriously, that's really a very important point. If you have a friend who …

- Is the jealous type
- Always has to be the center of attention
- Gets irrationally jealous if her significant other so much as glances at another woman
- Pretends to hate drama but always starts or stirs it up

… you might not want to invite her to dance with you.

I'm sure you know some women who can be pretty catty sometimes. Even the sweetest, nicest of delicate flowers—if pushed enough in the right circumstance and concerning her man—will resort to the most base, unbecoming actions, comments, and stunts she thinks will make her feel better and boost her standing in others' eyes. Unfortunately, these antics really just expose her own insecurities and make her feel worse.

Most women are self-conscious or insecure about their looks, but they really shouldn't be. Beauty is subjective. And believe me, different men have different tastes and love to admire the variety of women's shapes and sizes. But the one thing that impresses men over any "perfect" body is confidence! If you look like you're in love with your body, he will be, too.

You'll increase your own confidence if you're able to admit and be content with the fact that other women might be considered prettier than you. And that's okay, because you are simply a different type of woman. There will always be someone else who is prettier than you, who is a better dancer than you, or who has a better body or bigger boobs than you. That's life. Accept it and move on. When you allow yourself to say, "Okay, she's prettier than me," or, "Yeah, she's got a better body than me," and then let it go, you'll be so much happier. You'll release that negativity, and being "perfect" is one less thing you have to worry about. And the funny thing is, every other woman in the room is probably saying the same thing about you being prettier than her!

Lowering your ego is a tough thing to do, though. As a teacher, everyone expects me to be the best, but some girls do moves I can't do very well at all. Instead of feeling threatened by this—which is the female instinct—I openly admit, "I wish I could do it like that!" This public admission leaves me with great peace of mind because I'm able to accept that although I'm the teacher, I don't always have to be "the best."

When you put on a showcase that includes your friends, don't become threatened by them if you consider them prettier or if you think have a better body than you or can dance better than you—and don't let them feel threatened by each other, either. Celebrate your differences and have fun with each other!

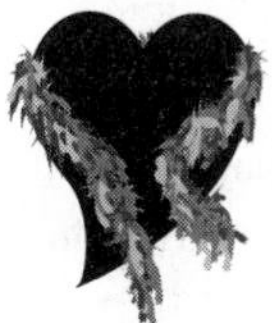

Feelin' the Love

Dancing for real people and hearing them clap and cheer for me made me feel like I was the hottest woman on Earth. And the tips at the end aren't bad, either!

—Marilyn, Gypsy Rose instructor

Besides, some men love the catfight thing and encourage it, finding it most entertaining and using their women as a source of amusement. Remember, dancing is all about us. We don't want to give the men that kind of power, do we? Nope.

Setting Some Ground Rules

Ground rules must be laid out at the beginning so all the girls are on the same page about the purpose of the show, learn how to deal with their own insecurities, feel comfortable dancing with other people's spouses watching, and remember that this is a show, not a contest.

As you bring up the rules, explain that you're not trying to be a killjoy, but you thought it would be really smart to set some ground rules for everyone so nothing bad or weird will happen. Or just show them this book. (Better yet, encourage them to get their own copy!)

It might feel weird to have to bring up these points, but trust me, it's better to talk about it now than having tension or cat fighting later.

Show vs. Contest

I highly frown on contests because that exalts one woman while making the others feel as if they weren't good enough. The purpose of a showcase is to make everyone involved feel great. Also contests give the impression that you're performing for your audience's approval, and *nothing* could be further from the truth! You are performing for *yourselves;* the audience are just lucky to be there.

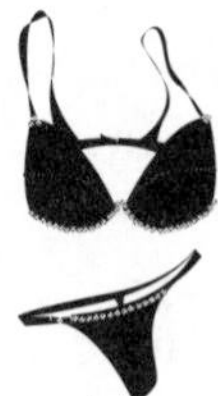

Behind the G-String

It doesn't matter if there's a less "experienced" girl, a "fat" girl, a "skinny" girl, or an "old" girl. As a matter of fact, the more variety, the better! It makes us all feel like we're special and good at what we do in our own way.

A contest also invites competition among friends, and nothing ruins a friendship faster or is pettier than women competing for male attention. That won't happen on my watch, ladies!

This is a female empowering show. You are putting on this great performance to please yourselves as strong, sexy women who are in control. You are not single entities here; you are a *team.*

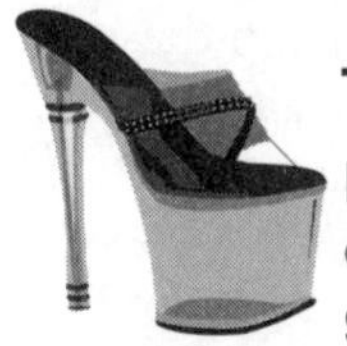

Trippin' Up

I danced with a girl named Jennifer at Snooky's who was drop-dead gorgeous. And she was the sweetest, nicest, most humble person, but a lot of dancers wouldn't even speak to her or gave her attitude because they felt her beauty was a threat to them. As a result, Jennifer felt very left out. Don't let this happen in your show.

How Far Do We Go?

I suggest no nudity at all or just topless if you want to go that far. This really depends on your relationship with everybody in the group.

You don't want to give it all away! It's actually sexier to tease with your bra and underwear than just take it all off. When he sees everything, it's like, "Yeah, okay." You're guaranteed to hold his attention if you let him think he's going to see something and he doesn't. And we all know—men want what they can't have.

How Raunchy Can We Get?

Just because you're doing a striptease doesn't mean you have to make it trashy. Save that stuff for the privacy of the bedroom. While you're dancing, go around "those places" delicately as I showed you how to do in earlier chapters. It's classier and reminds them that you don't have to touch there to feel sexy … you're sexy all over.

Can *I* Lap Dance *Her* Husband?

Remember what I said earlier about only inviting "normal" girls to dance with you? Here's where this really comes into play.

This question is one you should really discuss as a group, because if it isn't ironed out in the beginning, it can lead to much misery later (especially if alcohol is involved).

Can We Drink?

The wise answer to this is no, dancers shouldn't drink and your audience should only get a few beers, but not enough to get anyone drunk. And as dancers, you don't want to be drunk or heavily buzzed because you'll look stupid and the audience might laugh at you. Afterward, they'll remember, "Oh yeah, she was drunk" instead of, "Wow, she did a great job." Plus you'll be swinging around a pole and balancing on a chair. If you don't have all your senses, you could seriously hurt yourself. (I've seen it happen.)

Also after a few drinks you might not think clearly and see things that aren't really there. If your friend does a lap dance on your man, all in fun, drunk you might see her as trying to steal him or turn him on. Alcohol blows everything out of proportion and might cause the evening to end in disaster. Same thing with the guys. They won't think clearly if they see their woman dancing on another man.

If you want to have a truly good time, don't even serve alcohol, or at least serve it at the end of your showcase. It's only about an hour, and trust me, friendships will be saved if you avoid the booze before and during the show.

Making It Real

With the ground rules established and agreed upon, it's time to get to work! Set up a weekly (or more often if you want!) time for you all to get together at someone's house, preferably the one where the showcase will take place. During this time, you can all perform for everyone and get pointers on what works and what you need more practice on, including your striptease. Everyone should have a paper and pen to take notes during each other's dance so you can remember what looked really great and what might need some improvement.

At my recitals, each girl gets to dance to two songs of her own choice, but not back to back. Everyone is so nervous, but then after they do their first dance, they realize how much fun it was and their next dance is even stronger because they'll have done it before. It's almost as if the first song is a practice song. Each girl should do her stronger song first, that is, the one she's most confident with because she needs every ounce of comfort she can get when she first performs.

After you run through the lineup once, go through it again. If there's room and time, you can even coordinate a choreographed grand finale at the end. A particularly great sisterhood-team type song is "Lady Marmalade" from the *Moulin Rouge* soundtrack.

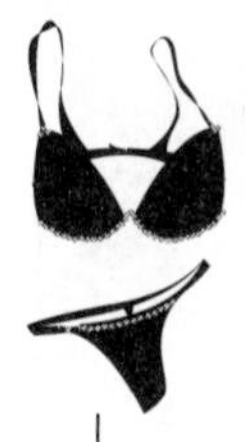

Behind the G-String

Any and all comments to each other should be positive and encouraging at all times. Remember you want to build each other up, not tear each other down!

Meanwhile, everyone can practice their moves with their songs at home. The more everyone dances, the better they'll be.

After a few weeks, or whenever you feel your group is ready, set a date for your recital. Everyone should be clear that this is a commitment, so no one can flake out the night before because "they just don't feel like it" or blow off rehearsals. This is all fun for you, but the more you treat it like a real show, the more it'll take on a life of its own and you'll all be so proud of yourselves because you made it all come together.

Goooooooooooooo Team!

Not only are you all a team as dancers, but you're a team as you set up the show, too. This means you'll have to ask, or assign, girls to do different things to bring it all together. Don't try to do it all yourself because this was your idea. Putting on a great show takes a lot more effort than you think.

In the following sections, I list some assignments you can give the girls. Of course, you don't have to do all of these; but if you do, your audience will be extremely impressed and the dancers will take this more seriously and become more to the show.

Turn It Up, DJ!

Throughout this book, I've talked about the importance of music, so it should come to no surprise to you that I've got DJ listed here. The DJ is in charge of collecting the girls' music and should be musically and electronically efficient. She'll need a lot of patience, too, because everyone changes songs a million times, even on the day of the showcase!

Each girl should have two songs. And it doesn't matter what anyone else thinks of those two songs—if it moves her and she can make it sexy. (Although everyone laughs at me when I mention the song, I can make Wham's "Wake Me Up Before You Go-Go" sexy. Really, I can dance to that song like it's nobody's business.) Just be sure to remind the girls that the song has to make them feel strong and sexy.

If you want to dance to your man's favorite song but you don't like it or it doesn't "do it" for you, choose another song that works for you. This is all about you, not him!

I find it's easiest to burn all the songs to one CD, in order, so that it's all in one place and the DJ doesn't have to fight with 20 CDs, remember whose song is whose, think about what number on the CD it is, get them in the correct order, etc.

The DJ should also have a small colored light so she can read her notes. (White lights are too distracting, no matter how small.)

You're Invited!

Naturally, you haven't told your sweetheart what you've been doing, which makes it that much more fun for you and increases the female sisterhood aspect of this craziness! But the day will come when he and the other guys must be told. Of course, you won't just say, "Hey, by the way, we're going to do a strip show next Saturday at Beth and Neil's house." Oh no, that won't do at all.

Brainstorm with everyone about invitation ideas. You all can design it together and put one girl in charge of having it made. Or you could ask the most creatively inclined girl to design it. She can use a invitation computer program and fun paper or cards from an office supply store. You could create a female-shaped card with a dress on, which could reveal a sexy bikini inside when opened. Really, anything creative is great, but so are simple invites.

Include this pertinent information on your invitation:

- The (cute!) name of your show
- The location
- The time
- What dancers are featured (Type or have the girls personally sign their stage names only.)
- RSVP e-mail address or phone number and the RSVP-by date

You should also include the following notes on the invitation. Feel free to change the wording as you like—or increase the amount of money the guys should bring!

> *Bring at least $30 in $1s and larger bills to tip the dancers.*
>
> *You must arrive promptly, 15 minutes before curtain. Latecomers will be turned away at the door.*

Receiving an invitation like this will pique any guy's interest—and have him running to the ATM!

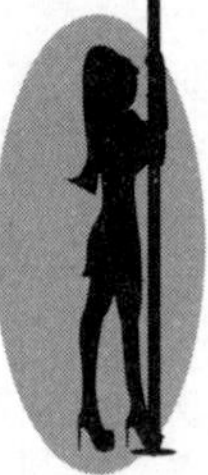

Slick Tricks

Make your man use his own money to tip, even if you have to go to the bank for him to be sure he's got enough small bills. But be sure it's *his* money—and don't give it back to him when the show's over!

Programs

You can make the programs yourself or have them professionally done at a printer. If you want to do them yourself, use some even-edge post cards from the office supply store. If you don't have an art program on your computer, you can use PowerPoint, which enables you to move pictures and text boxes around easily.

However you want to design and print your program, be sure to include the following information:

- Title of the show
- Date
- Time
- Stage names and songs
- Acknowledgments (DJ, food, etc.)

Make the programs a day or two before your showcase. Why wait so long? Because we women are prone to changing our minds at the last minute!

"Hello. Come Right In."

Have someone available to greet and seat your audience as they arrive so they know where to go and don't "accidentally" wander into the dressing room.

Be sure, however, that the greeter isn't wearing the costume she'll be using for her first song and that she's toward the end of the lineup so she doesn't have to rush to get ready when the show starts.

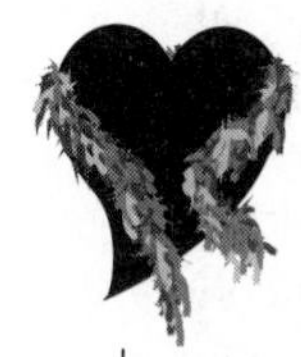

Feelin' the Love

I loved supporting and getting support from the other girls. I loved seeing all their different styles, talents, and attitudes. Some were nervous but then went on to give the performance of a lifetime.

—Cinnamon, student

"Please Welcome Coco to the Stage, Guys!"

Any show needs an MC to keep the audience informed and the show running smoothly. Your MC should be really bubbly and able to talk in front of an audience and have fun with it.

The MC should welcome the audience as a whole, thank them for coming, and tell them that hooting, hollering, and clapping during performances is highly encouraged. The MC will lay down the ground rules, too:

- Dancers can touch you, but you can't touch them.
- Each girl will go around after her song to collect her tip, so have your money out and ready.
- You can place your tips … (*wherever you agreed upon*).
- No talking during the performances.
- You can ask for change only between performances.

In addition, the MC has a few other things on her to-do list:

- Post a program in the costume room so everyone knows who's next.
- Introduce each girl by her stage name and say a few words about how good she is on the pole, what a cute butt she has, or something else fun.
- After each dancer finishes, the MC must lead the applause and remind her to collect her tips. (Girls in my recitals always forget because they're so caught up in the moment.)
- Determine when and if there will be an intermission and how long it will be.
- Announce each dancer at the end so she can do a quick walkthrough before everyone takes a group bow.

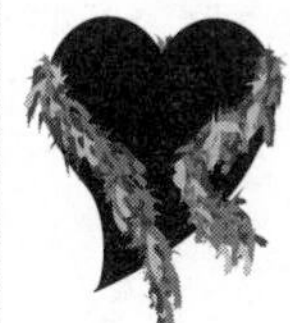

Feelin' the Love

Just before my name is announced, I get little butterflies in my stomach. Then I hear the music start, and I immediately become "Veronica" and all traces of the person everyone knows me to be vanish for the next 4 or 5 minutes.

—Veronica

"Has Anyone Seen My Shoe?"

One girl should be assigned to costume room duty, which means she'll be responsible for making sure everything is set for the big night. Here's a checklist she can follow:

- ❑ Mirrors—there can never be enough (A few full-length $10 mirrors from Wal-Mart will do. Place a few vertically for full-length views and a few horizontally for makeup.)
- ❑ Curling irons
- ❑ Hair spray
- ❑ Nail glue
- ❑ Small sewing kit
- ❑ Deodorant
- ❑ Disposable razors (We always miss a spot!)
- ❑ Fans or proper air conditioning
- ❑ Scissors

The costume queen should also be sure the costume room has easy access to a bathroom and into the show room itself, and that this access is covered so the audience can't see the girls coming and going.

Slick Tricks

Scissors are a must in the costume room, because the costume queen also doubles as the tag queen. Tag queens must look over each girl's costume and cut off any remaining tags. Nothing brings reality into a show more than when you see a bright white tag on a girl's bra, panties, or dress. This is a fantasy show; be sure all traces of the real world are nonexistent for 2 hours.

Sexy Snacks

You eat popcorn and candy at the movies, so why not serve some snacks at your showcase, too? But don't just dump some pretzels and soda on a side table. You've put in so much planning already. Have fun with the food display, too.

The snack queen is in charge of buying and displaying food, and she should be creative at it, particularly if she can bake things such as anatomically correct cookies, whoopee pies, etc. If there's a "nasty" bakery in your town, even better! You can also order those incredibly sophomoric but lots-of-fun anatomically correct candies online.

Soda is fine, but go a step further; sparkling apple juice in a champagne-type bottle is more fun. Again, I bring up a caution flag with the use of alcohol unless you supply only, say, a few beers, not enough to get anyone drunk during the show.

You *really* have to be careful with alcohol because it can not only lead to really bad mistakes and misinterpretations, but it's not safe for your girls to be swinging around a pole or attempting to balance on a chair backward if they're inebriated. At least try your first show alcohol-free, and of course the whole alcohol issue is contingent upon the security of your relationships with your friends and their spouses.

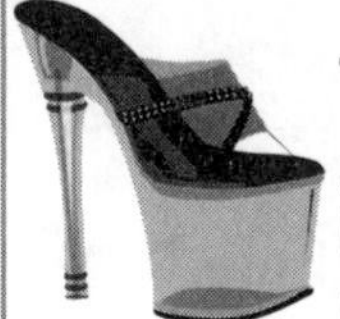

Trippin' Up

Although they might be fun for the ladies, refrain from offering your male audience lollipops of their own gender. That could get awkward. (It would pretty funny to see if any of the guys are secure enough in their manhood, shall we say, to dare eat one!)

Club Setup

Someone should be in charge of setting up the room you're going to use for the show. This means getting the colored light bulbs, black lights, chairs for the audience, and a chair for the chair dancing. The setup queen should also remove anything that could be accidentally hit or kicked and rearrange the furniture to create a clear wall (and remove plugs from the outlets so no one gets a cheap thrill when they slide down). She should also be sure the pole is far enough away so no one kicks the walls or an audience member (although if he's not a good tipper, he deserves it).

Your dancers will also want to watch each other dance. If possible, set up a viewing area of sorts, where the girls can watch the dancer onstage without being seen by the audience. It is very important that the other dancers can watch because they need to be hooting and hollering and clapping in support of the girl onstage and encourage the audience to do the same.

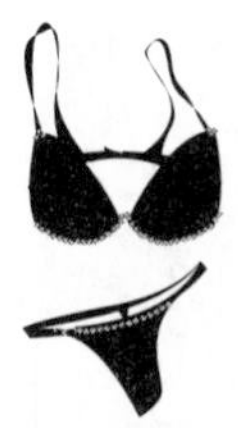

Behind the G-String

Refer to each other using stage names at all times. Your real names are of no importance anymore!

Fun Accessories

Assign a girl to pick up some fun and sexy accessories for all the girls. Most of the dancers will have gotten the necessary accessories with their costumes, but matching garters can be fun for all the girls. Check out the selection at www.wmsclothing.com. (They're great and much less expensive than what you'll find in party stores.)

If you want to make them really fun, personalize each of the garters with each girl's stage name. Most pet stores have machines that make pet tags. I use the large heart-shaped tags (*sans* the little bones) that cost $7.50. That's a little pricey but it's well, well worth it. Just follow the machine's directions to engrave the tags with the girls' stage names and sew the tags onto the garters. Give each girl her garter before the show.

This is just another small girl power bonding thing to do, but it'll really make you feel like you are truly a team!

Shake That Money Maker!

The tips aren't the focal point of your showcase, of course, but they do help! And it's also good for your audience to realize this isn't a free show, that they're expected to show their appreciation for your dance just like they would if they were at a real strip club.

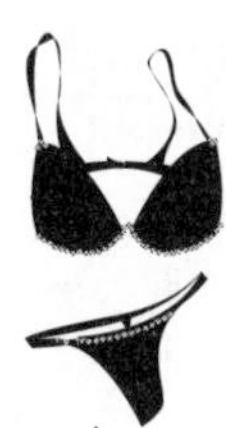

Behind the G-String

When men would sit at the stage and not tip the girl after she just danced for him, the girl would ask, "Do you work for free? Because I don't!" Then the dancer would kick the customer's beer all over him, as was custom.

There are two main times to collect tips when you're dancing: while you're dancing and after you're done. It takes a lot of practice to be able to collect good money while you're dancing, and it can interrupt your dance. (Mind you, if someone offers you money while you're dancing, take it!) Also, that breaks the spell of your dance and makes it more money-driven than empowerment-driven. You'll have more fun with the latter.

When your song is done and as everyone is clapping, begin your round and don't feel silly asking for tips. The audience knows they're expected to tip, and besides, you just gave them an amazing show and you are entitled to every dollar they give. Nobody dances for free!

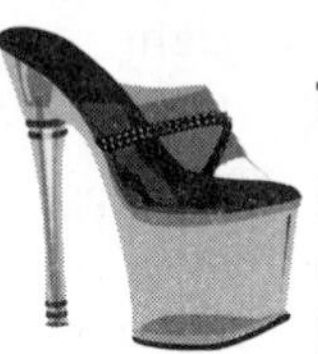

Trippin' Up

Never, ever, ask a girl how much money she made. That is rude and just invites catty competition. And if you see a girl drop a dollar as she's exiting the stage, always return it to her. Never keep it for yourself.

Garters are great to collect money in because he can easily slip it in and you run no risk of anyone trying to touch you, which hopefully you won't have in your showcase anyway. (This is where the team garter would be really neat.)

You can also collect money in your bra or underwear. When you do, treat the men like they're men at a club by protecting certain areas of yourself. Chances are, you won't have to worry about that in your showcase, but the fact that you're protecting yourself anyway sends a message, and they'll love that.

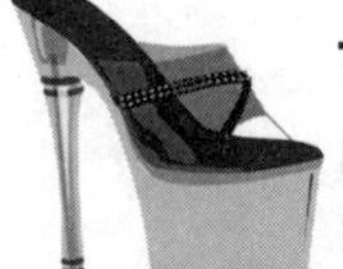

Trippin' Up

In clubs, some cheap guys like to rip a dollar bill, roll it up, and only give the dancer half. If someone tips you a rolled up bill at your showcase, just to challenge them and add some laughs, unroll the dollar bill right then, check to see that it's whole, and put it in your bra.

When you take money in your bra, you never want to just pull the chest strap out so he can put the dollar bill in because then his hands can wander. Here's how to do it: reach up with both hands underneath the chest strap of your bra so each hand is covering a breast. He then can place the dollar in your cleavage. Or you can just take the money with your fingers.

He can also place money in your bra's shoulder straps. Again, you never just want to hold the strap open. If he wants to place a dollar in your left shoulder strap, use your left hand to lift up the strap for him, and place your right hand over the strap where it meets the cup.

Protecting yourself when men want to put a dollar in your underwear is a little more important. Like with the bra, never, ever just pull out the sides of your panties. If someone wants to tip a dollar (or better yet, a $5) in your left hip, gently pull the side out with your left hand (I do a fancy finger roll in the side of the underwear that twists it once around my finger), and place your right hand, palm down, about an inch or so below your hip (over your underwear) so that were his hand to accidentally slide toward ground zero, your hand would stop it.

Lots of men also enjoy putting a dollar horizontally in the back of your underwear. He'll likely slip the dollar bill through and then hold on to it with both hands and try to slide it as far down as he can. That gets a little *too* personal. To avoid this, bunch a little of the fabric at the top of your undies with your thumb and forefinger and pull it out about an inch. Do the same thing with your other hand about 3 inches lower, resting on your butt.

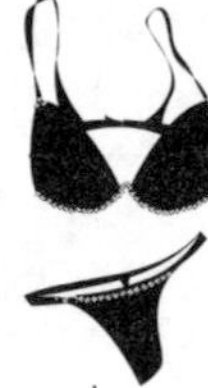

Behind the G-String

Some customers who sat at my stage when I was a dancer thought telling me what a beautiful body I had was a worthy substitute for tipping. I responded with "Thanks, but compliments don't pay my bills!"

Dancing for Mixed Audiences

Maybe your show isn't going to be just for your men; maybe you want to show your other girlfriends, or even you family members, what you can do.

Dancing for relatives can be creepy, unless you do it in the pure spirit of fun. I've had showcases where girl's parents have showed up, and my parents came to my first, really big recital. I must say, they were impressed. They knew this was all in fun and accepted me gyrating around in front of guys in my booty shorts and camisole.

Their focus, however, wasn't on me; it was on the whole show and the entertainment from the other dancers. Because we kept the show clean—as in no nudity and no touching yourself—none of us were embarrassed to have their parents or siblings there. It was even cleaner than a Las Vegas show, where many of the dancers in their large headdresses go topless. And that is what this is: a fun, entertaining, live show.

Although you might feel weird dancing in front of other women, don't. If it helps, keep this in mind: women are notoriously better tippers then men in a regular strip club, and the women you invite to your show may be the same, depending on your relationship with them.

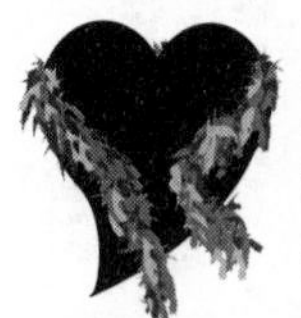

Feelin' the Love

When I'm dancing, I like to pay more attention to the women in the audience. They just aren't expecting any of us to give them a lap dance. The shocked, embarrassed, and otherwise uncomfortable faces they give you when you come right up and dance for them are priceless! I want them to see that I'm having a great time just goofing off and that dancing around like this doesn't have to be intimidating—they could do it, too!

—Meredith

It does feel funny dancing in front of a woman, especially if you're doing it for the first time, but you must take on the same attitude with them that you do with the men. They are at your stage, watching you perform. Therefore, they'll get the same show as everyone else. Look at your audience as equals, as if they are all just human beings with no gender.

If a female audience member looks particularly annoyed in a snobby kind of way, like she can't believe what you girls are doing, it's trashy and slutty and way beneath her, then by all means give that woman a lap dance! Get in her face, show her you're having fun. This is your moment, and no one in that audience, male or female, is going to ruin it for you. As one of my dancers, Veronica says, "The best part is that with the confidence of your stage personality, you can really get in their face and embarrass the heck out of them, then be able to look them in the eye when you see them the next day because you really were great."

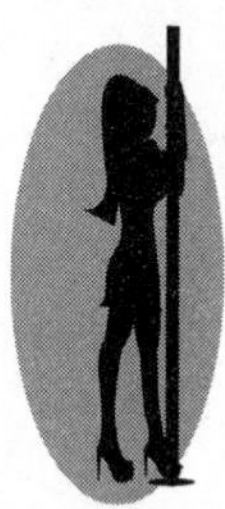

Slick Tricks

If you feel funny looking a person in the eye, look at his or her forehead instead.

However, if you sense that a female member of the audience is genuinely uncomfortable in an honest way, leave her alone. This is all in fun, but you don't want to make anyone feel uneasy—unless you sense that they're looking down on you. Then you really give it to them! Usually it's pretty easy to distinguish the two; just trust your gut instinct.

Finally, you are not *you* when you're dancing. You are someone else, your sexy alter ego. Put on that mask and remember it's all acting. You are the center of attention during your dance, so feed off the energy of the crowd to boost your adrenaline. This is *your* moment.

The Least You Need to Know

- The more effort you put into your showcase, the better the show.
- Support each other—this is a team effort.
- Be as creative as you can in your individual performances and the showcase in general.
- You're not performing for your audience; you're performing for yourself. Just have fun!

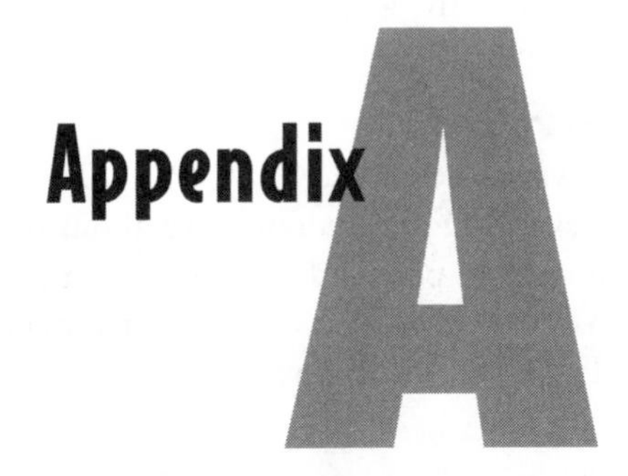

Where Can I Get It?

Now that you know what to do and how to do it, where do you actually get all the stuff? In this appendix, I've compiled a list of websites I frequently use so you can find the products I've mentioned in the book. (None of these websites or products paid me to list them; I'm just letting you know what works for me.)

Poles

Lil'Mynx Removable Dance Poles
www.stripperpole.com
I find the Lil' Mynx poles the best, and their customer service is impeccable. They've got colored poles as well as brass and chrome, and the best thing is their removable poles. (We used the Lil' Mynx removable pole in the DVD.) They're my first choice.

Mighty Grip
www.mightygrip.com
When your hands get too slippery or sweaty, you can apply a little of this powder to them to make them stick. This is great for first-time pole users whose nervous hands really sweat. (Plus, Mighty Grip has great customer service!)

Platinum Stages
www.platinumstages.com
Platinum Stages sells a free-standing pole that screws into a 4×4-foot stage. Although the pole doesn't attach to the ceiling, it's safe enough to use for upside-down tricks.

PoleDanzer
www.poledanzer.com
These removable poles use a fake smoke alarm to cover the area where the pole attaches to the ceiling.

X-Pole
www.xpole.co.uk
Several of my students rave about the X-Pole, a tension pole with a wide base at the top and bottom. The X-Pole is manufactured in England, but they ship to the United States.

Sexy Costumes, Shoes, and Lingerie

CatDancerz
www.CatDancerz.com
CatDancerz has a large variety of inexpensive costumes—you can spend hours going through the online catalogue. This is where I get all my costumes. The times I've called them, they've been very personable, and they ship immediately.

eBay
www.ebay.com
You can find costumes, shoes, and boots here for very little money. My students swear by eBay.

Teddy Shoes
www.teddyshoes.com
This store, located in Cambridge, Massachusetts, has the largest selection of the craziest kinds of shoes and boots known to man. Some of these shoes are just unbelievable!

WMS Wholesale
www.wmsclothing.com
This is a wholesale website, but no wholesale membership is required. I've found them to be the least expensive, especially for simpler costumes. Also, their shoes and boots are by far the best deal you'll get online. Their shipping is great, as is their customer service.

Makeup

Dermablend Coverage Cosmetics
www.Dermablend.com
Dermablend is great body makeup and covers every flaw you have. It stays on, too, so no worries about reapplying.

ERA Face
www.eraface.com
This aerosol makeup goes on incredibly smooth on your face. It's extremely light, too, so it's perfect for getting a great workout around the pole.

Sally Hansen
www.sallyhansen.com
I used Airbrush Legs makeup for my legs in the DVD, and it looks like I'm wearing nylons. I very highly recommended it!

Crazy Accessories

Cool Stuff Cheap
www.coolstuffcheap.com
To really liven up your dance area, check out this site. It's got really funky lights, disco balls—everything to really spice up your room.

High Heel Shoe Chair
www.highheelshoechair.com
I get so many comments on the high heel shoe chairs I have. They're incredibly comfortable, and chair dancing takes on a whole other dimension when it's on a high heel shoe chair! These chairs are also ideal for lap dancing because they make it easier for you to get to the floor and his body more easily accessible.

Appendix B

Exotic Dance Lessons in the United States

Exotic dance lessons are popping up all over the country—and the world—now that more women realize pole dancing isn't just for strippers anymore. Look around and you'll surely see several different kinds of studios—some run by women as an exercise and self-esteem class, others run by women who were real exotic dancers. My vote, naturally, is to go with the women who had to do this for a living. Then you'll get the real insight into the psychology of performing for a man as well as authentic moves and the real art of the tease. However, if you're looking for simply an interesting and fun way to workout, then by all means go to the nearest studio.

Here's a list of lessons offered in the United States, but so many are popping up that to find a studio near you, simply hop online and search for "pole dancing lessons" and your city, and you'll surely get results.

Arizona

Ecdysiastic Tendencies*
www.ecdysiastic.com

Reza Fitness Resort
www.rezaresort.com

California

Aphrodite Strip~N~Pole
www.aphroditestripnpole.com

Ecdysiastic Tendencies*
www.ecdysiastic.com

From Mind to Body
www.frommindtobody.com

Heart and Pole
www.heartandpole.com

Pole Position Fitnexx
www.polepositionfitness.com

S Factor
www.sfactor.com

Sedusa Studios
www.sedusastudios.com

Siren Studios
www.Sirenstudios.com

Slinky Productions*
www.LearnEroticDance.com

Soul Tree Motion
www.soultreemotion.com

Colorado

FlashDance Studios
www.flashdancestudios.com

Florida

Stripping Slim Fitness
www.StrippingSlimFitness.com

Illinois

Empowerment Through Exotic Dance
www.empowermentthroughexoticdance.com

Pilates Plus of Schaumburg
www.pilatesmindbody.com

Pole Appeal
www.poleappeal.com

Georgia

PoleLaTeaz
www.polelateaz.com

Maryland

Pole Primadonna
www.poleprimadonna.com

Xpose Fitness
www.xposefitness.com

Massachusetts

Gypsy Rose Exotic and Pole Dancing*
www.GypsyRoseDancing.com

Michigan

Feminine Arts Studio*
www.femininestudio.com

Pole Addiction
www.poleaddiction.com

Nevada

Exotic Dance School (Fawnia)*
www.ExoticDanceSchool.com

Studio Open
www.studioopen.com

New York

Art of Pole Dance*
www.dancepole.jp/lupoledance/EFrontPage.html

Exotic Dance Central*
www.exoticdancecentral.com

New York Pole Dancing*
www.poledancingnyc.com

Pole Lessons
www.polegirl.com

Ohio

Pole Kittens Fitness
www.polekittensfitness.com

Washington

Pole for the Soul
www.poleforthesoul.com

**Instruction by authentic exotic dancers.*

Index

D

E

F

G

H

I-J

K-L

M

N-O-P-Q

R

S

T

U-V-W

X-Y-Z

WARRANTY LIMITS

READ THIS ENCLOSED AGREEMENT BEFORE OPENING MEDIA PACKAGE.

BY OPENING THIS SEALED VIDEO PACKAGE, YOU ACCEPT AND AGREE TO THE TERMS AND CONDITIONS PRINTED BELOW. IF YOU DO NOT AGREE, DO NOT OPEN THE PACKAGE. SIMPLY RETURN THE SEALED PACKAGE.

This DVD is distributed on an "AS IS" basis, without warranty. Neither the authors, the publisher, and/or Penguin Group (USA) Inc./Alpha Books make any representation or warranty, either express or implied, with respect to the DVD, its quality, accuracy, or fitness for a specific purpose. Therefore, neither the authors, the publisher, and/or Penguin Group (USA) Inc./Alpha Books shall have any liability to you or any other person or entity with respect to any liability, loss, or damage caused directly or indirectly by the content contained on the DVD or by the DVD itself. If the DVD is defective, you may return it for replacement.